"The Ultimate Healing System"

BREAKTHROUGH IN NUTRITION, KINESIOLOGY AND HOLISTIC HEALING TECHNIQUES

Course Manual

The Ultimate Healing System

by Don Lepore

This research presentation is intended for use by licensed Medical Doctors, Osteopaths, Chiropractors, Doctors of Homeopathic Medicine, Nurses, Dieticians, Nutritionists and other health care practitioners.

Published by
Woodland Books
P.O. Box 1422
Provo, Utah 84603

ISBN 0-913923-63-X

Printed in the United States of America

TABLE OF CONTENTS

*M.R.T. - Muscle Response Testing

ABOUT THE AUTHOR

Dr. Donald J. Lepore, ND, DN, NMD is a nutritional research pioneer who has utilized kinesiology in his practice for the past ten years. He is a member of the NHF (National Health Federation), AANC (American Association of Nutritional Consultants), AHMF (American Holistic Medical Foundation), and the ANMA (American Nutritional Medical Association). He is presently New Jersey State Chapter President of the ANMA.

Presently, Dr. Lepore is director of the Life Extension Research Center in Jersey City, New Jersey. The center has a reputation of succeeding when all else has failed. Research is presently being conducted using biokinesiology, nutritional therapy which includes vitamins, minerals, herbs, amino acids, homeopathy and bath therapy approaches that are presented in this book.

DEDICATION

I dedicate this work to all the people who are needlessly suffering because of the lack of understanding by the majority of the present profession of health practitioners.

I dedicate this work to the practitioners (Medical or Holistic) who care enough about the healing of their clients to be broad-minded enough to be seeking alternative systems of diagnosis and healing.

TEXT TERMINOLOGY CLARIFICATION

(1) Metabolic Antagonist

I use the terminology "Metabolic Antagonist" instead of allergy because many of the medical profession believe allergies to be incurable. This I have found to be false!!

(2) Nutritional Antidote

This author believes that every Metabolic Antagonist has a Nutritional Antidote. And throughout this book these will be presented to you. Because of this information, many cases of people with Parkinson's Disease, Arthritis, Herpes, and many other so-called "incurables" have been successfully healed.

(3) Client

I will use this terminology instead of "patient." If you are a licensed medical practitioner please understand that it represents what you are accustomed to calling a "patient."

CHAPTER 1

THE LEPORE TECHNIQUE

The "Lepore" technique is basically a system which uses a refined "Muscle Response Test" technique to accomplish the following:

A.) Pinpoint the "Metabolic Antagonist".
B.) Measure the needed nutrient (Nutritional Antidote) which could be a vitamin, mineral, amino acid, herb, cell salt, or homeopathic remedy to neutralize the Metabolic Antagonist.
C.) Measure the needed support nutrients which are catalysts to assist in the absorption of the antidote.

Because it is an evolving test, Muscle Response Testing (M.R.T.) technique has different variations. My refining of the M.R.T. technique will demonstrate some differences from other published techniques. However, I have found that the changes I have instituted make the M.R.T. far more accurate and foolproof.

To perform the test:

Stand facing your client or the person to be tested.
Rub the client's thymus gland for fifteen seconds.
The thymus gland is about 2½ inches below the Adam's Apple to the right and left of the center, about 2 to 3 inches apart.

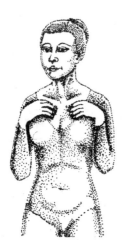

Figure 1

The purpose for this is to activate the thymus gland which in turn will "light up" the Acupuncture points of the body.

Next, rub the mastoid gland behind both ears (directly below the bony protuberance behind the ears).

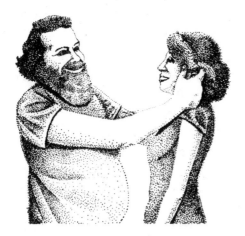

Figure 2

This *relaxes* the acupuncture points. This procedure activates and deactivates the points so that they are neutralized and are more accurate.

Now, ask the client to lift the left arm while you hold the right shoulder with your left hand and press on the left arm 1½ inches *above* the wrist. Use *only* two fingers of your right hand to ensure you do not overforce the client's arm. This is not a test of strength but a test of resistance.

Let's review:

1. Neutralize client:

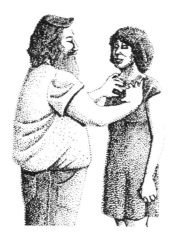

Figure 3

2. Hold client by right shoulder so as to stop him from falling down:

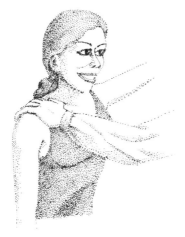

Figure 4

3. Place two fingers of your
    right hand about 1½
    inches above client's wrist:

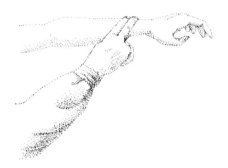

Figure 5

4. Push downwards, while client is resisting:

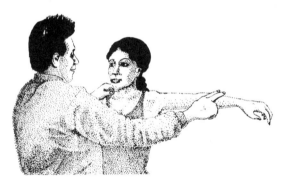

Figure 6

At this point the client's arm should *not* go down. The right arm should be at the side of the client.*

We do this to every client first:

(A) So the client feels the pressure we are going to exert on the arm.

(B) To test the client's arm to see if there is sufficient strength.

(C) If the client's arm goes down, (since you haven't placed any substance in the other hand) you are either pulling or pushing too hard, or the client has an arthritic arm (weak), or needs sodium.**

Now that you have the basic concept of the mechanics of the M.R.T., let us proceed to the Lepore technique.

---

*If client's left arm is arthritic, weak, or non-functional, use the right arm instead.

**This will be explained later. Please see page 77.

The next step is to test for allergic substances.
The substances I have on my test tray are:

(1) Brewer's Yeast
(2) Rice
(3) Wheat
(4) Fats (mayonnaise)
(5) Oatmeal
(6) Corn

(7) Citrus Fruit
(8) Peppers
(9) Tobacco
(10) Lettuce
(11) Milk
(12) Fish oil

The method for allergy testing is to place the container (plastic bag or glass vial) in the right hand of the client who then places that hand on own solar plexus (gut area — 1½ inches above the navel) and extends left arm. You press down on the client's left arm and if it remains rigid, ask the client to *drop the tongue to the bottom of the mouth*.

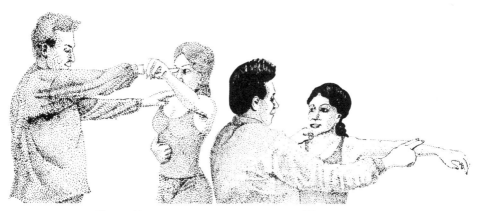

Figure 7   Figure 8

Then press again. If the arm remains rigid, the substance being tested is non-allergenic. If the arm goes down (gets weak), the substance *is* antagonistic (allergenic).

The client should keep the tongue away from the roof of the mouth during *all* testing. If the tongue touches the roof of the mouth, it will short-circuit the electromagnetic field to the acupuncture points and the test will not be *accurate*! For this reason, I usually tell my client to drop the jaw while being tested.

The *client's* arm will go down when the testing substance is antagonistic, or when the nutrient being tested is an overdose (too many milligrams) or insufficient (not enough milligrams).

The reason I have selected the previously mentioned substances, e.g., brewer's yeast, rice, wheat, fat, corn, citrus, and the "pepper group", is that many *natural* vitamins are made from these substances. (Many vitamin and mineral B-complex tablets and capsules are made from brewer's yeast.)

So many nutritionists read that brewer's yeast is a good source of B vitamins, etc., that they often prescribe it for their clients, who in turn get sick and nauseous because they are allergic to the pills. Many vitamin manufacturers are manufacturing "non-allergenic" pills. On the label they put, "No wheat, no soy, no yeast, no milk." But they *neglect to say "No rice"* because the pill is made from rice. They presume falsely that the rice is non-allergenic. We have found that many people are indeed allergic to rice. So how can these manufacturers claim to manufacture "non-allergenic" pills?

The most popular base for B-complexes (and vitamins and minerals) is brewer's yeast or rice bran.

The reason I test wheat is that it is highly allergenic in the summertime to many individuals. Additionally, some Vitamin E and octacosanol are manufactured from wheat.

The reasons for checking the client for commonly found allergies are:

A.) Zein (protein) coating on pills is made from corn.
B.) Vitamin C - made with rose hips - is not a true rose hip pill, but a rose hip base combined with a corn-derived "C".

Thus, anyone allergic to corn who takes these pills will "gag" on them because the pill affects the electromagnetic field at the throat and the throat will close automatically in order to save the person from being "poisoned" by the vitamin pill.

If you find yourself unable to swallow a pill, you are probably allergic to the coating or the base (filler or binder). One brand brags about its zein coating. The reason for the coat is that it gives it more shelf life.

In my tray I have citrus food.* Why? Because many people take citrus Vitamin C and are allergic to the citrus bioflavonoids. This tells me whether I should give them a super "C" complex containing bioflavonoids (which are usually manufactured from citrus), or a simple calcium ascorbate pill.

I test peppers because they are usually allergenic if the person smokes. I test milk because some pills like tryptophane are manufactured from milk. Tryptophane is meant to relax a client. Occasionally, it works the opposite for an individual who is allergic to milk.

*I use Homeopathic Antigens, but real fruits are okay. I used them for years, but they spoil.

A very popular vitamin company does not coat its pills because it uses a milk lactose base which extends the shelf life to fifty years, but what of customers who have a milk allergy and take these pills? They will become ill as a result of taking them and will be "turned off" to nutritional supplements!

Here we are promoting nutritional supplements and mistakenly poisoning our clients!

I test fish oil because many vitamin and mineral pills use fish oil as the source of vitamins A and D. Once again, if a client shows weak with fish oil, a multi-vitamin and mineral capsule with fish oil should not be used!

All of these substances were tested by the client clutching the substance in the right hand, and holding them to the solar plexus while the tester pushes down on the outstretched left arm.

Now to continue the Lepore Technique of M.R.T. and how to use it effectively to determine what nutrients the body needs.

CHAPTER 2

ALLERGIES AND ANTIDOTES

It is my personal feeling that this is probably the most important section of the book. From my experience in treating clients, I have found that many illnesses are caused by the body's inability to absorb nutrients because the *source* of these nutrients is hostile to the body.

We call this hostility "Metabolic Antagonism", which is just another way of saying "allergies". I prefer to use the term "Metabolic Antagonists" because many people in the medical profession consider allergies non-curable. We have found that this is simply not true. We have discovered that each substance that is a "Metabolic Antagonist" (or allergic substance) is caused by or attributed to a certain nutrient, or combination of nutrient deficiency. Furthermore, we have found that specific vitamins, minerals, and amino acid combinations are necessary for the complete absorption of particular foods.

For example: there are 23 different Vitamin B-complex factors. Yeast is promoted by the health food industry as a source of B-complex vitamins, but we have found that fifty per cent (50%) of our clients are allergic to the yeast. Why? The mineral important for the absorption of yeast is Zinc. Therefore, an allergy to yeast can be corrected by administering Zinc. Other vitamins which may also be lacking, and could subsequently cause a yeast allergy, would be Vitamins B-1 and B-6. Herbs which can be utilized to correct the yeast allergy are Pau D'Arco, Red Clover (rich in Zinc) and Comfrey. The amino acid necessary to alleviate a yeast allergy is Lysine, found in Comfrey.

The health food industry also uses rice as a base for multicap vitamins and B vitamins, but what many allergists and nutritionists do not realize is that a person can be allergic to rice. We found the antidotes to a rice allergy to be the mineral Manganese, the amino acids Arginine and Proline, and Vitamins B-6 (Pyridoxine) and B-12 (Cyanocobalamine).

A common allergy is the "wheat allergy". Vitamins such as Vitamin E are often made from wheat germ and are not absorbed properly by the person with a "wheat allergy". We have found the antidotes to wheat allergy to be Magnesium, the amino acid Histidine, and Vitamin F. Vitamin F is linoleic acid which exists in poly-unsaturated fats such as Safflower Oil, Olive Oil (which also contains Vitamin E), Castor Bean Oil, Sunflower Oil, and Peanut Oil. The herbs Black Walnut and Kelp are also helpful in correcting a wheat allergy, as they are naturally rich in Magnesium and other essential minerals. A lack of both Sodium and the amino acid Histidine will also cause an allergy to wheat.

Wheat allergies often occur in the summertime. The sun tends to burn up Vitamin F. If the sun should cause sunburn, the body will send all of its available Vitamin F to the sunburned area to correct it. Vitamin F is used as a skin regenerator. This is why people put oils on their bodies when in the sun! Many people, during the summer, will feel tired and exhausted. This is not only from the heat, which causes a Potassium and Sodium deficiency because of sweating, but is also due to a wheat allergy because the sun has burned up the body's supply of Vitamin F. It should be noted that a feathers/wool allergy will also respond to the (wheat) antidotes Magnesium, Histidine, Sodium and Vitamin F.

If and when you get sunburned, you should refrain from eating any wheat products, and this includes Italian pasta. I often tell people to eat Chinese food during the summer because rice is not affected by the sun. The food that grows in the tropics is not wheat, but coconut! Coconut contains a highly saturated fat which is the antidote to sunburn and a wheat allergy!

God did not permit foods that are antagonistic to man's existence to be grown in the area of consumption! So when you are in a different habitat zone, eat the foods from that area. They grow there especially to help man survive in that climate.

The next common allergy is the "Fat Allergy". This is quite an interesting allergy. Fats include Mayonnaise, Meat Fats, Ground Beef (Hamburgers), Pork, Hot Dogs, Cold Cuts, Milk Fats, Ice Cream, Butter, Margarine, Coconut Butter and ALL oils.

A fat allergy is usually caused by a lack of the mineral Sulfur. Sulfur is used to purify the blood and is also the antidote to the fat allergy. A lack of Sulfur can be caused by different things. One of the main causes is an overconsumption of fatty foods which depletes the body's sulfur and creates a fat allergy. Smoking and living in a polluted environment are two other significant factors. Many people with fat allergies actually have a Sulfur deficiency caused by smoking. Sulfur is used by the body to purify the tars, carbons, and other impurities which enter the body via smoking. Therefore, it is burned up quickly when a person is exposed to primary and secondary smoke pollutants. If the Sulfur is not replaced, the supply will gradually become depleted and can cause or lead to a fat allergy.

The symptoms of a fat allergy are a feeling of heaviness in the chest near the thymus gland almost as if someone were sitting on top of the chest, and a lot of phlegm in the throat, especially when a person arises in the morning. With a fat allergy there is usually congestion in the throat area where the Adam's Apple is located. The tonsils may also become inflamed. Tonsils are the "Sulfur Sack" of the body and, in my opinion, should rarely, if ever, be removed. Tonsils work to purify the blood, and when they become inflamed, it is a tell-tale sign that there is a lack of Sulfur and usually a fat allergy.

Sulfur can be obtained from many different sources. I have found the amino acids Methionine, Cysteine, Taurine, and Glutathione to be very good sources of Sulfur, and effective in correcting a fat allergy. The herbal sources of Sulfur include Sarsaparilla, Fenugreek, Eyebright, Dandelion, Burdock, and Fennel seeds; these are also effective in correcting a fat allergy. We have also used the Homeopathic Sulfur 1-x potency Cell Salts to help overcome and ameliorate this condition.

A fat allergy can be quite distressing due to the quantity of phlegm which seems to accumulate in the throat. However, we have found that the homeopathic Sulfur Cell Salts (1-x potency) can sometimes bring quick relief as they are dissolved in the mouth and not in the stomach. They go right to the throat, clearing it up within minutes in many cases. We have also found that *sunshine* helps correct a fat allergy. Exposure to the sun will help to burn up some of the fats in the system. Other suggested sources of Sulfur include bananas, eggs, garlic, and onions. The amino acid Threonine is also an antidote for a fat intolerance and should be tested also.

Another allergy is the "Corn Allergy". We have found it to be related to the wheat allergy, except that it occurs when there is also a lack of Potassium. Many times pills are coated with "Zein" coating, which actually is a corn-based coating. Pills such as these would not be absorbed properly by the person who is allergic to corn. Like the wheat allergy, the corn allergy can occur when there is a lack of Vitamin F, Magnesium, and the amino acid Histidine.

We have found that a lack of Iron can provoke an allergy to Oatmeal and Sesame. Many babies are fed Oatmeal, and sometimes get colic from it. This is an allergic response due to the low levels of Iron in the child. One of the best natural sources of Iron is the herb Yellow Dock. I prefer using Yellow Dock instead of inorganic Iron from the ground as many people cannot absorb inorganic Iron. Yellow Dock, on the other hand, yields *organic* Iron. The "oats" intolerance can also be corrected by Vitamin B-12 (Cyanocobalamin), amino acid Citrilline, and Folic Acid.

The next allergy to be discussed is the "Milk Allergy". We have found that a Milk Allergy can be corrected by the administration of Potassium. Milk and cheese can be allergenic if there is a deficiency of Potassium in the body. Once the Potassium level is brought up, the person will tolerate milk more readily. The "Milk" intolerance is also corrected by Aspartic acid and Vitamin D.

Another common allergy is the "Citrus Allergy". We have found that citrus fruits such as Oranges, Lemons, Grapefruit, Tangerines, Pineapple, Cantaloupe, and Tomatoes can be very allergenic when Pantothenic Acid (Vitamin B-5) is deficient.

Stress or trauma will cause the Adrenal Glands to burn up a great deal of Pantothenic Acid, which frequently results in an allergy to the citrus group. This can occur with both mental and emotional stress. I have seen a person's Pantothenic Acid level change with a five minute discussion of personal problems and distresses. The need for Pantothenic Acid had lowered after the client had talked about problems and relieved some of the distresses. My conclusion: In a relaxed state the adrenals do not burn up Pantothenic Acid as rapidly as they would in a stressful situation when more is needed to survive. Therefore, stress and/or trauma can actually create a citrus allergy situation. The mineral antidote for citrus allergy is Calcium. The amino acid antidote for citrus is Serine.

When there is a deficiency in Niacinamide/Niacin, a person could become allergic to the food group which consists of Peaches, Pears, Peppers, Plums and Nectarines. I call this the Niacinamide/Niacin group. Smoking can also cause an allergy to this food group as Nicotine and Niacin or Nicotinic Acid are opposite molecules and Nicotine displaces Niacin in the body.

Many people who smoke create hiatal hernias because they deprive the body of Niacinamide/Niacin and Sulfur, thus causing allergies. We have found that the hiatal hernia can be caused by a lack of Niacinamide/Niacin and a lack of Sulfur.

Many nutritionists are aware of the allergenic properties of the "Nightshade Vegetables" such as Potatoes, Tomatoes, Eggplant, Peppers, and Tobacco. Allergies to these foods can often cause arthritis or aggravate existing arthritis. Many nutritionists believe that the way to correct the allergies is to have the person eliminate these foods from the diet. The awareness that these foods can be antagonistic is good, but the theory of diet elimination is not sound.

We have found that an allergy to Peppers (along with Peaches, Pears and Plums) is caused by a deficiency in Niacinamide/Niacin, and an allergy to tomatoes (and citrus fruits) is generally caused by a Pantothenic Acid deficiency. By administering these two vitamins, the client can correct the allergy and eat the formerly allergenic foods without suffering any adverse reactions. One of the best sources of these two vitamins is a product called "Royal Jelly" which contains 500 mg. of Pantothenic Acid and 500 mg. of Niacinamide in one 100 mg. capsule. We have found this to be the best source of these nutrients, as it is natural and better absorbed. The mineral antidote for this Pepper Series is Phosphorus. The amino acid antidote for this series is L' Glutamine.

We have seen that many health disease conditions are caused by allergies. Even greens such as Celery, Cabbage, Cucumbers, Lettuce, Green Beans, Parsley, and anything green can be allergenic when there is a lack of Potassium. Greens, however, can also be very important, especially in the summertime when people are lacking Sodium. During the summer we have found that people lack not only Potassium but Sodium as well, as both are lost through perspiration. Perspiration causes a loss of three times more Potassium than Sodium.

When a person's Sodium and Potassium levels have been depleted, we have found that they become allergic to everything. This may be why people tend to eat more salads in the summer. The salad has the Sodium needed to correct the allergic condition that arises when the heat is excessive. When there is a Sodium deficiency, "Greens" are very important as they contain the vital organic Sodium that is needed to help correct this allergic condition.

Many times people will go to the beach for the day and return home feeling exhausted. This is usually due to the loss of Sodium and

Potassium and the loss of Vitamin F which is burned up by the sun. If the person has a hot dog on the way home, there might be an allergic reaction to the fat in the hot dog. The wheat bun may also affect the individual because of a wheat sensitivity due to the loss of Vitamin F from the sun. What is needed during the hot summer days is a tremendous number of salads and foods that are rich in Potassium such as Bananas (which ironically grow in the tropics). Bananas are a miracle food containing a large amount of Potassium, Sulfur, and digestive enzymes. Incidentally, bananas are the only food containing an important brain neuro-transmitter—serotonin.

Another very good source of Potassium is Bee Pollen which contains approximately 300 mg. of Potassium per 500 mg. capsule. Alfalfa, which contains two parts Potassium to one part Sodium, is also a good source. These shall be discussed in detail later in the book.

It should be noted that if a person is lacking Sodium, all foods *except* Sodium-bearing foods will become allergenic. This is one of the reasons respiratory disorders such as bronchitis, asthma, or lung problems will manifest. When the person is allergic to almost all foods, the allergic reaction from the foods eaten can cause an "asthmatic condition" or a respiratory problem.

If a person should become Potassium depleted, milk, cheese and all foods containing Sodium would become allergenic. Of all the vitamins and minerals, Potassium and Sodium tend to be the most unstable since they are burned up so quickly. Heat, or any activity causing you to perspire, will cause a loss of Potassium and Sodium. Perspiration contains Potassium, Sodium, Uric Acid, Ammonia and Chloride. Hence, when you are sweating, you are losing all these important minerals. Stress will also cause a loss of Potassium and Sodium because stress affects the Adrenal Glands which create more of a need for these two minerals.

I have taken the time to build "FOOD BLOCK" allergies, or categories of different foods which are related to the specific food allergy. These groups, or food blocks, are governed by different vitamins and minerals. For instance, when I talk about an allergy to rice, this also means that a person would be allergic to the rice allergy food group, which consists of cinnamon, blueberries, grapes, strawberries, watermelon, wine and pumpkin. The mineral Manganese is the antidote to this allergy and if missing, an allergy to these foods would occur. The amino acids Arginine and Proline are the antidotes to the "rice" allergy. Vitamin B-12 is the antidote vitamin.

When I speak of a "Yeast Allergy" the following foods are included: barley, cherries, millet, potatoes, prunes, raisins, rye and walnuts. The antidote to the yeast allergy is Zinc which neutralizes the allergy to these foods. I call this group of unrelated foods the "Yeast Allergy Food Group" so I don't have to list each individual food, thereby saving time. The amino acid is Lysine, while the vitamins B-1 and B-6 are the antidote vitamins to the "yeast" group.

The "Citrus Group" includes oranges, lemons, limes, grapefruit, tomatoes, pineapples, tangerines and cantaloupe. An allergy to these foods (citrus allergy) can be neutralized by Pantothenic Acid, also known as Vitamin B-5, Calcium, and the amino acid Serine.

After I have identified the Metabolic Antagonist (allergy), I administer the needed antidotes—the amino acid, vitamin, and mineral for a period of four days while the client avoids the antagonistic substance. The client returns to be rechecked on the fifth day to see (A) if the Antagonist substance is neutralized, and (B) to adjust the amount of the antidotes' quantity. For example, for a "wheat" allergy I would determine through the M.R.T. what amount of Magnesium is needed. Let's say they need 5x200 mg. 6x500 mg. of Histidine and two capsules of Safflower Oil are also needed. In four days (on the fifth day) the wheat allergy could show OK - but it's only an abatement, not a cure. Then we would retest the nutrient amounts. The test may now show 1x200 mg. of Magnesium, 1 of Histidine, and 1 capsule of Safflower Oil. The client would take the *new* test amounts for one or two more weeks then return for another retest. By then, the allergy should be abolished. This has always worked for us.

On the next page is a chart to clarify the antidotes to the allergies.

CHART I.
"Food Allergens and Their Neutralizing Nutritional Antidotes."

FOOD	VITAMINS	MINERAL	AMINO ACID	HERB
1. Yeast Series Barley Cherry Millet Potatoes Prune Raisins Rye Walnuts	Thiamin (B1) Pyridoxin (B6)	Zinc	Lysine (Comfrey)	Pau D'Arco Red Clover Comfrey
2. Rice Series Cinnamon Curry Blueberry Grapes Straw- berries Water- melon Wine Pumpkin	Pyrdoxine Cyanoco- balamin (B12)	Manganese	Arginine Proline	Yucca Beet Powder
3. Wheat Feathers Wool Dust Detergents Cat & Dog Dander	Essential Fatty Acids (F) - (Linoleic)	Magnesium	Histidine	Black Walnut Kelp Spirulina
4. Corn	Essential Fatty Acids	Magnesium Potassium	Histidine	Black Walnut Kelp, Bee Pollen

FOOD	VITAMINS	MINERAL	AMINO ACID	HERB
5. Fat Series Meat Fats Vegetable Milk Fats Cosmetics	Biotin (H) Carnitine (Bt)	Sulfur	Methionine Cysteine Taurine Glutathione Threonine Carnitine	Sarsaparilla Eyebright Fenugreek Dandelion Burdock Fennel Seeds
6. Oatmeal Sesame	Folic Acid Cyanoco- balamin, C	Iron	Citrilline	Yellow Dock
7. Milk (Cheese)	D	Potassium	Aspartic Acid Asparagine	Bee Pollen Alfalfa Hawthorne Berry
8. Citrus	Pantho- thenic Acid (B5)	Calcium	Serine	Royal Jelly Comfrey
9. Peppers Peaches Pears Plums Nectarines	Niacinamide	Phosphorus	L'Glutamine	Royal Jelly

CHAPTER 3

THE VITAMIN KINGDOM

HOW TO TEST FOR NUTRIENTS

To test the nutrients we will use the acupuncture points on the body. This will be done by placing two fingers of the client's right hand onto the appropriate acupuncture nutrition points.

Some books say use one finger, and others, three. I prefer two fingers because it permits the other finger to hold the nutrients in the palm.

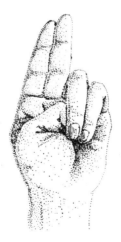

Figure 9

This will become clearer to you as we progress.

VITAMIN A

Right Eyelid

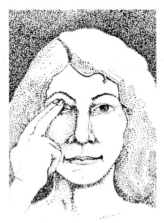

Figure 10

Vitamin A comes in two different forms:

(1.) Fat soluble (fish oil)
(2.) Water dispersible (Beta-Carotene, Lemon Grass)

We prefer the water dispersible type, for there is less danger of over-dose.

*RDA: 5,000 I.U. for adults
        3,000 I.U. for children

Therapeutic Range:

As much as test shows.

Beneficial Effects:

Vitamin A counteracts night blindness and weak eyesight; aids in the treatment of many eye disorders; builds resistance against respiratory disorders; plays a vital role in nourishing skin and hair, teeth, bones and gums; protects against the damaging effects of polluted air; and increases the permeability of blood capillaries contributing to better tissue oxygenation.

*Recommended Daily Allowance

Signs of Toxicity:

Nausea, vomiting, diarrhea, hair loss, headaches, flaky, itchy, and "blotchy" skin, blurred vision, bone pain, and liver enlargement. In order to counteract a Vitamin A overdose, take one gram of Vitamin C (Ascorbic Acid) every hour until symptoms disappear.
Note: Women on the Pill need more A.

Food Sources:

Colored fruits and vegetables, carrots, green leafy vegetables, liver, eggs, milk, and fish liver oil.

Author Observation:

Cold weather and too much Vitamin C will use up Vitamin A.

Raw Juice Sources:

Carrots, escarole, kale, parsley, pimento, spinach, sweet potatoes, turnip greens and watermelon.
Vitamin A is more effective when taken with:

Vitamin B complex	Helps preserve stored Vitamin A.
Vitamin C	Helps protect against toxic effects of Vitamin A. Helps prevent oxidation.
Vitamin D	1 part Vitamin D to 10 parts Vitamin A.
Vitamin E	Acts as an antioxidant.
Vitamin F	When Vitamin F dosage is increased, increase supply of Vitamin A.
Calcium	When Vitamin A dosage is increased, increase supply of Calcium and Phosphorus.
Phosphorus	When Vitamin A dosage is increased, increase supply of Calcium and Phosphorus.
Zinc	Helps in the absorption of Vitamin A.

Vitamin A effectiveness is diminished by:

Mineral Oil
Lack of Vitamin D in the body.

VITAMIN B

The B vitamins can be tested by placing the pill(s) in the right palm while touching the tongue with two fingers or by just holding the vitamin pill(s) in the palm and placing the palm in the "solar plexus" area* of the body. The tongue is a little more sensitive, but the solar plexus is more practical.

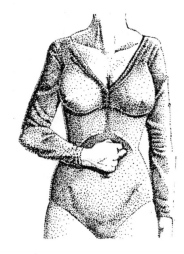

Figure 11

B-1	Thiamine	B-13	Orotic Acid
B-2	Riboflavin	B-15	Pangamic Acid
B-3	Niacin	B-17	Laetrile
B-5	Pantothenic Acid	Biotin	(Vitamin H)
B-6	Pyridoxine	Choline	
B-9	Folic Acid	Inositol	
B-12	Cobalamin	PABA	

The B vitamins are "synergistic". In other words, they are more potent together than when used separately. During stress, illness, and surgery, the need for the B vitamins increases.

Overconsumption of sugar and alcohol also destroys the B vitamins. Diabetics and alcoholics often need more of the B vitamins than most people. All B vitamins are water soluble. Any excess is excreted and not stored in the body. The B vitamins must be replaced daily.

*Gut area of torso

Food Sources:

Colored Fruits and Vegetables, Carrots, Green Leafy Vegetables, Liver, Eggs, Milk, and Fish Oil.
The B complex vitamins are more effective when taken with:

- Vitamin C
- Vitamin E
- Calcium
- Phosphorus

VITAMIN B-1: (Thiamine)

RDA 1.0 milligrams
Therapeutic doses up to 100 milligrams

Beneficial Effects:

Vitamin B-1 is an anti-beriberi.
An anti-aging nutrient.
Aids digestion, particularly of protein.
Helps stabilize emotions, and relieves irritability and depression.
Helps produce Hydrochloric Acid in the stomach.
Helps correct constipation by improving Peristalsis.
Helps prevent Edema.
Helps the heart muscle, brain, and entire nervous system.
Is also a catalyst in the cure for yeast and wheat allergies.

Food Sources:

Brewer's Yeast, Blackstrap Molasses, Brown Rice, Organ Meats, Eggs, and Nuts.

Raw Juice Sources:

Asparagus and avocado.
Note: The heat from cooking destroys this vitamin. Vitamin B-1 is also destroyed by caffeine, alcohol, food-processing, estrogen, sulfa drugs, air, and water.
Vitamin B-1 is more effective when taken with:

Vitamin B-complex	Vitamin E
Vitamin B-2	Vitamin C (helps protect against
Folic Acid	oxidation)
Niacin	Manganese
	Sulfur

VITAMIN B-2: (Riboflavin)

RDA: 1.6 milligrams for men
       1.3 milligrams for women

Beneficial Effects:

Useful in the treatment of bloodshot eyes, abnormal sensitivity to light, itching and burning eyes, and cataracts.

Useful in the treatment of skin conditions and mouth sores, inflammation of the mouth, sore burning tongue (magenta colored tongue), and cracks on lips and corners of mouth.

Useful in correcting oily hair, oily skin, and premature wrinkles on the face and arms.

Can also correct splitting nails, and such aging symptoms as a "disappearing" upper lip.

Food Sources:

Brewer's Yeast, Wheat Germ, Rice Polishings, Blackstrap Molasses, Organ Meats, Eggs, and Nuts.

Raw Juice Sources:

Beet greens, kale, and spinach.
Note: Light, especially ultraviolet light, and alkalies are destructive to vitamin B-2.
Vitamin B-2 is more effective when taken with:

Vitamin B-complex
Vitamin B-6 (B-2 and B-6 doses should always be the same.)
Vitamin B-3
Vitamin C (helps protect against oxidation.)

VITAMIN B-3: (Niacin, Niacinamide, Nicotinic Acid)

RDA: 18 milligrams for men
       Small amounts for women and children

Therapeutic Dosage:

As a part of a megavitamin therapy, Niacin is sometimes given in dosages of 5000 milligrams per day.

Beneficial Effects:

Niacin mellows the personality!
Raises the irritability threshold.
Relieves depression.
Neutralizes allergic reaction from peppers, pears, peaches, plums, and nectarines, thereby removing headaches, indigestion and skin problems.
Sometimes useful in alleviating toothache and backache.
Niacinamide is similar in effect and therapeutic value to Niacin, but does not cause flushing, tingling and itching.
After my clients have confidence in my system, I often start them on a Niacin program (3 × 500 mg. per day). I do not use, nor suggest my students use, Niacin in the beginning of a nutritional program because women clients think they are having "hot flashes".
The advantage of taking Niacin instead of Niacinamide is that the skin complexion improves from the "flushing".
I often use Niacin to help smokers stop smoking. This works because Nicotine is the opposite (mirror image molecule) of Nicotinic Acid (Niacin).
By substituting Niacin for Nicotine, the craving for cigarettes will stop. Smoking also displaces Niacin by substituting Nicotine for the Niacin in the brain which causes allergies to the foods previously mentioned and will create a "Hiatus Hernia" effect in the stomach.
Many Hiatus Hernia conditions are merely an allergic reaction to certain foods (peppers, pears, peaches, plums, and nectarines).
We have found that Novocaine, Procaine, and the substance GH-3, and KH-3 to use up Pantothenic Acid. So if you are using any of these you should also use a Panothenic Acid supplement. *After* a dental visit where Novocaine was used a Panathonic Acid supplement will normalize your B-5 level. If B-5 is taken before the dental visit, the Novocaine will not work so easily!
When you find yourself grouchy, you should check your Niacin level. This can be done by holding one or more Niacin pills in the right hand on the solar plexus and extending the opposite arm to be "pumped". Another person should pump the extended arm. If the arm goes down when "pumped", it could mean that the amount is too much or too little.

Best Natural Source:

Royal Jelly
100 mg. of Royal Jelly contains 500 mg. of Vitamin B-3
Note: I have yet to see a Niacin "flush" reaction from anyone using
Royal Jelly.
Vitamin B-3 is more effective when taken with:

Vitamin B-complex
Vitamin B-1
Vitamin B-2
Vitamin C

VITAMIN B-5: (Pantothenic Acid)

RDA: From 50 to 5,000 milligrams

Beneficial Effects:

Will stop a "Citrus Allergy" (lemon, lime, orange, tangerine, grapefruit, tomato, pineapple, and cantaloupe).
Is involved in all the vital functions of the body.
Stimulates the Adrenal Glands and increases production of Cortisones and other Adrenal hormones.
Is an anti-stress vitamin, and helps to avoid premature aging.
Helps hair loss, and can change gray hair back to its natural color.
Can correct Hypoglycemia (low blood sugar).
Can also help to correct painful and burning feet, adrenal exhaustion, and emotional sensitivity that can cause asthmatic attacks.

Best Sources:

Bee Pollen and Royal Jelly
1-500 mg. capsule of Bee Pollen contains 50 mg. of Pantothenic Acid.
1-100 mg. capsule of Royal Jelly has the equivalent potency of a 1500 mg. pill of manufactured Pantothenic Acid, and is readily absorbable and a non-allergic source.
Vitamin B-5 is more effective when taken with:

Vitamin B complex
Vitamin B-6
Vitamin B-12
Biotin (Aids in the absorption of B-5)

Folic Acid (Aids in the absorption of B-5)
Vitamin C (Helps protect against oxidation)
Sulfur

Note: An overdose of Pantothenic Acid (B-5),e.g., taking 1,000 mg.
over a nine month period without balancing with the mineral
Sulfur, will cause a sore throat, and a feeling of heaviness on the
upper chest, along with an allergy to fats.

Pantothenic Acid displaces Sulfur in the body, so I recommend taking
the Sulfur containing amino acids Methionine, Cysteine, and Taurine,
as a balancer.

VITAMIN B-6: (Pyridoxine)

RDA: 2 milligrams for children
2.5 milligrams for lactating and pregnant women

Therapeutic Doses:

Up to 1,000 milligrams

Beneficial Effects:

Vitamin B-6 feeds the Pituitary gland to aid in the balancing of the
body's electrolytes - Potassium and Sodium.

Fights Anemia, Edema, mental depression, skin disorders, sore
mouth and lips, halitosis, nervousness, Eczema, kidney stones, loss of
muscular control, migraine headaches, and senility.

Vitamin B-6 helps in the absorption of Vitamin B-12

Is also a catalyst in the healing of a Wheat Allergy.

Aids in the absorption of amino acids (protein)

NOTE: An overdose of Vitamin B-6 can trigger *vivid dreams*.

Food Sources:

Brewers Yeast, Wheat Bran, Wheat Germ, Liver, Kidney, Heart,
Cantaloupe, Cabbage, Blackstrap Molasses, Milk, Eggs, Beef, Green
Leafy Vegetables, Green Peppers, Carrots, Peanuts, and Pecans.
Vitamin B-6 is destroyed by cooking and food processing.

Vitamin B-6 is more effective when taken with:

Vitamin B-Complex   Vitamin C
Vitamin B-1   Magnesium

Vitamin B-2
(Should be taken in balance with B-6)
Vitamin B-5
(Should be taken in balance with B-6)

Potassium
Linoleic Acid
Sodium

VITAMIN B-12: (Cobalamin, Cyanocobalamin) (Hydroxycobalamin)

RDA: 3 micrograms for adults
      Less for children
Only vitamin that contains essential mineral elements.

Beneficial Effects:

Vitamin B-12 is essential for the production and regeneration of red blood cells, prevents anemia, promotes growth in children, prevents such eye problems as burning, excessive watering, and even Cataracts and some types of diminished sight, involved in many vital metabolic and enzymatic processes.

Therapeutic Doses:

I have successfully administered up to 15,000 micrograms per day for one week, reducing it down to 10,000 mcg. the second week, and 5,000 mcg. the third and fourth weeks.

Because B-12 is difficult to assimilate when taken orally, many medical doctors will administer it in the form of an intravenous injection. I find this to be a questionable procedure because many times the injection may carry with it some of the needle cleaner, or sterilizing substance such as sodium hydroxide. This may also be injected into the body, and if a patient's Potassium level is low, the person may have an allergic reaction which some may believe to be a reaction from the B-12, but actually is from the substance that was used to sterilize the needle.

I prefer to use a timed-release B-12 pill that bypasses the stomach and opens in the small intestines. I do not usually recommend timed release pills, but in the case of B-12 it is sometimes better since the timed-release capsule will bypass the stomach where the B-12 can be destroyed by stomach acids. There is also the sublingual approach, which some nutritionists prefer. With the sublingual approach, a lozenge is absorbed in the mouth into the saliva glands, passing directly into the blood stream.

Vitamin B-12 should also be combined with Calcium during absorption to benefit the body properly.

A deficiency in Vitamin B-12 may cause a sore mouth, loss of mental energy, difficulty in concentration, a feeling of numbness or stiffness, soreness and weakness in the legs and arms; reduced sensory perception, difficulty in walking, and impotency in men.

Natural Sources:

Milk, Eggs, Liver (Desiccated Liver is an excellent source), fortified Brewer's Yeast, Peanuts, Bananas, Sunflower Seeds, Comfrey Leaves, Kelp, Concord Grapes, Raw Wheat Germ and Bee Pollen.
Vitamin B-12 is more effective when taken with:

Vitamin B-Complex	Inositol
Vitamin B-6 (helps increase absorption)	Potassium
Vitamin C (helps increase absorption)	Sodium
Choline	Calcium
Folic Acid	

VITAMIN B-13: Orotic Acid

RDA: Not known

Beneficial Effects:

Essential for the biosynthesis of Nucleic Acid.
Vital for the regenerative processes in cells.
Metabolizes Folic Acid and Vitamin B-12.
Can possibly prevent certain liver problems and premature aging.
Can possibly aid in the treatment of Multiple Sclerosis.

Vitamin B-13 is destroyed by water and sunlight.

Food Sources:

Root Vegetables, and is also present in the "Whey" portion of milk (The liquid portion of sour or curdled milk).

VITAMIN B-15: (Pangamic Acid or Calcium Pangamate; DiMethylGlycine)

RDA:
Vitamin B-15 is an antioxidant. It increases the body's tolerance to hypoxia (insufficient oxygen supply to the tissues and cells.) B-15 helps extend cell lifespan, regulates fat metabolism, neutralizes a craving for liquor, stimulates the glandular and nervous systems, and also lowers blood cholesterol and aids in protein synthesis. It is also helpful in the treatment of heart disease, angina and asthma.

We have found B-15 exceptionally helpful to a smoker who is trying to stop smoking. It gives the client the extra oxygen needed which tarred lungs cannot supply to the cells. This is also an important supplement for residents of big cities and high density pollution areas.

Food Sources:

Whole Grains, Seeds, Nuts, and Whole Brown Rice
Vitamin B-15 is destroyed by water and sunlight.
Vitamin B-15 is more effective when taken with:

Vitamin B-Complex
Vitamin C
Vitamin E

Vitamin B-17: Laetrile (Nitrilosides, Amygdalin)

RDA: *5 to 30 Apricot Kernels eaten throughout the day.

Beneficial Effects:

It is used as an anti-cancer nutrient in controlling cancer and as preventive therapy. Made from the seeds or kernels from various fruits, e.g., Apricots and Peaches. B-17 is legal in only a few states, having been prohibited by the F.D.A. on the grounds that there is a Cyanide content which could be poisonous to the consumer. In fact, there is a cyanide molecule bound up, but it is released only in the presence of cancer cells. Vitamin B-12, cyanocobalamin also has a cyanide molecule bound up with cobalamin. Vitamin B-17 is helpful in reducing high blood pressure, cataracts and sickle cell anemia.

*As stated in the *Nutritional Almanac*.

Food Sources:

Apricot kernels, Cherry kernels, Peach and Plum kernels, Apple Seeds, Raspberries, Cranberries, Blackberries, Lima Beans, Mung Beans, Flaxseed, Millet and Buckwheat, Kasha and Caszava beans. Vitamin B-17 is more effective when taken with:

Vitamin A	Vitamin B-15	
Vitamin B-Complex	Vitamin C	Vitamin E

BIOTIN: (CoEnzyme R, or Vitamin H)

RDA: 150-300 micrograms

Beneficial Effects:

Helps the synthesis of Ascorbic Acid and is essential for normal metabolism of fats and protein. Also is a preventative treatment for baldness, can help hair growth, and helps keep hair from turning gray. Can alleviate Eczema, Dermatitis, Dandruff, Seborrhea, skin disorders, lung infections, Anemia, loss of appetite, mental depression, drowsiness, and hallucinations.

Food Sources:

Nuts, Brewers Yeast, Beef Liver, Egg Yolk, Milk, Kidney, and Unpolished Rice.

NOTE: Biotin can be synthesized in the body by intestinal bacteria. Raw egg white prevents absorption of Biotin by the body. Raw egg white contains Avidin, a protein that prevents Biotin absorption.

Biotin is more effective when taken with:

Vitamin B-Complex
Vitamin B-12
Folic Acid
Pantothenic Acid
Vitamin C
Sulfur

CHOLINE

The Choline M.R.T. point is located at the back of the head:

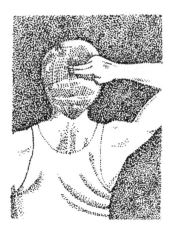

Figure 12

Choline is a member of the B-complex family, and is also a "Lipotropic Factor" (fat emulsifier).

Choline teams up with Inositol (available in Lecithin) to utilize fats and cholesterol. Lecithin helps to digest, absorb, and carry fats in the blood and the fat soluble vitamins A, D, E, and K.

Choline is one of the few substances able to penetrate the so-called blood brain barrier (which ordinarily protects the brain against fluctuations in the daily diet) to go directly into the brain cells to produce a chemical that aids the memory.

Choline is necessary for the synthesis of the nucleic acids DNA and RNA. Choline minimizes excessive deposits of fats and cholesterol in the liver and arteries, and also helps eliminate poisons from the body by aiding the liver and gall bladder functions.

Choline can combat hardening of the arteries (Arteriosclerosis) and also, Alzheimer's Disease. Choline is also helpful in reducing High Blood Pressure and in treating kidney damage, Glaucoma and Myasthenia Gravis. Choline combined with other nutrients has been known to aid hair growth and prevent baldness. Choline is part of the nutritional regime to help combat tardive dyskinesia, along with Manganese, Zinc, and Niacin.

RDA: Not yet established.

Best Sources:

Liquid or granular Lecithin (Usually derived from soybeans), Brewer's Yeast, Wheat Germ, Egg Yolks, Liver, and Green Leafy Vegetables.

CHOLINE is more effective when taken with:

Vitamin A	Folic Acid
Vitamin B-Complex	Inositol
Vitamin B-12 (Helps to synthesize Choline)	Linoleic Acid
	(Vitamin F)

NOTE: Migraine headaches in the back of the head can usually be corrected by the administration of Choline. The commercial products are Choline tablets: Phosphatidyl Choline (A "Super Lecithin"), Choline Chloride and DMAE (DiMethyl-AminoEthanol Bitartrate). Also, please beware if using Choline Chloride liquid, as it should be diluted with juice or water and should not be continued for more than 21 days at a time because the Chloride tends to irritate the digestive system.

The memory can also be corrected by the administration of choline. And it should be noted that choline is depleted in the brain by coffee. No wonder so many Americans are absent-minded!!

To test the Choline point, place the two fingers of the right hand at the rear of the head while extending the left arm to be "pumped". If extended arm goes down when it is pressed (or pumped), the Choline point is weak and Choline is needed.

FOLIC ACID

RDA: 400 micrograms for adults

Therapeutic Doses:

1,000 micrograms

Beneficial Effects:

Folic Acid is essential to the formation of red blood cells. It also aids in protein metabolism for division of blood cells. Folic Acid is necessary for the growth and division of all body cells and for the production of RNA and DNA. It helps build antibodies to prevent and heal infection. Also helps prevent premature graying of the hair, and correct skin disorders such as Grayish-brown skin pigmentation.

Folic Acid will help reproductive disorders such as avoiding spontaneous abortion, difficult labor, lowers the infant death rate, and improves lactation. Folic Acid is essential in the utilization of sugars and amino acids (protein). It can act as an analgesic for pain and can also prevent canker sores. Also helps ward off Anemia when grouped with Vitamin B-12.

NOTE: Sunlight destroys Folic Acid. Vitamin C increases the excretion of Folic Acid.

Food Sources:

Deep Green Leafy Vegetables, Organ Meats, Oysters, Salmon, Milk, Carrots, Egg Yolks, Cantaloupe, Apricots, Pumpkins, Avocados, Bean, Rye, and Wheat.

Folic Acid is more effective when taken with:

Vitamin B-complex
Vitamin B-12 (Cyanocobalamin)
Biotin
Vitamin B-5 (Pantothenic Acid)
Vitamin C   Helps protect against oxidation.

INOSITOL

The M.R.T. point for Inositol can be found at the base of the skull and can be checked by touching the right hand fingers to the point while having someone press down on the extended left arm.

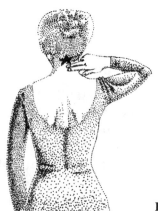

Figure 13

RDA: Not yet established

Inositol is another member of the B-Complex family and a "Lipotropic Factor" (fat emulsifier). Inositol combines with Choline to form Lecithin which nourishes the brain cells and also lowers Cholesterol levels. It promotes healthy hair by preventing fall out, aids the heart, and burns up fat.

We have found that it can also help reverse the symptoms of degeneration in the Myelin Sheathing of the nerves which can cause Paralysis of the lungs, hands, and limbs.

Deficiencies in Inositol may cause baldness, eczema, eye abnormalities, constipation, and high blood cholesterol.

Food Sources:

Lecithin, Brewers Yeast, Wheat Germ, Unprocessed Oatmeal and Corn, Milk, Nuts, Citrus Fruit, and Liver.

Inositol is more effective when taken with:

Vitamin B-Complex
Vitamin B-12
Choline
Linoleic Acid

PABA: (Para-aminobenzoic Acid)

The Muscle Response Testing point for PABA is like all the other "B" vitamins. It can be tested by placing the PABA in the palm of the

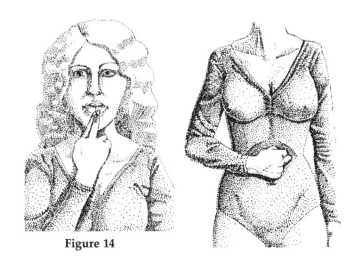

Figure 14   Figure 15

hand while touching the tongue and extending the other arm to be "pumped", or by holding the PABA in the hand to the Solar Plexus and extending the other arm.

RDA: Not yet established

Function:

PABA stimulates the metabolism and all vital life processes. PABA prevents skin changes due to aging. PABA helps sustain natural hair color and had been used in combination with Biotin, Folic Acid, Pantothenic Acid, and Choline to restore graying hair to its natural color with success.

Applied as a lotion or salve to the skin, it is an excellent sun screen and skin rejuvenator. PABA is also helpful for a variety of skin disorders including Eczema and Lupus Erythematosus.

A deficiency of PABA can cause extreme fatigue, Eczemea, Anemia, gray hair, reproductive disorders, infertility, vertigo, and loss of libido.

Food Sources:

Brewers Yeast, Whole Grain Products, Milk, Eggs, Yogurt, Wheat Germ, Molasses, and Liver.

PABA is also synthesized by freindly bacteria in the intestines if the intestines are healthy.

NOTE: If you are taking Penicillin, or any Sulfa drug, the PABA intake should be increased.

VITAMIN C

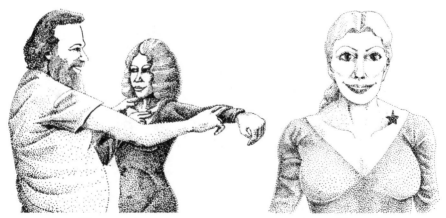

Figure 16   Figure 17

The Vitamin C acupuncture point is in the hollow between the left breast muscle (pectoral muscle) and left shoulder muscle (deltoid muscle) just below the collarbone on the left side.

There are two types of vitamin C: (a) water dispersible (the most popular) and (b) fat soluble.

Vitamin C from corn, rose hips, citrus, and acerola hips is all water soluble, as is ascorbic acid.

Vitamin C from Palmatate is fat soluble.

A 500 mg "corn" (water soluble) is equal in strength to a 325 mg palmatate (fat soluble).

In utilizing Vitamin C, note that there is a different reaction from different sources of "C."

If the label reads 1,000 mg of Vitamin C *with* rose hips it is usually a corn C in a base of rose hips. No way can a 1,000 mg Vitamin C pill be of rose hips in a one-tablet size!! This is a natural C but if you are allergic to *corn*, this could be a disastrous situation. The same thing would happen if you took a "Citrus C" (orange, lemon, lime, or grapefruit flavored) and were allergic to the citrus.

The body does not absorb the vitamin when the base is allergic. In my practice, I use a water dispersible "Calcium Ascorb" because it is the least allergic form of Vitamin C.

Vitamin C plays an important role in the formation of collagen, which is important for the growth and repair of tissue cells, gums, blood vessels, bones, and teeth. It also helps the body to absorb Iron in addition to acting as a catalyst in the absorption and utilization of other nutritional substances.

Vitamin C accelerates healing after surgery. It helps decrease blood cholesterol and lowers the incidence of blood clot formation in the veins. It will also prevent Scurvy.

Many nutritionists prefer time release capsules to ordinary pills and capsules. I DO NOT PREFER THEM!!

In my work with people who have had *Colostomies (the use of a plastic bag as a feces remover), I have seen that the time released pills or capsules pass into the bag and *do not dissolve*!!

How many people without colostomies have excreted time release pills undissovled in their bowel movements??

---

*COLOSTOMY: The surgical procedure when it is necessary to remove the rectum, usually for cancerous tumors; the lower colon is cut across and is diverted through an artificial anus made in the skin of the abdomen. A special apparatus is placed over the opening so a plastic bag can be applied in which the feces collect and can be emptied out.

I prefer a "Buffered" Vitamin C such as the Calcium Ascorb, taken about three hours apart to insure body absorption!!

Many nutritionists use a "Super C" with Bioflavonoids. I do not prefer this type of vitamin combination at the beginning of a program because I believe that many manufacturers use "Citrus Bioflavonoids" which most clients are initially allergic to. The reason is that in this stressful society, the Adrenal Gland is constantly being bombarded with stressful situations that burn up Pantothenic Acid, the antidote to a Citrus Allergy.

Also, our Western civilization consumes a lot of sugar in the average diet which burns up the B-Complex vitamins (of which Pantothenic Acid is a part), thereby creating the "Citrus Allergy".

Peppers are a source of Vitamin C, but will also become allergic in the presence of a Niacinamide deficiency. Niacinamide is another B vitamin that is destroyed by sugar. Niacin, also known as Nicotinic Acid, is displaced in the brain by Nicotine which is absorbed during cigarette smoking.

So again, I feel that the best source of Vitamin C would be a buffered Calcium Ascorb pill or "C"-Ascorb powdered crystals that can be mixed into a beverage that the individual is not allergic to. Sometimes a manufacturer of a "C-Ascorb" will use a sodium Ascorb. This can either be very useful, or dangerous! If a person's Potassium level is very low, there will be an allergic reaction to the *Sodium* C-Ascorb. However, it can also be useful if a person is low in Sodium, such as in the summer when the body is excreting Sodium through perspiration, thereby needing the extra Sodium. Again, always test each type of Vitamin C to find out what is best for the individual.

Do not purchase "bargain" Vitamin C from a pharmacy, for these are synthetic! They are usually non-allergic, but they are also non-absorbable!! A good natural 500 milligram Vitamin C will test twice as strong as a bargain brand synthetic. So where is the bargain if you need twice as much? Since they are Lavorotary and the body is Dextropotary, only 20% of the synthetic form is absorbable.

Did you ever plug a 110 appliance into a 220 electrical outlet? I did! It burned out the motor in 5 minutes! So why do we want to pollute our own bodies with synthetics?

Chemists will tell you there is no difference between natural and synthetic vitamins. In a test tube maybe! But not in your stomach! I'll go into this more thoroughly in Chapter

NOTE: Vitamin C is burned up by cigarette smoking. Each cigarette uses up to 25 mg. of Vitamin C. Polluted air and carbon monoxide from exhaust fumes will also burn up Vitamin C.

TOO MUCH Vitamin C will displace the mineral SULFUR. So when taking Vitamin C be sure to take an adequate amount of Sulfur along with it.

Vitamin C is more effective when taken with:

All vitamins and minerals	Calcium (Helps body utilize C)
Bioflavonoids	Magnesium

Food Sources:

Citrus Fruits, Rose Hips, Tomatoes, Green Pepper

Raw Juice Sources:

Cabbage, Parsley, Green Peas, Green Peppers, Pimento Rutabaga, Tomato, Turnip Greens, Watercress, Cantaloupe, Green Mint, Lemons, Lime, Orange, Raspberries, Rose Hips, Strawberries, Watermelon.

VITAMIN D

(Calciferol, Vio Sterold Ergosterol)
Known as the "Sunshine Vitamin".

The Vitamin "D" point (acupuncture point) is in the area where the left leg comes into the trunk of the body. It is in the fold where a pants crease would be if you were to wear shorts or pants.

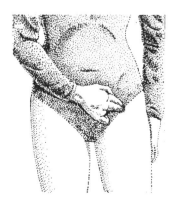

Figure 18

The provitamins D are found in both plant and animal tissue. Vitamin D-2 (Calciferol) is a synthetic. Vitamin D-3 is the natural form as it occurs in liver oils.

RDA: 400 I.U.

Vitamin D is a fat soluble vitamin and can be acquired through exposure to sunlight, or orally through food or food supplements.

Vitamin D is very important for Calcium and Phosphorus absorption, to strengthen bones and teeth. It also aids in assimilation of Vitamin A.

I prefer to obtain my Vitamin D from the sunlight because it's the direct way. Less calories too! Twenty minutes a day should give the adequate R.D.A.

People who work during the day, or who must wear heavy uniforms (Nuns) may not be getting a sufficient amount of Vitamin D, and therefore, should use food supplements of Vitamin D.

City dwellers who live in smog-covered urban areas also need Vitamin D supplements.

Ironically the vitamin manufacturers take Vitamin A capsules and radiate them with artificial ultra-violet light to produce a Vitamin D pill. Instead of taking this kind of supplement, try to get out in the sunlight. Ultraviolet sunlight acts on the oils of the skin to produce the vitamin, which is then absorbed into the body.

Vitamin D can help eye problems (conjunctivitis, Myopia, and cataracts).

Food Source:

Anything that grows in the sunlight, Fish liver Oil (Cod Liver oil, remember?).

Sardines, herring, salmon, Tuna, Milk and Dairy products.

(It should be noted there is more D in the milk in summertime because the cows themselves are out of the barns. So summer milks and cheeses are richer in Vitamin D than winter products.)

Someday they might even put skylights on the barn roofs!

It should be noted that too much D can cause over-calcification of the body. A strong Magnesium intake can dissolve (neutralize) this over-calcification.

Vitamin D is more effective when taken with:

Vitamin A   10 parts Vitamin A to 1 part Vitamin D
Choline   Helps prevent toxicity
Vitamin C   Helps prevent toxicity

Vitamin F
Calcium
Phosphorus

NOTE: An overdose of "D" can cause diarrhea, and the desire to sleep all day especially in a darkened area. This can be antidoted by administering a "dry" E vitamin 400 I.U. every half hour till the symptoms disappear.

VITAMIN E

The vitamin E point is in the hollow between the right breast muscle (pectoral muscle) and the right shoulder muscle (deltoid muscle) just below the collarbone. (This point is exactly the same as the Vitamin C point, but on the opposite side of the body.)

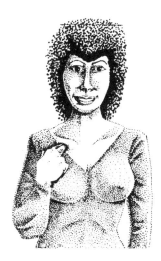

Figure 19

RDA: 15 I.U. for men
     12 I.U. for women

Vitamin E is fat-soluble and stored in the liver, fatty tissues, heart muscles, testes, uterus, blood adrenal and Pituitary glands. Yet 60 to 70 percent of daily doses are excreted in the feces. Unlike other fat-soluble vitamins, E is stored in the body for a relatively short time; similar to Vitamins B and C.

Vitamin E is composed of compounds called Tocopherols, (alpha, beta, gamma, delta, epsilon, zeta, eta, and theta). Alphatocopherol is the most effective. Vitamin E prevents fat soluble vitamins (A and D) and unsaturated fatty acids (F) from being destroyed in the body by oxygen.

Vitamin E oxygenates the tissues and markedly reduces the need for oxygen intake. Vitamin E will also prevent rancidity when added to other substances.

Vitamin E strengthens muscles (especially the heart) and dilates the blood vessels. This combination helps to prevent heart disease and helps to relieve Angina Pectoris.

Vitamin E relieves muscle spasms, helps to heal scar tissue, and when used internally and externally, prevents scar tissue formation from burns and sores. Vitamin E *retards* the aging process by retarding cellular aging due to oxidation. Vitamin E has been successfully used to treat male and female infertility, and also protects the lungs against air pollution by working with Vitamin A. It also *prevents* and *dissolves* blood clots.

In my own research, I have administered up to 2,000 I.U. of Vitamin E to clients over a three month period. What I have discovered is that it specifically nourishes the Pituitary gland which then functions at a more proficient level, thereby affecting the entire endocrine system! This permits the glands to manufacture hormones and regenerate the body!

To insure this specific effect, I group Vitamin E with the herb Gotu Kola, Alfalfa, the amino acids Ornithine and Tryptophan, Vitamin B-6, and Pituitary Glandular.

Food Sources:

Wheat Germ, Soybeans, Vegetable Oil, Broccoli, Brussel Sprouts, Leafy Greens, Spinach, Whole Grain Cereals, and Eggs.

Raw Juice Sources:

Spinach, watercress, lettuce, celery, parsley, turnip leaves, and wheat germ oil.

NOTE: Vitamin E does not cause high blood pressure. If anything, it lowers it. Those who have experienced high blood pressure from Vitamin E were probably allergic to the wheat germ or soy!!

Vitamin E is more effective when taken with:

Vitamin A
Vitamin B-complex
Vitamin B-1 (Thiamine)
Inositol: Helps body utilize Vitamin E
Vitamin C: Helps protect against oxidation
Vitamin F
Manganese: Helps body utilize Vitamin E
Selenium

VITAMIN F

(Polyunsaturated Fats)
(Linoleic, Linolenic and Arachidonic Acid)

The Vitamin F acupuncture (MRT) point is above the collar bone on the right side of the body. It is at the base of the neck between the collarbone and the neck (on the sterno muscle ½ inch above the collarbone).

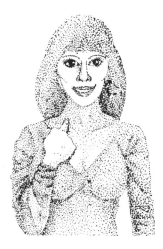

Figure 20

Vitamin F is a fat-soluble vitamin consisting of the unsaturated fatty acids. Unsaturated fatty acids usually come in the form of liquid vegetable oil, while saturated fatty acids are usually found in solid animal fat. Unsaturated fatty acids are important for tissue respiration in vital organs, making it easier for oxygen to be transported by the bloodstream to all cells, tissues, and organs.

Vitamin F also helps maintain resilience and lubrication of all cells and combines with protein and cholesterol to form living membranes that hold the body cells together.

Vitamin F regenerates the skin!! A lack of Vitamin F could cause ulcerations on the lower limbs.

In my own research, I have found Vitamin F to be an antidote to a wheat and corn allergy. That is the reason we butter our bread!!! (And corn muffins).

We have found that wheat (and corn) allergies are abundant in the summertime.

Also, a sunburn could cause the Vitamin F in the body to become deficient, thereby causing an instantaneous wheat (and corn) allergy.

So, if and when you get sunburned, put safflower oil (or olive, sunflower, peanut, or almond oil) on the skin and let it absorb into the pores.* It will help regenerate the skin. I use safflower because it has the highest polyunsaturated fat content.

Have you ever heard of a "swimmer's ear" infection? It is not an infection from the water, but a wheat allergy caused by the sun. It is not an infected right ear, but an *inflamed* ear. (The left ear is governed by a rice allergy).

To test this theory, put the pinky of your right hand into the right ear. Then pull down on the left arm. The arm will go right down. Now, hold a sufficient amount of safflower capsules in your hand (this amount can be determined by placing the capsules in the right hand and holding it

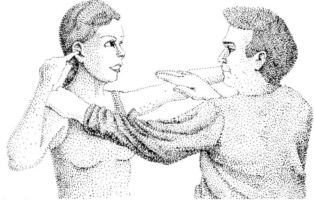

Figure 21

*This also stops the wheat allergy instantaneously.

to the solar plexus while pumping the left arm down, adding or taking away capsules until the arm gets rigid.) Place the pinky of the right hand containing the safflower capsule into the right ear again. Now pump the arm. It should stay rigid!

Now, take a piece of wheat in the right hand and hold it to the solar plexus. If there is an allergy, the left arm will go down. (Remember to keep the tongue away from the roof of your mouth.)

Now take the wheat and the safflower pills used for the ear test and place them together in the right hand. Hold them over the solar plexus point and the arm should stay rigid because the safflower neutralized the wheat. (It should be noted that Vitamin F works wonderfully with Vitamin E).

Food Sources:

Safflower oil, sunflower oil, peanut oil, corn oil, (vegetable oils in liquid form).
Vitamin F is more effective when taken with:

Vitamin A
Vitamin C
Vitamin D
Vitamin E
Phosphorus

VITAMIN G

Is another name for Riboflavin (B-2). Please see Page 24.

VITAMIN H

Is another name for Biotin. Please see Page 31.

VITAMIN K
(MENADIONE)

The test point for Vitamin K is one half inch to the left of the navel.

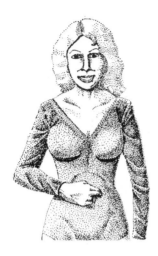

Figure 22

RDA: Not yet established.

Suggested adequate dosage is 300 mcg.

There are three types of K: K-1 and K-2 are formed by natural bacteria in the intestines, K-3 is a synthetic.

Vitamin K is fat soluble, and is often called the clotting factor because it is essential in the formation of prothrombin, a blood-clotting substance. Vitamin K helps to prevent internal bleeding, hemorrhage, and nose bleeds. It aids in reducing excessive menstrual flow.

If a deficiency exists, Celiac Disease, sprue, diarrhea, and colitis might be symptomatic. A Vitamin K deficiency can be caused by X-Rays and radiation.

Food Sources:

Yogurt, alfalfa, egg yolk, safflower oil, soybean oil, kelp, green vegetables, and fish and liver oil.

Raw Juice Sources:

Cabbage, kale, cauliflower, and spinach.

VITAMIN P

Bioflavonoids, Citrin, Hesperidin, Quercitin, Rutin, Vitamin P is considered to be part of the Vitamin C complex.

The Bioflavonoid point is below the collarbone on the left side of the body, beneath the outer edge of the bony protuberance.

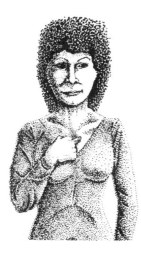

Figure 23

RDA: None established. Usual dosage is 25-150 Mg. per day.

Vitamin P (Bioflavonoids) is also called the capillary permeability factor (P stands for permeability). The prime function of bioflavonoids is to increase capillary strength and regulate absorption. Bioflavonoids prevent capillary hemorrhaging, and stop the appearance of purplish or blue spots on the skin.

Bioflavonoids work synergistically with Vitamin C and prevent Vitamin C from being destroyed by oxidation. Bioflavonoids also help build resistance to infection.

Bioflavonoids help to alleviate: Hypertension, respiratory infection, hemorrhoids, varicose veins, hemorrhaging, bleeding gums, eczema, psoriasis, cirrhosis of the liver, hemorrhages of the retina, radiation sickness, arteriosclerosis, coronary thrombosis, and helps in the treatment of edema and dizziness due to disease of the inner ear.

In our research with different people, we have found that it is wise to *avoid* Bioflavonoid enriched Vitamin C pills in the beginning of the program because many people are allergic to citrus fruits. It is a common problem in this stress-laden world. Distress attacks the Adrenal Glands and thereby burns up their main nutrient which is Pantothenic Acid (B-5). Pantothenic Acid is the antidote for a citrus allergy. So until this condition is straightened out, we refrain from using a Bioflavonoid

Vitamin C. When the Pantothenic Acid level in the body becomes normal, then we use what is called a "Super C with Bioflavonoids".

Even if a client needs Bioflavonoids, we refrain from administering them until the citrus allergy is abated (at least three weeks into the program).

Food Sources:

The white segment part of citrus fruit (Lemon, Oranges, Tangerines and Grapefruit), Strawberries, Prunes, Buckwheat, Apricots, Blackberries, Cherries and Rose Hips.
Bioflavonoids (Vitamin P) are more effective when taken with:

Vitamin C

NOTE: If Bioflavonoids are needed, a pain may occur on the left chest where the "P" point is. It is often mistaken for a heart pain, but it is not. By administering Vitamin P the pain will stop.

VITAMIN T

Vitamin T can be tested by holding your hand to the Solar Plexus and pumping the extended arm:

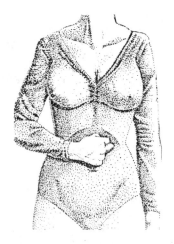

Figure 24

RDA: None established

Vitamin T helps in blood coagulation and in the formation of platelets in the blood. Vitamin T combats Anemia and Hemophilia. It is also useful in improving a fading memory.

Food Sources:

Sesame Seeds, Sesame Butter, Tahini, Egg Yolks.

VITAMIN U

Vitamin U can be tested by holding the hand to the Solar Plexus:

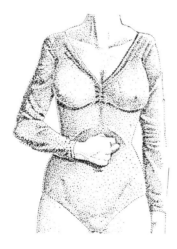

Figure 25

MDR: None known

Vitamin U is the vitamin-like factor found in some vegetables, notably raw cabbage. Vitamin U promotes healing activity in peptic ulcers, particularly in duodenal ulcers.

In our research we found that Vitamin U helps to remove the allergic reaction to tobacco smoke. If a person is a non-smoker and cannot tolerate smoke, it could indicate a Vitamin U deficiency, which would also cause a person to be more affected by the pollution in the air. Vitamin U can be considered an anti-cancer vitamin. Therefore, it is indispensable to inhabitants of urban areas where there is a great percentage of cancer victims.

Food Sources:

Raw cabbage, Alfalfa, Raw cabbage Juice, Homemade Sauerkraut.

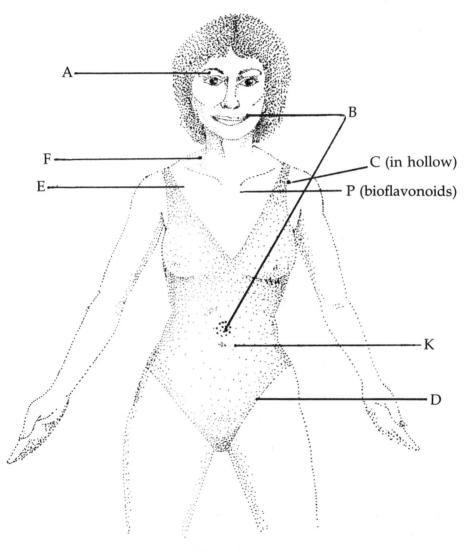

Figure 26

CHAPTER 4

THE MINERAL WORLD

ELEMENTAL VS. CHELATED

Minerals are either Elemental or Chelated. The elemental form is the element in its most basic form. The Chelated mineral is an elemental element suspended (held as if by a claw) in an Amino Acid or another organic compound to facilitate the absorption of the mineral by the body.

Chelation (pronouced key-lay-shun) is taken from the Greek word meaning claw. A chelate is a specific type of complex in which only minerals with a valence (combining capacity) of two can be chelated.

Iron, Zinc, and Calcium (which all have a valence of 2) can be chelated. Potassium (valence of 1) and Phosphorus (valence of 3 and 5) *cannot* be chelated, only complexed.

Selenium, Chromium, Molybdenum, Vanadium, and Nickel have multiple valences including the valence of 2, so they can both complex and chelate with amino acids.

When non-chelated minerals (for example mineral sulfates or mineral gluconates) reach the intestine, the sulfate or gluconate portion is removed and the elemental mineral is chelated by the body for absorption provided sufficient amino acids are available for the chelation to take place.

Chelated minerals help side-step this part of the digestive process because they are already bonded with naturally associated amino acids. This insures the body's absorption of the minerals.

It should be noted that 100 mg. of a chelated mineral may only have 10 mg. of the elemental mineral. Always be aware of what you are testing!!

Also, chelated bases are usually milk or soy, which might cause an allergic reaction in your client should there be a milk and/or soy allergy. Always test the specific pill that the client will be taking during the program because all pills are not the same. Different manufacturers use different bases.

For example, a very famous manufacturer uses milk lactose to fill up the capsules which are half filled with an amino acid. It makes the capsule appear large and full, and therefore, more impressive market-wise. (We prefer the smaller more potent capsules). We have found these to cause an allergic reaction in a person with a milk intolerance.

Once a client brought me a Potassium Gluconate pill which had a label stating that the pills contained "600 mg." of Potassium, but on the side of the label the Potassium content was 99 mg. *elemental* Potassium. This person thought he was taking 600 mg. of elemental Potassium, but he was not!!

MINERALS

Calcium
Chlorine
Chromium
Copper
Fluorine
Germanium
Iodine
Iron
Magnesium
Manganese
Molybdenum
Phosphorus
Potassium
Selenium
Silica
Sodium
Sulfur
Zinc

CALCIUM

The Calcium point is located in the hollow of the left shoulder which can be found behind the Clavical bone on the Trapezius muscle. It is similar to where the Vitamin F point is found, only it is on the other shoulder.

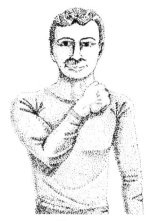
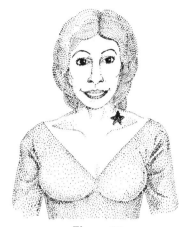

Figure 27   **Figure 28**

RDA dosage 800 - 1400 mg.
(Depending on age)

Therapeutic Dosage:

Can be up to several times more than the RDA.

Function:

Calcium is the body's most abundant mineral. Ninety-nine percent of the Calcium in the body is deposited in the bones and teeth; the remainder is found in the soft tissues.

The complete Calcium content of an organism is entirely renewed in approximately six years. To be able to sustain the right Calcium equilibrium in the body, a person needs a satisfactory daily intake.

Calcium is essential for proper heart action and also for normal clotting of the blood. Calcium is of extreme importance in pregnancy and lactation.

Calcium helps maintain a balance between Sodium, Potassium and Magnesium. Calcium is also essential for the proper utilization of Phosphorus and Vitamins A, C and D.

Calcium can help to alleviate Insomnia, so I usually schedule Calcium (Bone Meal, Oyster Shell, or Calcium Orotate) at bedtime because it is a natural sedative!!

Deficiency Symptoms:

A deficiency of Calcium can cause muscle cramps, numbness and tingling in arms and legs, porous or fragile bones (osteomalacia or osteoporosis), brittle nails, joint pains, tooth decay, nervousness, mental depression, irritability, and also Parkinson's Disease.

Toxic Effects:

Excessive Calcium has been known to cause over-calcification of the bone joints and kidney tissue (which can be corrected by administering Magnesium over a period of time).

Food Sources:

Milk, cheese, most raw vegetables especially dark leafy vegetables such as endive, lettuce, watercress, kale, cabbage, dandelion greens, and brussel sprouts. Other good sources are sesame seeds, oats, almonds, walnuts, millet, sunflower seeds, and tortillas.

In my research, I do not use Calcium Lactate. I will usually start my client on Comfrey (the herbal source of Calcium), and then after about one or two weeks, I switch to Bone Meal or Oyster Calcium and sometimes Calcium orotate or Asporotates.

The reason for the utilization of Comfrey at the beginning of the program is that it is also a digestive aid. This usually helps to "break down" (thereby assisting assimilation) other nutrients being administered in the program. After a few weeks, when the amount of the nutrient needed decreases, then you would switch over to bone meal and/or Oyster Calcium.

I do not use Calcium lactate because many of my clients have "milk allergies", or an intolerance to milk. One of the biggest causes of a Calcium deficiency is a milk or dairy allergy which we have found to be caused by a Potassium deficiency and an absence of an enzyme called Lactase.

When a person burns up their Potassium through stress, trauma, or even perspiration and does not replenish it, they will become intolerant to dairy products, which usually manifests itself as a Sinus condition, cold, or flu. Potassium can be replenished through the use of carrot juice, bee pollen, and alfalfa, all of which are excellent sources.

When there is an intolerance to milk, the person will no longer absorb the Calcium in the milk and cheese products that are staples in the western man's diet. This brings about dental and bone problems in old age. Bones can be regenerated, but it takes months! So, prevention in this case is worth a pound of cure.

When Comfrey is being used, the Phosphorus point should also be checked as Comfrey does not contain Phosphorus. Phosphorus can be found in bone meal along with Magnesium and Vitamin D. Dolomite is supposed to be a combination of Calcium and Magnesium in perfect balance, but we have found the amount of Magnesium contained in Dolomite to be insufficient. We advise administering Magnesium independently of Calcium. Magnesium should be administered side by side with Comfrey throughout the day, but it should be noted that Comfrey should not be administered with *any* Calcium product as the comfrey could cause the Calcium (if the calcium is in excess) to "clump" in the kidney, causing stones to form.

When there is a lack of Calcium in the body, the first skeletal area to show a loss is the jaw bone. Teeth can also become loose, leaving the dentist to believe that the gums are at fault. This is not correct! With a lack of Calcium the jaw bone actually thins out so that the roots of the teeth no longer fit causing the teeth to become loose.

To correct this problem, all bone growth nutrients (Calcium, Phosphorus, Magnesium, and Fluoride) should be increased, finding the correct amounts by using the M.R.T. method to find the proper balance of each nutrient. Massaging the gums with the finger will also increase circulation of the area bringing with it the nutrients necessary for regeneration.

The other area affected by a Calcium deficiency is the Coccyx bone area in which a dull ache may occur. The Coccyx bone is not a left over tail from prehistoric man, but is actually a Calcium warehouse. When a bone (toe, finger, or even hairline) is cracked, Calcium is sent from the Coccyx bone to repair the damaged area, making a person feel pain not only in the damaged area, but also in the Coccyx bone. To remedy this condition, increase the person's Calcium intake.

Bone meal, because of its similarity to the composition of the human bone, is the preferred Calcium supplement. The Phosphorus level should also be checked if the bones have been injured. Calcium is the inner bone, and helps to manufacture bone marrow which in turn manufactures red blood cells; white Phosphorus is the outer bone which makes up tooth enamel, outer bone, etc.

Calcium is more effective when taken with:

Vitamin A   Helps in absorption.
Vitamin C   Helps in absorption.

Vitamin D   Helps in the reabsorption of Calcium in kidney troubles,
and in the retention and utilization of Calcium.
Vitamin F   Helps make Calcium available to tissues.
Iron   Helps in absorption.
Magnesium   2 parts Calcium to 1 part Magnesium.
Manganese
Phosphorus   2.5 parts Calcium to 1 part Phosphorus.
Hydrochloric acid

CHLORINE

Chlorine can be tested by holding to the Solar Plexus:

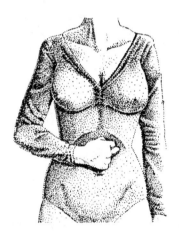

Figure 29

RDA dosage 500 mg.

Function:

Chlorine is an essential mineral occuring in the body mainly as a
compound with Sodium and Potassium. Chlorine compounds such as
Sodium Chloride, or salt, are found primarily in fluids within the cell.
Chlorine is a general cleanser of the organism, expelling waste matter,
helping to clean the blood, and having a tendency to reduce excessive
fat.

Chlorine unites with Hydrogen and other elements to form
Hydrochloric Acid, which is needed for proper protein digestion and

mineral assimilation. Chlorine also helps the liver in its detoxifying activity. Chlorine is an acid forming element.

Deficiency Symptoms:

Lack of Chlorine can cause impaired digestion of foods, obesity, goiter, miners disease, hypoactive adrenals and meningitis.

Food Sources:

Tomatoes, Celery, Iceberg Lettuce, Kelp, Spinach, Cabbage, Kale, Parsnips, and Radish.

Raw Juice Sources:

Asparagus, Carrots, Celery, Red and White Cabbage, Cucumbers, Lettuce, Radish, Spinach, Collards, Ripe Olives, Tomatoes, Sauerkraut, Kale.

NOTE: It is my theory that heart conditions have become prevalent since the turn of the century because of the chlorination of drinking water (tap water). This happens because the Chlorine unites with the Potassium and Sodium already in the body and carries this electrolyte compound out of the body through the urine and sweat. I believe that we should drink only pure mineral water that has not been chlorinated. (Also see Chapter 14 on "Drinking Water.")

Swimming in a chlorinated pool could also be detrimental. Have you ever gone swimming in a chlorinated pool and felt exhausted afterwards? It wasn't just the exercise of swimming that did it! After soaking in a pool for a while, the Chlorine will be absorbed through the pores of the skin leaching the Potassium and Sodium from the body and causing an electrolyte depletion.

All muscles (the heart included) run on Potassium. A lack of Potassium and Sodium can cause exhaustion, lack of appetite, and instantaneous food allergies which can also cause ear inflammations.

Swimming in a salt water (Sea Salt) pool or the ocean would have a different effect on the body. The salt water would saturate the body with organic and inorganic minerals that are contained in the water, thereby nourishing the body through the pores with the minerals that the body needs.

CHROMIUM

Chromium can be tested by holding to the Solar Plexus: (see figure 29, page 56).

Function:

Chromium is *not* a trace mineral, but is an essential mineral. It is an integral part of many enzymes and hormones and works well as a co-factor with insulin to move glucose from the blood into the cells. It is needed for proper sugar metabolism in the body, and is usually needed by diabetics.

Chromium is influential in reducing plaque build up in Arteriosclerosis.

Deficiency Symptoms:

A severe Chromium deficiency could be a contributing cause of Diabetes, high or low blood sugar, hardening of the arteries, and heart disease.

NOTE: Most nutritionists would recommend G.T.F. (Glucose Tolerance factor) as a Chromium source. But I use *straight* elemental Chromium because I have found many of my clients to be allergic to the yeast base that is the normal base for G.T.F.

Natural Sources:

Normally present in natural mineral water, brewer's yeast, liver, *raw* sugar, and cane juice.

All white sugar sweets should be avoided, as they not only burn up the B-Complex vitamins, but burn up Chromium as well.

COPPER

Copper can be tested by holding to the Solar Plexus: (see figure 29, page 56).

RDA: 1 mg. to 1.5 mg. Infant
      1.5 mg. to 2 mg. Child
      2.5 mg. Adult

Function:

Copper is necessary to the central nervous system. Copper contributes to hair and skin color and also stimulates the brain. High concentrations of this mineral are found in the liver, brain, kidneys, and heart.

The elements Molybdenum, Zinc, and Sulfur are antagonistic to copper and so have an adverse effect on copper's absorption. Since copper is needed to assist in the formation of hemoglobin, a deficiency of copper could lead to Anemia because copper must be present with Iron to form hemoglobin.

Copper also promotes blood cell production in bone marrow, and also helps form the cover which surrounds elastin, the chief component of elastic muscle fibers through out the body. Copper also increases tissue respiration.

Deficiency Symptoms:

A deficiency of Copper may cause anemia, loss of hair, impaired respiration, graying of hair, low blood pressure, eczema, enlargement of the prostate gland, and sexual indifference.

Food Sources:

Leek, garlic, artichoke (globe), parsley, and beet root.

Foods rich in Copper are generally those rich in Iron. Especially good sources are: almonds, beans, peas, green leafy vegetables, whole grain products, prunes, raisins, pomegranates, and liver.

NOTE: Copper will burn up Sulfur in the system. When using Copper, be sure to also give adequate amounts of Sulfur to balance out the amount of Copper.

Copper is more effective when taken with:

Cobalt
Iron
Zinc

FLUORINE

Fluorine can be tested by holding to the Solar Plexus: (see figure 29, page 56).

RDA: Not known

Function:

Fluorine is essential for bone and tooth building. Fluorine works with silicon to harden and preserve bones, preventing Osteoporosis. Fluorine discourages growth of acid-forming bacteria, thus reducing tooth decay.

Deficiency Symptoms:

A lack of Fluorine can cause tooth decay, failing eyesight, cataracts, falling hair, brittle finger nails, spongy and bleeding gums, and tuberculosis of the lungs.

Toxicity Symptoms:

Fluorine toxicity may occur when the content of Fluorine in drinking water exceeds two parts per million. It may cause mottling, which is discoloring, and brittleness of tooth enamel. Mottling occurs only during tooth development, not after the enamel has been formed.

Natural Sources:

Organic Fluorine is found in steel-cut oats, sunflower seeds, milk, cheese, carrots, garlic, beet tops, green vegetables, and almonds.

Raw Juice Sources:

Cabbage, cauliflower, garlic, sauerkraut, spinach, sprouts, watercress, endive, chervil, blackeyed beans, avocado, juniper berries, quince, sea cabbage.

Fluorine is normally present in sea water and naturally hard water.

GERMANIUM (OXIDE)

RDA: Not known

Germanium can be tested by placing the pills in the palm of the hand, which then is placed in the Solar Plexus area.

Pump the opposite arm; add or take away pills in the palm being held over the solar plexus area until the opposite arm, which is being pumped, becomes rigid.

Germanium is a trace mineral salt which will stimulate the formation of Red Blood Cells on account of its influence upon the Bone Marrow. Its clinical use in various forms of anemia has met with beneficial results. Germanium enables the blood's malignant cells to attract oxygen and so normalize themselves. Germanium has been effective in curing cancer.

Food Sources:

Korean Ginseng, Garlic, Barley and in the Chinese Herbs Sanzukon, Kashi, Hishi.

IODINE

The M.R.T. acupuncture point for Iodine is located in the hollow of the throat under the "Adam's Apple" (which is also the Thyroid point). RDA: 150 mcg. (.15 mg.)

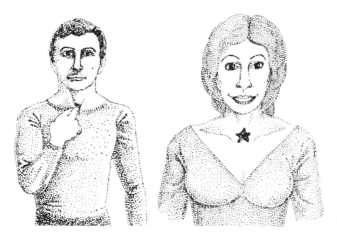

Figure 30

Function:

Iodine is needed to combine with Tyrosine (an amino acid) in the manufacture of Thyroid hormones.

Iodine is an essential part of the hormone Thyroxine. Thyroxine regulates the body's production of energy in the cells and promotes growth and development. Iodine helps to prevent rough and wrinkled skin and regulates the rate of metabolism, energy production, body weight, and development of reproduction glands (female). Iodine also increases the metabolism of Calcium.

Deficiency Symptoms:

Iodine deficiency may cause enlargement of the Thyroid gland (Goiter), imbecility, inferior mental activity, falling hair, dry skin and hair, anemia, fatigue, lethargy, loss of interest in sex, slow pulse, low blood pressure and a tendency towards obesity.

An Iodine deficiency can also cause sterility and a deformed body. A prolonged deficiency can cause Cretinism, thyroid cancer, high blood cholesterol, and heart disease.

Insufficient Iodine will also cause poor circulation of the blood and Lymphatic system, and can also lead to an excessive build up of estrogen in the body which can contribute to the development of cancer of the breast.

Food Sources:

The Best Dietary Sources of Iodine are Kelp, Dulse, and Other Seaweed. Other Good Sources are: Swiss Chard, Turnip Greens, Garlic, Watercress, Pineapples, Pears, Artichokes, Citrus Fruit, Egg Yolks, and Seafood.

Raw Juice Sources:

Artichokes, Carrots, Garlic, Green Grapes, Sea Lettuce, Dulse, Mushrooms, Bartlett Pears, Pineapple, Avocado, Potato Skin, Chives, White Onions, Broccoli, Chard, Celery, Lettuce, Kale, Red Cabbage, Savory Cabbage, Strawberries, Tomatoes, Watercress, Asparagus, Brussel Sprouts, Chervil.

IRON

The iron M.R.T. point is located in the "crease" between the leg and the torso on the right (opposite the Vitamin D point), where a pants leg creases when you sit down.

RDA: 0.35 mgs. for infant per pound of body weight
0.25 mgs. children, per pound of body weight
9 mgs. boys, five to eleven years old
11 mgs. girls, five to eleven years old
13 mgs. boys, over eleven years old

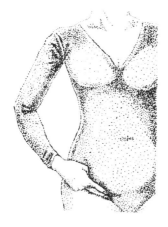

Figure 31

15 mgs. girls, over eleven years old
12 to 14 mgs. men
15 to 17 mgs. women
17 mgs. women, before menopause
13 to 20 mgs. pregnant and nursing women
12 to 14 mgs. women, after menopause

Function:

The Iron in the blood forms an indispensable basic constituent of the red blood cells (hemoglobin). The complete and optimal assimilation of Iron is closely correlated to Copper in its metabolism. Thus, an adequate quantity of Copper in our diet is an indispensable precondition for proper Iron assimilation, as well as an adequate intake of chlorophyll, the green coloring matter of vegetable and plant leaves.

Women need about one and a half times more Iron than men because of their basic biological needs due to menstruation, gestation, and lactation.

The major function of Iron is to interact with Copper and protein to form hemoglobin, the coloring matter of red blood cells. Hemoglobin transports oxygen in the blood from the lungs to the tissues where oxygen is used for energy.

Iron is also necessary for the formation of myoglobin, which is found only in muscle tissue. Myoglobin, transports oxygen to muscle cells where it is used for the chemical reactions involved in muscle contraction. Vitamin C also enhances Iron absorption.

Deficiency Symptoms:

A lack of iron can cause anemia, pale skin, abnormal fatigue, brittle nails, shortness of breath, depression, a red inflamed tongue, low blood pressure, sciatic rheumatism, dizziness, and a loss of interest in sex.

When Iron is low in the body, a headache will usually occur on the right side of the head, half way between the eye socket and the temple, and can expand to above the eyebrow behind the eyeball. This headache will immediately disappear upon the intake of Iron.

The headache will occur in this area:

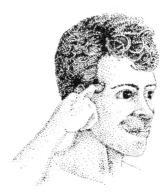

Figure 32

Note: Too much Iron can cause a headache on the right side of the head in the same spot but will disappear upon the intake of zinc.

Natural Sources:

Liver, molasses, kelp, the herb Yellow Dock, and beets. Most green vegetables also contain Iron.

Raw Juice Sources:

Wild blackberries, head lettuce, asparagus, currants, pears, plums, spinach, sun-dried raisins, black mission figs, strawberries, cherries, okra, dandelion leaves, beets, concord grapes, kale, artichokes.
NOTE: A lack of Iron can cause allergies to: Oats (oatmeal) and sesame.

NOTE: Extremely dark stools do not mean constipation, but an overdose of Iron. Coffee and tea drive Iron out of the body. Sometimes the Iron in the foods is not assimilated because of a lack of H.C.L. (hydrochloric acid) in the body which is necessary to digest the Iron.

Iron is more effective when taken with:

Vitamin B-12 Helps Iron function in the body.
Folic Acid

MAGNESIUM

The Magnesium M.R.T. acupuncture point *is* the navel! Insert a finger into the navel and pump the other arm.
RDA: 350 to 700 mgs.

Function:

Half of the Magnesium in the body is combined with Calcium and Phosphorus in the bones, assuring the strength and firmness of the bones and teeth. The remainder of the Magnesium is in the muscles, red blood cells, and other soft tissue.

Magnesium is an important catalyst in many enzyme reactions, especially those involved in energy production. Magnesium also helps in the utilization of Vitamins B and E, fats, Calcium, and other minerals.

Magnesium is regarded as effective in reducing cholesterol levels and in that respect, is considered helpful in preventing heart attacks. It is also useful in the treatment of nervousness, neuromuscular problems, and depression. Magnesium helps to produce Lecithin in the body.

We have found in our research that calcification of the kidneys, bladder, or prostate gland can be corrected by administering Magnesium. We have also found that Magnesium can help to correct an allergy to wheat and corn. Magnesium can also help clear up ringing in the ear.

Deficiency Symptoms:

When Magnesium is deficient, kidney stones, or kidney or bladder calcification can occur as well as gall bladder stones. A lack of Magnesium could also cause muscle cramps, arteriosclerosis, heart attack, epileptic seizures, nervous irritability, confusion, depression, impaired protein metabolism, and premature wrinkles. A lack of this mineral can also cause over-calcification of the joints (rheumatoid arthritis), diabetes, and constipation.

Food Sources:

Kelp, almonds, cashews, dulse, soybeans, raw and cooked green leafy vegetables, figs, apples, safflower, and sesame.

Raw Juice Sources:

Oranges, lemons, grapefruit, tangerines, limes, plums, spinach, dandelion leaves, mustard greens, lettuce, apples, grapes, savoy cabbage, pomegranates, sugar beet tops, cherries, corn, peaches, and pears.

Magnesium is more effective when taken with:

Vitamin B-6
Vitamin C
Vitamin D
Calcium 1 part Magnesium to 2 parts Calcium
Phosphorus
Protein

MANGANESE

The Manganese M.R.T. point is approximately 2½ inches below the Iodine point (hollow of neck area) on top of the Thymus gland.

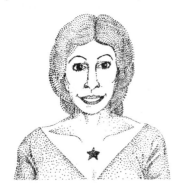

Figure 33

RDA: Not known

Function:

Manganese is an important component of several enzymes which are involved in the metabolism of carbohydrates, fats, and proteins.

Manganese is an essential element concentrated in the tissues of the bones, liver, pituitary gland, kidney, pancreas, spleen, heart, brain, and intestines. Manganese improves eyesight. Manganese also helps Iron carry oxygen from the lungs to the cells of the body, thereby promoting tissue respiration.

Manganese strengthens connective tissue and is helpful in correcting the effects of Myasthenia Gravis. Manganese can also arrest Tinnitus and stop an allergic reaction to rice and the "Rice Group".

Many times in our research, a lack of Manganese was found to cause Arthritis in the hands and feet where connective tissue is so important.

Deficiency Symptoms:

Diabetes, problems with the left ear (Tinnitus), male and female sterility, impotence in men, sexual indifference, loss of muscular strength (Myasthenia gravis), allergic reaction to rice and the "rice group foods".

Food Sources:

Whole grain cereals, wheat germ, nuts, beans, egg yolk, sunflower seeds.

Raw Juice Sources:

Chives, watercress, endive, nasturtium, almonds, chestnuts, walnuts, parsley, peppermint leaves, wintergreen, acorns, blackeyed beans, butternuts, french beans.

Manganese is more effective when taken with:

Vitamin B-1 (Thiamine)
Vitamin E
Calcium
Phosphorus

NOTE: Manganese counteracts the effects of opium because it is a brain and nerve tonic.

MOLYBDENUM

The M.R.T. acupuncture point which we use for Molybdenum, is the Solar Plexus point. Hold the Molybdenum in the palm of the hand over the Solar Plexus while extending the left arm to be pumped. See figure 29, page 56.

Molybdenum is involved in the metabolism of toxic aldehydes. Molybdenum takes part in the final stages of the metabolism of purines into uric acid. In man, Molybdenum is found primarily in the liver and kidneys.

Molybdenum is considered to be antagonistic to Copper, thus, may have protective action in Copper poisoning.

Molybdenum is involved with proper carbohydrate metabolism.

Deficiency Symptoms:

Sexual impotence in older males and esophageal cancer.

Food Sources:

Brown rice, whole cereals, millet, buckwheat, brewer's yeast, legumes, and naturally hard water.

PHOSPHORUS

The M.R.T. acupuncture point is on the front of the lower left torso, between the hip bone and pubic bone (where a pants crease would extend upward from the left leg). (The same as the iron point but on the opposite leg).

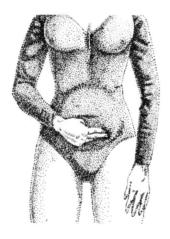

Figure 34

RDA: 800 mg. for adults

Function:

Phosphorus is the second most abundant mineral in the body. Phosphorus is an essential mineral related to Calcium metabolism and is controlled mostly by the Parathyroid glands.

Phosphorus is necessary in the synthesis of RNA and DNA and it is important for bone and teeth construction. The ratio between Phosphorus and Calcium should be two parts Phosphorus to five parts Calcium.

Phosphorus is important in synthesizing Lecithin and Cerebrin which are both needed by the brain. In the brain, there are approximately fifteen million cells. These cells need a generous supply of Phosphorus. Phosphorized fats constitute the solid matter of the brain.

The Phosphorus compounds (Lecithin) are found everywhere in the tissues, lymph, and other liquids of the organism, as well as in the white and gray matter of nerve and brain tissue (Phosphorus comprises 16-18% and is involved in the higher mental functions).

Phosphorus stimulates hair growth, prevents the blood from becoming too acid or alkaline, helps maintain the density of bone structure. Phosphorus is the *outer* bone and the enamel coating on teeth. Therefore, a deficiency in Phosphorus can cause Arthritis.

Deficiency Symptoms:

A lack of Phosphorus can cause Rickets, Insanity, Loss of Memory, Failing Eyesight (especially in the left eye), Falling Hair, Cataracts, Sciatic Rheumatism, Neuralgia, Neuritis, Tooth Decay, Spongy and Bleeding Gums, Lung Tuberculosis, and Indifference to Sex.

Food Sources:

Rice Bran, Wheat Bran, Pumpkin and Squash Seeds, Wheat Germ, Rice Polishings, Sunflower Seeds, Brazil Nuts, Safflower Seeds.

NOTE: We believe Phosphorus is destroyed by excess sugar in the blood stream. Just sucking on a piece of candy will permit the sugar to enter the blood stream via the saliva glands and destroy the Phosphorus in the blood causing dental decay and bone degeneration!! We also have found that this sugar can affect the vision of the left eye.

Phosphorus is more effective when taken with:

Vitamin A
Vitamin D
Vitamin F
Calcium 1 part Phosphorus to 2.5 parts Calcium
Iron
Manganese
Protein

POTASSIUM

The Potassium M.R.T. acupuncture point is the point ½ inch behind the hollow in the right cheek where the jaw bone starts to connect up.

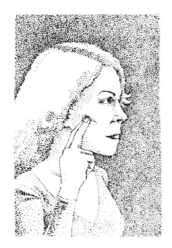

Figure 35

Place the "pointer" finger in the hollow of the jaw, and where the "index" finger touches you will find the correct point (on the right side of the face).

Function:

As far as I am concerned, Potassium is one of the most important and least understood minerals. It is an electrolyte which carries the electrical acupuncture "Ch'i" energy that nurtures and activates muscles and organs. Potassium is an essential alkaline base forming mineral.

Potassium and Sodium are responsible for maintaining proper fluid balance within the body's cells. Potassium controls more of the internal fluids of the cells (Intracellularcation) while Sodium controls more of the surrounding or external fluid of the cells.

Potassium regulates heart muscle action and arterial blood pressure. We have found that the diastolic pressure (lower number) can be reduce as much as 10 to 20 points in 15 minutes after drinking an 8 ounce glass of "Potassium Broth" such as carrot juice. (Also see Chapter on Carrot Juice). Using a Sphygmomanometer (a blood pressure gauge), we have experimented by taking a person's blood pressure before drinking carrot juice, and then re-checked it 15 minutes after drinking the juice to find that the diastolic pressure reading had actually dropped as much as 20 points!

Potassium helps carry our enzyme reactions throughout the body. Potassium regulates blood pH and is important in the formation of Glycogen in the liver, muscles, and cartilage. Potassium assures the elasticity of muscles, and helps maintain different elements in solution, it is also an important constituent of the right brain.

When a stroke affects the right side, it is usually due to blood clotting related to a lack of Potassium. Bell's Palsy on the right side is usually a Potassium deficiency affecting the muscles of the face and body on the right side (left side of the body is influenced by the Sodium level).

Potassium helps the kidneys to eliminate waste matter, therefore assisting in eliminating blood impurities. Potassium is vital in preventing heart attacks (combined with Magnesium) by strengthening the heart. Potassium feeds the entire endocrine system, and thus aids in the increase of glandular secretions.

Deficiency Symptoms:

A lack of Potassium will cause a milk and milk product (cheese) allergy. Lack of Potassium will also cause Edema if the Sodium level is too high in proportion to the Potassium level.

Lack of Potassium can also cause auto-intoxication because Potassium is the carbon transporter from the cells via the blood stream to the lungs where the oxygen meets with the carbon and carries it out of the body as carbon dioxide.

A lack of Potassium will cause high blood pressure (diastolic) and a weakened heart. Walking around with a Potassium deficiency (causing a weak heart) is like driving a new Cadillac without gas!! It will die!! So will you!!

According to Japanese military doctor Sagen Ishizuka, the amount of

Potassium and Sodium in foods consumed determines body strength, ability to adapt to climate and weather changes, and man's mentality. He is *so* right!! I would like to add man's productivity to that list.

Potassium is the main constituent of soft tissue, and can be considered the key mineral for maintaining naturally good health. Lack of Potassium can cause damage to the heart muscle and lead to heart attacks. Lack of Potassium can also cause Sciatica on the right side.

NOTE: Diuretics, Prednisone, ACTH, and Digitalis will deplete Potassium levels. Also, sweating in a hot climate will cause a loss of Potassium, three times the amount of Sodium lost. The loss of these two electrolytes can cause instantaneous allergies to most "non-green vegetables" which would cause diarrhea and nausea (Montezuma's Revenge). It should also be noted that in his book "The New Handbook of Prescription Drugs", published by Ballantine Books #29271, Richard Brack, M.D. F.A.P.L., describes the potential negative effects of Potassium Chloride U.S.P. on page 284: "We feel that this pharmaceutical type of mineral pill should never be used."

In our research we utilize Bee Pollen and Alfalfa concentrate capsules as a source of natural Potassium. Each 500 mg. capsule of Bee Pollen contains approximately 300 mg. of Potassium. Each 500 mg. capsule of Alfalfa-Concentrate contains 600 mg. of Potassium along with some Sodium in a perfect balanced ratio of two parts Potassium to one part Sodium. These natural sources of Potassium happen to be totally absorbable and without any side-effects!!!

The heart is a "Potassium Vehicle" in a Sodium sea. The (Yin) right side of man is governed by Potassium, and the (Yang) left side of man is governed by Sodium. A lactating woman's milk secreted from the right breast has a predominate Potassium composition, while the milk secreted from the left breast has a predominate Sodium composition.

A baby who nurses always on one breast may need that specific nutrient because the mother may be deficient in that nutrient. When a baby changes breasts, it may be changing not for physical comfort, but to obtain the nutritional balance it seeks!!

Food Sources:

Potatoes (especially peelings), oranges, tomatoes, bananas, dulse, kelp, parsley, soybeans, rice bran, apricots, and dates.

Raw Juice Sources:

Carrots, Dandelion leaves, beet tops, blueberries, cabbage, coconut, endive, lettuce, mint leaves, parsley, spinach, pineapples, swiss chard, artichokes, brussel sprouts, grapes, green peppers, leek, rhubarb, celery turnip leaves, wild black cherries, yellow tomatoes.

A facial modality that can help you self-determine your Potassium need is seen when the *right* corner of the mouth dips downward. This would indicate that Potassium is needed (since the right side is governed by Potassium).

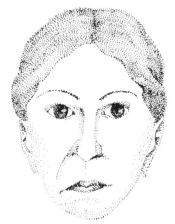

Figure 36

If the left side is dipping downward, your immediate need is for Sodium.

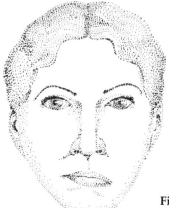

Figure 37

If both sides dip downward, the Potassium and Sodium are both low.

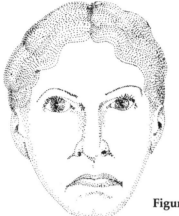

Figure 38

If the right nostril is clogged, this could also indicate a need for Potassium. A clogged left nostril will mean a need for Sodium.

A lot of phlegm in the throat, especially in the morning, accompanied by swollen tonsils (sore throat), indicates that there is a Sulfur deficiency.

Potassium is more effective when taken with:

Vitamin B-6
Sodium

SELENIUM

Selenium can be tested by holding to the Solar Plexus: See figure 29, page 56.

RDA: Not yet established
50 mcg. to 150 mcg. is the usual spectrum of dosage.

Function:

Selenium is an anti-oxidant, which means that it prevents the hemoglobin in red blood cells from being damaged by oxidation.

Selenium prevents, or at least slows down, aging and hardening of the tissues through oxidation. Selenium inhibits the formation of free radicals.

Selenium provides protection against Mercury toxicity, in particular, Methyl Mercury (the industrial waste type). Men have a greater need for Selenium, for it is utilized in the manufacture of semen. Almost half of a man's body's supply is concentrated in the testicles and portions of the seminal ducts adjacent to the prostate gland.

Selenium can also alleviate hot flashes and menopausal distress. Selenium is helpful in the treatment and prevention of dandruff (Selson Blue shampoo is Selenium based).

There are different forms of Selenium. Regular selenium is a yeast base and can be highly allergic if the client has a yeast allergy. In our research, we prefer to use Sodium Selenate, which is difficult to find in many health food stores. Another form is Sodium Selenite, which is more available.

It should be noted that Selenium is synergistic with Vitamin E, another anti-oxidant. The two taken together make both more effective. When taking Sodium Selenite, do not take it with Vitamin C, for they will burn each other up.

Selenium can help regenerate the liver after damage, especially by Cirrhosis. Selenium is essential for the function of the enzyme Glutathione Peroxidase.

Deficiency Symptoms:

Selenium deficiency can cause liver damage, muscle degeneration, premature aging, heart disease, and muscular dystrophy. Prolonged severe deficiency may lead to development of cancer, especially in the gastrointestinal tract.

Toxicity Warning!

Selenium toxicity, or Selenosis, can result from drinking contaminated water, or the excessive exposure to photoelectric equipment and xerography (a certain type of photocopying process which emits a form of Selenium into the air).

"Selenium occurring naturally as either a red powder or a gray crystal, is amon the most poisonous elements in the universe, and yet, in pure form, it is an essential trace mineral for animal and man."

Indications of a Selenium toxicity are loss of hair, brittle fingernails, irritability for no known reason, and Amyotrophic Lateral Sclerosis (a degeneration of the spinal cord which results in paralysis).

Food Sources:

Onions, milk, eggs, kelp, garlic, mushrooms, organically grown foods, seafood, most vegetables, and brewer's yeast.
Selenium is more effective when taken with:

Vitamin E

SILICON
(Silica, Silicea)

Silicon can be tested by holding to the Solar Plexus: See figure 29, page 56.
RDA: Not known

Function:

Silicon is found in nature as white sand, quartz, flint, etc. It is the stiffening element in bamboo, cane, and the stems of certain grasses.

In the body, Silicon is found in the connective tissues, including those within the brain and nervous systems. Silicon is essential for building strong bones and for normal growth of hair, nails, and teeth.

Silicon is beneficial in all healing processes and protects the body against many diseases, such as: Tuberculosis, irritation in the mucous membranes, and skin disorders.

Silicon enables the system to throw off accumulated pus; hence, it is used to correct boils, pustules, and hardened glands. Silicon is the lancet mineral of biochemistry.

Deficiency Symptoms:

Lack of Silicon can cause soft brittle nails, aging symptoms of the skin such as wrinkles, thinning and loss of hair, poor bone and teeth development, insomnia, osteoporosis, carbuncles, boils, abscesses, and chronic fatigue.

Silicon deficiency and Epilepsy are said to be analogous. A lack of Silicon causes inability to connect one's thoughts, bad memory, and nervous disorders.

Food Sources:

Young green plants, horsetail, alfalfa, nettles, kelp, bamboo, sugar cane, flaxseed, apples, strawberries, grapes, beets, onions, parsnips, almonds, peanuts, sunflower seeds, and steel-cut oats.

Raw Juice Sources:

Calimyrna figs, lettuce, strawberries, mustard greens, white onions, parsnips, olives, asparagus, dandelion greens, cabbage, cucumbers, radishes, alfalfa.

SODIUM

The M.R.T. point for Sodium is located one half inch behind the hollow on the left cheek where the jaw bone starts to connect up. This can be found by placing the "pointer" finger in the hollow of the jaw. The correct point is found where the index finger touches (on the left side of the face).

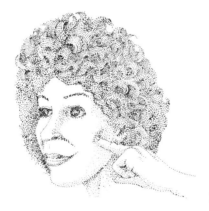

Figure 39

Function:

Sodium is the most misunderstood mineral. Sodium is a blood electrolyte, and is responsible for making blood minerals soluble. Without sufficient Sodium, the blood could clot causing a stroke on the *left* side.

Sodium contributes to the formation of saliva and other digestive enzymes while maintaining the correct amount of water in the body. Excessive sweating, vomiting, or high fever could cause a loss of

Sodium which would cause a loss of water. Dehydration would result, therefore disrupting the fluid balance surrounding the cells. The eyeballs would change fluid content and thereby change the inner pressure affecting the eye lens focus.

Sodium is an alkaline and will neutralize acidity in the blood and aid the lymphatics. Sodium is needed for proper muscle contraction, and also sustains the contractibility of mammalian muscles.

The two minerals, Potassium and Sodium, must be in correct balance for the body to function normally. The amount of Sodium ingested is regulated in the body by the Adrenal hormone: Aldosterone, which controls the kidneys. Therefore, when there is a high intake of sodium, the rate of excretion is high, and if the intake is low, the excretion rate is also low.

When the heart or the kidneys are not functioning normally, the sodium concentration within the cells rises. The cell cannot pump fast enough to eliminate this excess, and water is retained. This results in edema or swelling of the body tissue. This usually is caused by insufficient Potassium.

A low Sodium diet is often erroneously advised for the treatment of edema. The thing to do is to elevate the Potassium level which would not diminish the amount of Sodium, but reduce Sodium's potent hold on the fluid. By increasing the Potassium level, the "fluid holding power" of Sodium would be reduced without a loss of Sodium. The body would then reduce its Edemic condition, not by lowering the Sodium in the body, but by increasing the Potassium to balance out the electrolytes which should have a ratio of one Potassium to one Sodium. By doing this, the body would then normalize.

Many Physicians who recommend a "low sodium diet" are unknowingly complicating the problem because a low Sodium diet can lead to a stroke or Bell's Palsy on the left side of the body.

Sodium is necessary to hold the body's Calcium and Magnesium in solution, while also preventing over-coagulation of the blood, thus protecting against blood clots in the brain and elsewhere which can cause a stroke!

The greatest crime Physicians are guilty of is administering Diuretics (water pills). These pills not only take the fluid out of the body, but also the Sodium, Potassium, and minerals that might be in the solution, therefore starving the body of essential nutrients!

It should be noted here that there is a difference in organic Sodium that exists in vegetables such as celery, okra, and spinach as compared to the insoluble, inorganic commercially produced table salt.

Table salt is produced by exposing the Sodium Chloride to high temperatures approximately 1500°F, to solidify the salt crystals, while additives and adulterants are used to glaze the salt crystals so that the salt will be free pouring under moist atmospheric conditions.

Such salt is not completely soluble in water or the blood stream and it will adhere to the walls of the arteries. This is not the Sodium we recommend for man's needs! We suggest vegetables and fruits as the prime source of Sodium.

If table salt is to be used, we suggest the use of powdered rock salt, kosher salt, or sea salt which have been found to be completely soluble in water and compatible for human absorption.

It should be noted that Sodium retards aging by neutralizing waste products and filtering poisonous substances out of the blood stream through the Lymphatic system. Sodium also aids in the elimination of Carbonic Acid and halts fermentation.

Deficiency Symptoms:

When there is a Sodium deficiency a person may become allergic to almost everything. That is why on hot sweltering days (when Sodium is lost through perspiration) people will lose their appetite, but may desire to eat things such as salad which is usually high in Sodium!!

One of the most obvious results of a low-Sodium situation is depression and crying for no logical reason. The tears are the Saline fluid leaving the eyes because there is insufficient Sodium to hold in the fluid. When this happens over a period of time, the eyeball will become compressed by the eye muscle. The eye muscle's outer pressure on the eye becomes greater because the fluid inside is less and vision distortion will result!! This is correctable and vision can be restored by increasing the Saline solution by ingestion of carrot and celery juice! (Please see chapter on juice therapy.)

When there is a lack of Sodium, the body starts to perspire excessively and starts to dehydrate causing dry parched lips, and can result in constipation. If the Sodium level drops lower because of excessive perspiration, then everything will become allergic causing diarrhea and gas in the intestinal tract.

A deficiency of Sodium can cause Arthritic pains, especially on the left side in the left knee, and Sciatica on the left side from the Sciatica point down the left leg, sometimes causing numbness in the toes and foot.

A lack of Sodium can be a cause of Diabetes by preventing absorption of enough oxygen to burn up food carbons. A deficiency in Sodium can cause nausea, muscular weakness, heat exhaustion, mental apathy, and respiratory failure.

A deficiency of Sodium could cause allergic reactions to all foods. When this happens, the blood pressure's higher number (systolic) will *rise*, causing high blood pressure. This can be brought down 20 to 40 points in fifteen minutes by administering a six ounce glass of celery juice to the patient (celery juice is high in Sodium).

A Sodium deficiency could cause Sciatica pain on the left side. However, if both Potassium and Sodium are deficient, the *whole lower back* could ache!!!

Food Sources:

Kelp, Irish moss, olives, dulse, celery.

Raw Juice Sources:

Celery, Carrots, Okra, Spinach, Strawberries, Apples, Asparagus, Beets, Cucumbers, Gooseberries, Plums, Radishes, Swiss Chard, Turnips.

A way to visually see a Sodium deficiency, is to look at the lips of the person. If the left corner is lower than the right, a Sodium deficiency exists!!

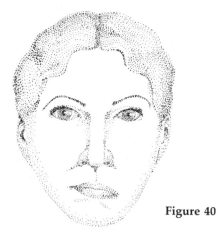

Figure 40

Sodium is more effective when taken with:

Vitamin D
Potassium
Sodium effectiveness is diminished by:
Lack of chlorine
Lack of potassium

SULFUR

The M.R.T. acupuncture point for Sulfur can be found on the throat on both sides of the Adam's apple or, on the Solar Plexus.

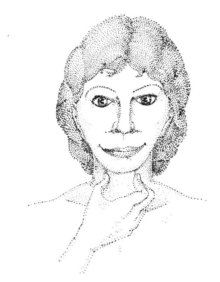

Figure 41

Function:

Sulfur plays a very important role in the body in the form of complex organic compounds. This mineral is present in all body cells. It is concentrated in the skin, hair, and nails, and is known as the beauty mineral.

Sulfur aids in dissolving acids in the body, improves circulation, normalizes heart action, and acts as an oxidizing agent on the blood.

Sulfur is essential in the formation of the amino acids Cysteine, Methionine, Lysine, Glutathione, and Taurine for the replacement of proteins in the organism. If our regimen contains sufficient protein of the right kind, Sulfur will be automatically furnished in the right amounts, but if our diet contains too many fats or Copper, Sulfur will be burned up.

Sulfur is the antidote to a fat allergy. It also increases bile function having a cleansing effect in the digestive tract. Sulfur is needed for the synthesis of Collagen, and the formation of body tissue. Sulfur contributes to the perspiration balance in the pores of the skin and also prevents the drying out or aging of the skin.

Sulfur helps maintain youthful elastin in the skin, and is also helpful in skin problems, especially Eczema. DMSO (Dimethyl Sulfoxide) can be a supplementary source of topical Sulfur.

RDA: None established

Deficiency Symptoms:

A lack of Sulfur can cause poor growth of nails and hair, Dermatitis, Eczema, Auto-Intoxication caused by a fat allergy, constipation, and improper bile secretion.

In our research, we have found that the Tonsils are the Sulfur sack of the body through which the blood is purified. When you wake up in the morning with a throat full of phlegm, this is a tell-tale sign that your sulfur is low and that you should not be eating any fats; for at this point, an allergic reaction could set in. Fats include: meat fats, cream, butter, all dairy products, and *all* oils, including margarine. An allergic reaction could bring about fever and extreme exhaustion. The condition would resemble the flu with a lot of phlegm in the nose and throat.

Another tell-tale sign of a Sulfur depletion is when the voice begins to drop in pitch (not volume). As the Sulfur in the body is depleted, the voice will get lower and deeper each day.

The things that are antagonistic to Sulfur are fats, Pantothenic Acid, and Copper. When administering either Pantothenic Acid or Copper, *always* balance it with the appropriate amount of Sulfur. By placing them together in the palm of the hand and by using the M.R.T. technique, you will be able to determine how much of each (together) the body can take.

When using this method, Sulfur when alone, may show strong for one unit, but when placed side by side with a B-5 (Pantothenic Acid) pill, it may test for two (double) or more units.

In our research, we don't use Pantothenic Acid pills, we use Royal Jelly which is very rich in Pantothenic Acid. For a source of Sulfur we use the herb Sarsaparilla which is rich in Sulfur, and the amino acids Methionine and Cysteine. We also use Homeopathic Sulfur $1\times$ when the client does not have a milk allergy.

Food Sources:

Garlic, onions, radishes, turnip, horseradish, kale, watercress, cabbage, cranberries, and eggs.

Raw Juice Sources:

Red Cabbage, Carrots, Chestnuts, Coconut, Figs, Nuts, Oranges, Spinach, Brussel Sprouts, Chervil, Cranberries, Dill, Endive, Mustard Greens, Leeks, Marjoram, Nasturtium, Red Raspberries, Loganberries, Sorrel, Rhubarb, Turnip Greens, Watercress, Cauliflower, Onions, Parsnips, Peaches, Radishes, Rutabaga, Apples, Asparagus, Cherries, Cucumbers, Gooseberries, Grapes, Horseradish, Potatoes, Ruebuck Berries, Blackberries, Dewberries.

Sulfur is more effective when taken with:

Vitamin B Complex
Vitamin B-1 (Thiamine)
Biotin
Vitamin B-5 (Pantothenic Acid)

Sulfur's effectiveness is diminished by:

Insufficient protein

ZINC

The M.R.T. point for Zinc is located on the front of the lower right torso, midway between the hip bone and pubic bone in the area where a pants crease would extend upward from the right leg.

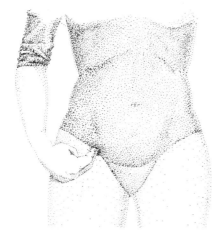

Figure 42

RDA: 15 mg.

Function:

Zinc is an essential mineral found in most tissues of the body; the kidney, liver, pancreas, and spermatozoa having the highest concentrations of Zinc. Zinc influences the entire hormonal system and all the glands, especially the Prostate gland.

Zinc is essential for the formation of RNA and DNA, and also for the synthesis of body protein. Zinc affects tissue respiration by its participation in Carbonic Amyldrase which transports Carbon Dioxide from the tissues to the blood.

Zinc is essential for growth and normal functioning of the sex organs and for normal function of the Prostate gland. Zinc increases the rate of burn and wound healing. Zinc tends to normalize insulin in the blood and so is recommended in some types of diabetes. Zinc is considered useful in reducing cholesterol and in the treatment of Cirrhosis of the liver.

Deficiency Symptoms:

A lack of Zinc could cause retarded growth, birth defects, hypogonadism or undeveloped gonads (sex organs), enlargement of the Prostate gland, impaired sexual functions, loss of fertility, lowered resistance to infection, slow healing of wounds, and skin diseases.

Lack of Zinc could also cause white spots on finger and toe nails, and poor sense of taste and smell. A Zinc deficiency can cause hair loss, dandruff (Zincon shampoo contains Zinc), apathy, and a loss of interest in learning.

In our own research, we have found a lack of Zinc to be the cause of an allergic reaction to Brewers Yeast, barley, cherry, millet, potatoes, prunes, raisin, rye, and walnuts. As the Zinc intake is increased to what the body needs, the allergic reaction disappears!!

Many Brewers Yeast based B-Complexes, and multi-vitamin and mineral supplements are allergic unless there is sufficient Zinc in the body prior to ingestion.

Food Sources:

Lean beef, calves liver, beef liver, soybeans, pumpkin seeds, sunflower seeds, brazil nuts, cashews, tuna fish, peanuts.
Zinc is more effective when taken with:

Vitamin A
Calcium
Copper
Phosphorus

Zinc's effectiveness is diminished by:

Lack of Phosphorus

Mineral Relativity Wheel

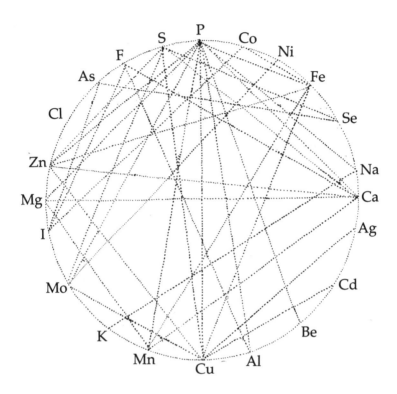

Aluminum - Al	Magnesium - Mg
Arsenic - As	Manganese - Mn
Beryllium - Be	Molybdenum - Mo
Cadmium - Cd	Nickel - Ni
Calcium - Ca	Phosphorus - P
Chlorine - Cl	Potassium - K
Cobalt - Co	Selenium - Se
Copper - Cu	Silver - Ag
Fluorine - F	Sodium - Na
Iodine - I	Sulfur - S
Iron - Fe	Zinc - Zn

Figure 43

MINERALS

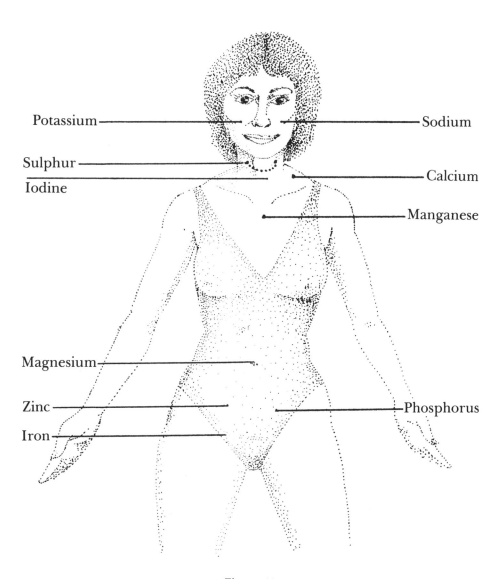

Potassium

Sulphur

Iodine

Sodium

Calcium

Manganese

Magnesium

Zinc

Iron

Phosphorus

Figure 44

CHAPTER 5

THE AMINO ACID WORLD

PROTEIN
AMINO ACIDS

Protein is an essential component of all living matter because of it's water content and because the body, including skin, muscles, hair, nails, internal organs, and the brain, is made primarily of protein.

Protein is composed of amino acids, of which there are 25 prominent ones presently known. Nine of the amino acids are essential and cannot be produced in sufficient quantities by the human body. They must be supplied by the diet. These amino acids are: Histidine, Isoleucine, Leucine, Lysine, Methionine, Phenylalanine, Threonine, Tryptophane, and Valine.

The non-essential amino acids are also needed, but they can be constructed within the body, chiefly in the liver, by transformation of one amino acid to another. Amino acids compete with one another; therefore, man needs an adequate total number of amino acids, plus an ample supply of essential amino acids.

Most animal protein foods, such as eggs, milk, and meat, contain all of the essential amino acids, and are therefore classified as high quality proteins.

A number of plant foods are deficient in one or more of the essential amino acids. All cereal grains are deficient in Lysine. Rice and corn also lack the amino acids Threonine and Tryptophan. Peas, beans, and other legumes are deficient in Methionine and Tryptophan. Soybeans and seed oil are low in Methionine. Gelatine is considered pure protein, but lacks Tryptophan.

By combining different foods with complementary amino acids, it may be possible to obtain a satisfactory amino acid balance. Because of the necessary reactions between amino acids and their dependence upon each other for these reactions, a diet containing only a small amount of one essential amino acid will reduce the utilization of other amino acids.

All amino acids must be present at the same time before they can be utilized as protein. In other words, the chain is only as strong as its weakest link! The excess amino acids that cannot be used as protein because of insufficient complementary amino acids are used as energy, excreted as urea, or are converted to carbohydrates or fat. Amino acids cannot be stored for future use as protein.

Amino acids are broken down and released in the intestinal tract during ingestion of food protein and are carried by the bloodstream to the body cells where they are used for growth, repair, muscles, red blood cells, body tissue, and general maintenance.

The body is continuously degrading and resynthesizing proteins and other nitrogenous compounds. In fact, more protein is turned over daily within the body than is ordinarily consumed in the diet. Some of the amino acids released during the breakdown of tissue proteins are re-utilized, but the metabolic products of amino acids (Urea, Creatine, Uric acid, and other nitrogenous products) are excreted in the urine. Nitrogen is lost in feces, sweat and other body secretions and excretions, and additionally in sloughed skin, hair and nails. Therefore, dietary amino acids are required continuously to replace these losses even after growth has ceased.

During cellular anabolism (build up), amino acids join together by peptide bonds to form specific proteins. With cellular catabolism (breakdown), proteins and amino acid chains are broken up into fragments.

Amino acids are classified:

D: Dexyrorotational, which means they bend polarized light (light through a prism) to the right; these are usually synthetic.

L: Laevorotational, which means they bend polarized light to the left. The "L" classifications are derived from natural sources, and is usually the group which is generally ingested. The "D" form is a mirror image of the "L" form and has different functions.

DL-Phenylalanine (a mixture of both forms) functions as a pain killer. The most used form is the "L" series, so many distributors of amino acid supplements simply drop the "L" so that "L-Lysine" would then become just plain "Lysine".

Amino acids function together in a unique balance. Any upset in this balance can lead to a variety of disorders. These disorders are not only the direct result of a missing amino acid, but can also be the indirect result of another amino acid becoming too concentrated.

For example, gelatin is an imbalanced protein high in the amino acid Glycine. If Glycine levels become too high we produce excessive uric acid which can lead to gout.

When the amino acids serve as precursors to other chemicals in the body, these chemicals may exist in a balanced relationship. Such is the case for the brain neuro-transmitters: Serotonin, Dopamine and Norepinephrine. All three of these chemicals require certain amino acids for their synthesis.

By altering the amount or ratio of the precursor amino acids, one can upset the balanced interrelationship among these neurotransmitters. If left unadjusted, this unbalanced relationship can lead to behavioral disorders which can be corrected by the therapeutic use of specific amino acids.

PROTEIN/AMINO ACID TESTING TECHNIQUES

There are two methods which can be used to test for amino acids. One way is by grasping the hair and holding it between the fingers making certain that the hand does not touch the scalp. While doing this, use the

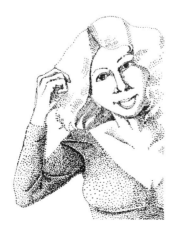

Figure 45

M.R.T. method of testing. If the pumped arm goes down, place the amino acid complex pill into the hand that was used to touch the hair and continue to add one pill at a time (still grasping the hair) until the pumped arm becomes rigid. If you over-dose, the pumped arm will again go down.

I prefer to test the amino acid complex and then test each individual amino acid. This can be done by placing the capsule (or pill) in the palm of the hand while holding the hand to the Solar Plexus area. You can add capsules until the pumped arm becomes rigid. Again, if you over-dose the arm becomes weak again.

I use both methods to test my clients because I use one to double-check the other.

ESSENTIAL AMINO ACIDS

These are the amino acids that *cannot* be produced in the body:

L-HISTIDINE:

L-Histidine is needed by the red and white blood cells, bones and gastrointestinal tract. We have found in our research that L-Histidine can counteract a wheat or corn allergy which can ordinarily cause an inflammation of the right ear. Also, a lack of this substance can cause Tinnitus (ringing) in the right ear. Many physicians misdiagnose an inflamed ear from an allergic reaction as an infected ear (For more information please see Chapter on Tinnitus.).

Histidine is the amino acid from which the biochemical substance Histamine is derived. Both histidine and histamine chelate trace minerals such as Copper and Zinc. Because of Histidine's chelating properties, it is sometimes used in the treatment of Rheumatoid Arthritis to remove heavy metals such as copper, which tends to overload in the tissues.

Histidine can be used to treat hallucinations and paranoia. Histidine is also used to improve sexual orgasm, impotence and loss of sexual power.
Glands affected by Histidine:

Adrenal
Pineal

Complementary Vitamins:

Vitamin B-5 (Pantothenic Acid)
Vitamin C
Vitamin B-3 (Niacin)
Vitamin E

Complementary Minerals:

Potassium
Bromine
Sodium
Chloride
Chromium
Zinc

Food Sources:

Histidine is readily available from most protein foods.
NOTE: Histidine has a tendency to displace Arginine, so the two
        should be administered together.

L-ISOLEUCINE:

L-Isoleucine is an essential amino acid which is needed for proper hemoglobin formation. Isoleucine participates in hydrophobic interactions. An imbalance among Isoleucine, Leucine and Valine can create a build up of certain metabolites in the urine, creating the disease called "Maple Syrup Urine Disease" (branched chain Ketoaciduria).

This disease is caused by an enzyme defect diagnosed by the presence of a sweet odor in the urine. If Isoleucine, Leucine and Valine are not taken in a well-balanced proportion, a nutritional conflict will occur among these three amino acids.

Three carbons of Isoleucine are converted to succinate, an intermediate in the Krebs Cycle. The Krebs Cycle is stage three of the process of respiration by which aerobic cells obtain energy from the oxidation of glucose by molecular oxygen. Isoleucine is also needed for muscle functions.

A lack of Isoleucine can cause flu symptoms, as well as gravel and hemoglobin in the urine.

Glands and organs affected by Isoleucine:

Thymus
Lymph
Hypothalamus
Eyes
Pineal
Kidney

Complementary Vitamins:

Vitamin A
Vitamin B-3 (Niacin)
Vitamin C
Vitamin B Complex
Vitamin B-15
Vitamin E
Vitamin B-12

Complementary Minerals:

Chrome
Zinc
Calcium
Selenium
Magnesium
Sulfur

Food Sources:

Chicken, Fish, Beef, Soybeans, Eggs, Cottage Cheese, Liver, Baked Beans, Legumes, and Milk.

L-LYSINE:

Lysine is an essential amino acid which can be used to alleviate a feeling of helplessness, fatigue, nausea, dizziness, anemia, and depression.

Lysine helps to assure adequate absorption of the mineral Calcium, thereby promoting bone growth. Lysine helps form collagen, the protein which makes up the matrix of bone cartilage and other connective tissue. Before Lysine can be utilized for the formation of collagen, it must be converted to another form.

This conversion process is regulated by Vitamin C. (This shows the fascinating inter-relationship of the various nutrients). One relatively recent use for Lysine is its use in the symptomatic treatment of Herpes Simplex, which has become a major Venereal disease in the United States.

We have found in our research, that Lysine can also help as the amino acid antidote to a Brewers Yeast* allergy, and can also help correct Hypoglycemia. Lysine is necessary for binding the Co-enzymes Pyridoxal Phosphate, Lipoic Acid, and Biotin to enzymes.

Homesickness is sometimes a result of a Lysine deficiency. A lack of Lysine can cause destruction of "electric current" carrying fibers, causing loss of muscular integrity.

In our research, we have found that Lysine displaces Methionine. Therefore, the two should be taken together.

Glands and Organs Affected by Lysine:

Pancreas
Solar Plexus
Spine
Hypothalamus
Eye
Pineal
Thyroid
Brain
Adrenals

Complementary Vitamins:

Niacin
B-Complex
Vitamin C
Vitamin B-5 (Pantothenic Acid)
Vitamin B-6
Vitamin A
Vitamin B-15
Vitamin E
Vitamin B-2
PABA

*Brewers Yeast Series includes: Barley, cherry, millet, potatoes, raisin, rye, prunes, walnuts.

Complementary Minerals:

Chromium
Zinc
Rubidium
Iodine
Sodium
Calcium

Food Sources:

Lysine is found in all high-protein foods, such as fish, chicken, eggs, garbanzo beans, and milk. The herb Comfrey is also rich in Lysine. Strict vegetarians should use a Lysine supplement.

L-LEUCINE:

Leucine is an essential amino acid that is reported to lower blood sugar. Leucine helps wound healing of the skin and bones. Leucine is also used to treat "Maple Syrup Urine Disease".

If Leucine, Isoleucine, and Valine are not taken in a well balanced proportion, a nutritional conflict might occur among these three amino acids.

A lack of Leucine might cause digestive problems, colon spasms, and the inability to gain or lose weight. Leucine has also been used to correct a congested liver or a damaged kidney.

Complementary Vitamins:

Vitamin A
Vitamin B Complex
Vitamin B-2
Vitamin B-12
Folic Acid

Complementary Minerals:

Copper
Manganese
Calcium
Selenium

Glands and Organs Affected by Leucine:

Thymus

Lymph
Tonsils
Appendix
Skin
Stomach

Food Sources:

Chicken, fish, beef, soybeans, eggs, cottage cheese, liver, baked beans, and milk.

L-METHIONINE:

Methionine is an essential amino acid because it is a Sulfur-containing amino acid by which Cysteine, Cystine, and Taurine (non-essential amino acids) can be manufactured in the body.

Methionine is a member of the "Lipotropic" team which includes Choline and Inositol. Its primary function as a Lipotropic is to prevent excessive accumulation of fat in the liver. Methionine increases the liver's production of Lecithin, which prevents a cholesterol build up.

Methionine, and the other sulfur containing amino acids, function as antioxidants, free radical deactivators, neutralizers of toxins, and as aids to protein synthesis.

The sulfur amino acids (of which Methionine is the essential amino acid) serve a useful role as natural carriers of the trace mineral Selenium which is a potent protector against Cancer, and a major compound for slowing down the aging process. Methionine will also stimulate hair growth.

In our research, we have found that the sulfur amino acids are the antidotes to a "fat allergy" which would manifest itself by a sore throat (enlarged tonsils). If the tonsils have ignorantly been removed, no soreness would be present. (Please read chapter on Sulfur.)

Glands Affected by Methionine:

Thymus
Lymph
Adrenal

Complementary Vitamins:

Vitamin A
Vitamin C

Vitamin B-12
Vitamin B-5 (Pantothenic Acid)

Complementary Minerals:

Chromium
Zinc

Food Sources:

The best sources of Methionine are egg yolks, garlic, onions, and sarsaparilla.

L-PHENYLALANINE:

L-Phenylalanine is an essential amino acid because it is the precursor of Tyrosine. Both Phenylalanine and Tyrosine are used by the brain to manufacture Norepinephrine, a neurotransmitter.

A neurotransmitter is a chemical which transmits signals among neurons and allows them to communicate. Norepinephrine requires a number of nutrients for its synthesis: Protein, oxygen, Iron, Vitamin B-6, Vitamin C, Copper and the amino acid Tyrosine.

Phenylalanine supplements may improve learning and memory, on one hand, and reduce certain types of depression on the other. Phenylalanine is helpful in a variety of depressions including the depressive phase of a Manic-Depressive illness, endogenous schizophrenia, and the Post-amphetamine depression withdrawal syndrome.

Patients with depression may have a functional decrease in the activity or concentration of central nervous system catecholamines, a class of neurotransmitters which includes: Dopamine, Epinephrine and Norepinephrine. Most drugs used for treating depression have catecholamine-like activity, or they increase catecholamine concentrations in the central nervous system.

Phenylalanine inhibits appetite by increasing the brain's production of the neurotransmitter Norepinephrine (NE). Phenylalanine causes the brain to release the hormone CCK (Cholecystokinin) which has been shown to inhibit eating in experimental animals.

Norepinephrine is rendered inactive by the enzyme Monoamine Oxidase (MAO). As Homosapiens get older, approximately forty-five years of age, the levels of "MAO" increase to a point where greater than normal amounts of norepinephrine are necessary to initiate transmission. Therefore, the older we get, the more important it becomes to provide all the necessary ingredients for the synthesis of norepinephrine; especially the amino acid Phenylalanine.

Deficiency Symptoms:

A lack of Phenylalanine could cause swollen glands, Thyroid trouble, formation of rectal calculi (causing a disturbed anal area), depression, and tumors arising from a serous or mucous surface.

Too much Phenylalanine can cause irritability, insomnia, or headaches.

NOTE: When using Phenylalanine, one should monitor one's blood pressure. Phenylalanine has been known to raise the blood pressure.

Glands and organs affected by Phenylalanine:

Parathyroid
Hypothalamus
Eye
Pineal

Complementary Vitamins:

Vitamin A
Vitamin B-3 (Niacin)
Vitamin C
Vitamin B Complex
Vitamin B-15
Vitamin E

Complementary Minerals:

Calcium
Selenium
Magnesium
Sulfur

DL-PHENYLALANINE:

"DL"-Phenylalanine is different than "L"-Phenylalanine in that it is a racine mixture consisting of equal parts of the "D" and "L" isomers.

Function:

DL-Phenylalanine inhibits the carboxypeptidase and enkephalinase. These enzymes hydrolyze endorphins and enkephalins, which function as excitory transmittor substances that activate portions of the brain's analgesic system. In other words, Phenylalanine intensifies and prolongs the body's natural pain killing process.

DL-Phenylalanine is as effective as Imipramin (Monoamine Oxidase inhibitor) in decreasing depression and has fewer side effects. DL-Phenylalanine is· effective in relieving pre-menstrual depression, and in potentiating the effects of acupuncture and electrical transcutaneous nerve stimulation.

L-THREONINE:

Threonine is an essential amino acid which functions as a lipotropic factor that prevents fatty build up in the liver.

Threonine, along with many other amino acids, is an important constituent of collagen, elastin, and enamel protein. Threonine may be converted to aceyl - CoA are intermediate of the Krebs Cycle.

The kreb cycle is stage III of the process of respiration by which aerobic cells obtain energy from the oxidation of glucose by molecular oxygen.

Deficiency Symptoms:

A lack of Threonine can cause a "fat allergy" which would also show itself as indigestion, intestinal malfunction, and a sore throat, as if a "cold" were coming on.

A lack of Threonine can cause female ovarian cysts or fluid on the ovary(s) as well as female-dysmenorrhea (painful and difficult menstruation), and intermittent spotting. Lack of Threonine can also cause an inflamed uterus.

Glands and organs affected by Threonine:

Thymus	Peyer's Patches
Lymph	Skin
Tonsils	Stomach
Appendix	

Complementary Vitamins:

Vitamin A

Vitamin B Complex
Vitamin B-2
Vitamin B-12
Folic Acid

Complementary Minerals:

Copper
Manganese
Calcium
Selenium

L-TRYPTOPHAN:

Tryptophan is an essential amino acid. Tryptophan is a precursor to Serotonin, an inhibitory neurotransmitter, which decreases the activities of neurons, thereby inducing sleep.

Serotonin controls emotions, perception of pain, promotes calmness, and lifts depression and anxiety. There are usually lower than normal levels of Serotonin in patients who have migraine headaches, and since Tryptophan is the precursor of Serotonin synthesis, then Tryptophan is usually effective in treating migraine sufferers.

Tryptophan produces Nicotinic Acid (Niacin, Vitamin B-3) which counteracts the effect of Nicotine in cigarettes. Tryptophan reduces blood pressure via blood vessel dilation and reduces blood fats and cholesterol. Tryptophan also raises blood histamine levels. Tryptophan is a growth hormone stimulant and aids in the utilization of B-complex, especially Vitamin B-6.

Deficiency Symptoms:

A lack of Tryptophan can cause insomnia, schizophrenia, arthritis, joint dysfunction and dermatitis on the dorsal surface of one's hands and the back of the neck.

Glands and organs affected by Tryptophan:

Parathyroid
Lymph
Thymus
Lung
Spleen

Complementary Vitamins:

Vitamin A
Niacin (B-3)
Vitamin E

Complementary Minerals:

Calcium
Selenium
Magnesium
Sulfur

Food Sources:

Tryptophan is present in high quality protein foods such as: fish, chicken, eggs, beef, soybeans, and milk.

To test Tryptophan, place the pills in one hand and place that hand in a fist position in to the Solar Plexus area of the body while extending the other arm. When the proper amount of Tryptophan pills are in the hand, the other arm will become rigid. See figure 29, page 56.

The way to test your clients to see if they need Tryptophan, Valerian, Calms Forte, Lobelia, or other relaxants, is to test the nerve center which is found in the back of the neck.

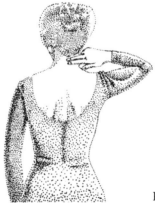

Figure 46

If the nerve center shows weak after placing the fingers at the back of the neck and pressing down on the extended arm, the next thing to do is find out how many pills will make the arm rigid. To do this, place the pills in the palm while touching the fingers to the back of the neck and pumping the extended arm. Add or subtract the amount of pills until you get the exact amount that makes the extended arm rigid.

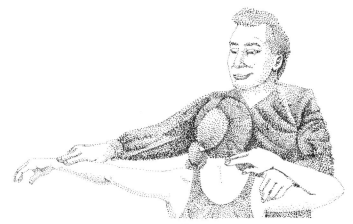

Figure 47

When you find the exact amount needed, you have reached the minimum/maximum of the needed antidote for the condition. When trying to rebuild and relax the nervous system, administer the proper amount of the proper antidote at bedtime so that the person sleeps soundly and awakens refreshed.

L-VALINE:

L-Valine is an essential amino acid. Three of Valine's carbon atoms are converted to succinate, an intermediate in the Krebs Cycle. The Krebs Cycle is stage three of the process of respiration by which aerobic cells obtain energy from the oxidation of Glucose by molecular oxygen.

Valine, along with Leucine and Isoleucine, are used to treat "Maple Syrup Urine Disease" (Branched chain ketoaciduria). If Valine, Isoleucine, and Leucine are not taken in a well balanced proportion, a nutritional conflict might occur among these three amino acids.

Deficiency Symptoms:

A lack of Valine can cause an inflammation of the lower part of the throat and rectum.

A lack of Valine can also cause cell deterioration and spitting up of blood as well as abnormal reddening of the skin (Erythema). Erythema is a redness of the skin that occurs in patches. Among the possible causes of a Valine deficiency are inflammation of the skin, heat, sunlight, exposure to cold, or excessive drinking of alcoholic beverages.

A lack of Valine could cause mental and emotional upsets, nervousness, and insomnia.

NOTE: Valine with Alanine, Serine and Cystein make up the amino properties of human insulin.

Glands and organs affected by Valine:

Thymus	Duodenum
Lymph	Heart
Tonsils	Liver
Appendix	Spleen
Peyer's Patches	Thyroid
Skin	Posterior Pituitary

Complementary Vitamins:

Vitamin A
Vitamin C
Vitamin E
Vitamin B Complex

Complementary Minerals:

Copper
Manganese
Magnesium
Sulfur

NON-ESSENTIAL AMINO ACIDS

Because an amino acid is called non-essential, does not mean it is not important. It means that the non-essential amino acid can be manufactured in the body if the essential amino acids are present. Example: Lysine and Methionine create Carnitine. Methionine and Serine create Cysteine.

The non-essential amino acids are: Alanine, Arginine, Aspartic Acid, Asparagin, Cysteine and Cystine, Glutamic Acid, Glutamine, Glycine, Hydroxyproline, Proline, Serine, and Tyrosine.

ALANINE:

Alanine is easily synthesized in the body from Acetaldehyde or enzymatic decarboxylation of L-Aspartic acid.

Deamination of L-Alanine produces Pyruvic Acid, an important intermediate in the Krebs Cycle. The Krebs Cycle is stage three of the process of respiration by which aerobic cells obtain energy from the oxidation of glucose by molecular oxygen. Alanine is also used as a food seasoning.

A lack of Alanine could give the following symptoms:

A.) A feeling of burn-out
B.) Convulsions
C.) Mental deterioration
D.) Spastic movements
E.) Hyper-muscular contractions
F.) Sweats at night
G.) A tic
H.) Twitches

The lack of L-Alanine could be caused by an improper diet, and/or insufficient rest.

Glands and organs affected by L-Alanine:

Thymus
Hypothalamus
Eye
Pineal
Thyroid
Brain

Complementary Vitamins:

Vitamin C
Vitamin A
Niacin (Vitamin B-3)
Vitamin B-Complex
Vitamin B-12
Vitamin B-15
Vitamin E
Vitamin B-2
PABA
Pantothenic Acid (Vitamin B-5)

Complementary Minerals:

Chromium
Zinc

Calcium
Selenium
Magnesium
Sulfur

L-ARGININE:

L-Arginine is a semi-essential amino acid synthesis from L-Ornithine. Arginine is synthesized in the body, but not fast enough to cover all the requirements of the tissues.

Arginine forms citrulline by hydrolysis. Arginine is able to block the formation of tumors, and also causes the release of a growth hormone which is an immune system stimulant. Arginine has also improved immune responses to bacteria, viruses, and tumor cells. Arginine is also a wound healing promoter and is involved in the regeneration of the liver.

Arginine increases the amount of growth hormone, thereby increasing muscle mass while decreasing the amount of body fat. Researchers have found that L-Arginine improves most defense mechanisms; therefore, it may play an important role in the care of severely injured or ill patients.

Arginine is the circulatory stimulant of the urea cycle. It promotes the detoxification of ammonia. The urea cycle takes place in the liver and utilizes ammonia to produce urea, an excretion product. Ammonia is poisonous to living cells.

In our research, we have found Arginine to be the amino acid which is the antidote to the rice food allergy series*. We have found Arginine to relieve Tinnitus in the left ear. See chapter on Tinnitus.

Deficiency Symptoms:

A lack of Arginine can cause sterility because Arginine comprises 80% of seminal fluid. A lack of Arginine can cause intestinal problems, inflammation, especially of the veins, and is also believed to be a cause of cellulite.

Glands and organs affected by Arginine:

Hypothalamus

---

*Rice food series allergy includes an allergy to cinnamon, blueberry, grapes, watermelon, wine, and pumpkin.

Eye
Pineal
Thymus
Lymph
Tonsils
Appendix
Peyer's Patches
Skin
Parathyroid

Complementary Vitamins:

Vitamin A
Niacin (Vitamin B-3)
Vitamin C
Vitamin B Complex
Vitamin B-15
Vitamin E

Complementary Minerals:

Calcium
Selenium
Magnesium
Sulfur

Food Sources:

Peanuts

NOTE: Arginine supplements should be balanced with Lysine to avoid a Herpes Syndrome eruption.

NOTE: Arginine has been found to inhibit the growth of several cancerous tumors. It has been found that Arginine significantly inhibited the growth and development of mammary tumors. Arginine in some manner inhibits cellular replication of Ehrlich ascites tumor cells. Arsenic is a toxic metal (used in pestacides) that provokes cancer formation by inhibiting Arginine and Zinc metabolism, according to a study by Dr. Nielson in 1983. Arginine was found to stimulate Lymphocytis by increasing their number and response to mitogens. Arginine helps to stimulate the thymus.

Arginine Toxicity

An overdose of Arginine can cause watery diarrhea.

L-ASPARAGINE

L-Asparagine is a non-essential amino acid because it can be synthesized in the body from Aspartic acid. Its chemical structure is identical to that of Aspartic acid, except one side chain is linked to ammonia, making it an Amide. Asparagine is necessary for the metabolism of toxic ammonia in the body.

Asparagine serves as an amino donor in a certain type of transamination in the liver. Asparagine participates in the metabolic control of the functions of the cells in the brain and the nervous system. Asparagine is used in the treatment of the brain and nervous system.

Deficiency Symptoms:

A lack of Asparagine will cause Gall Bladder dysfunction and liver trouble.

Glands and organs affected by Asparagine:

Thymus
Lymph
Liver

Complementary Vitamins:

Vitamin A
Niacin
Choline
Inositol

Complementary Minerals:

Chromium
Zinc

Food Sources:

The natural source of Asparagine in which it is available in abundance is Asparagus Juice!!

L-ASPARTIC ACID:

L-Aspartic acid is a non-essential amino acid produced in the body by the enzymatic addition of ammonia to fumaric acid.

Function:

Aspartic acid is used to form Threonine, an essential amino acid for the body. Aspartic acid aids in the disposal of ammonia in the body. Aspartic acid detoxifies ammonia from the body. Ammonia is poisonous to living cells.

Aspartic acid also increases resistance to fatigue by increasing stamina. Aspartic acid has nitrogen as one of its elements. The nitrogen derived from Aspartic acid is used to form Ribonucleotides, precursors of RNA and DNA.

Aspartic acid is used in drugs to protect the liver and promote the functions of the cells in the body. Aspartic acid is also used as a mineral transporter. Aspartic acid can also neutralize a "milk" allergy.

L-CARNITINE:

L-Carnitine is a non-essential, non-protein amino acid derived by the transformation in the body of Lysine and Methionine, with the assistance of Vitamin C, B-6, and B-3 (Niacin).

Carnitine is found in concentration in muscle and organ meats only. Carnitine is not found in any vegetable. Vegetarians should take note of this fact. Biosynthesis of Carnitine by humans occurs in the liver with the major storage site being the Skeletal muscle.

In my research, I have found that Carnitine is important to correct a "Fat" allergy condition. It is one of the antidotes for this allergy. Carnitine has an important regulatory effect on fat metabolism in the heart and skeletal muscle. It transfers fatty acids across the membrane of the mitochondria of cells. In the absence of Carnitine, fatty acids build up around the cell and are poorly metabolized.

Recently, on a vacation in Mexico after being exposed to the sun at poolside, I applied Vitamin F (Safflower oil) to my skin to regenerate it. After doing this, I noticed that my need for Carnitine increased. When I stopped applying the oil, my need for Carnitine decreased. This was observed over a two week period by daily muscle testing. So, if one is using such oils on the skin, even in a weekly rubdown, the Carnitine level should be checked. The symptoms would be either a sore throat, heaviness on the Thymus area, and a possible pain over the heart area. These symptoms will disappear in 45 minutes with the administration of Carnitine (or Methionine and Lysine).

Carnitine introduced into tissue cultures has been shown to stimulate fat metabolism, encouraging the clearance of fatty acids and triglycerides.

The amount of Carnitine needed is different in men than it is in women. Men have a higher blood Carnitine level than women. High levels of Carnitine are also found in the epididymis of the testes in men.

The Spermatozoa of a man who is depleted in Lysine become infertile on account of a potential Carnitine deficiency.* This is the first tissue to show deficiencies in men who have been deprived of Carnitine or Lysine. Adequate levels of Carnitine are necessary for energy metabolism within the sperm for proper motility and fertility.

Carnitine prevents Ketones from building up in people who are susceptible to Ketosis. Ketosis is the accumulation of Ketone bodies, or fat waste products in the blood. These ketones can cause the blood to become acid and lead to the loss of Calcium, Magnesium and Potassium in the urine. Ketosis, when uncontrolled in poor weight loss diets or diabetes, can be life-threatening.

CITROLINE

Citroline is a non-essential amino acid because it can be manufactured in the liver by Lysine. Citroline will convert to Arginine then to Ornithine in the kidney. This series of interactions serves to convert a highly toxic compound, ammonia, into a non-toxic compound, urea, which will be excreted from the body in the form of urine. In our research we have found that the absence of Citroline can cause a malabsorption of Iron. So in our practice when we find a client "unable" to absorb Iron, prior to their association with us, we have found them to be in need of Citroline. Upon the addition of the needed amount of Citroline, within weeks, a person who had an Iron deficiency, can be normalized. Citroline is an "OAT" allergy antidote.

L-CYSTEINE and L-CYSTINE:

L-Cysteine and L-Cystine are non-essential amino acids. Cysteine and Cystine are interconvertable. Cysteine is created in the body from Serine and Methionine.

---

*Methionine and Lysine make Carnitine.

Cysteine is an effective antioxidant and scavenger of free radicals. Free radicals are chemically reactive molecules which can damage proteins, fats, and nucleic acids (RNA and DNA). Cysteine helps minimize the random cross linking of cells caused by free radicals which can result in aged skin, hardening of the arteries, accumulation of age pigments (age spots), arthritis, and mutagenic disorders such as cancer.

Cysteine may also act as a membrane stabilizer and serve as a protectant at the cellular level against the adverse effects of heavy smoking and heavy drinking.

Acetaldehyde is a major toxicant common to both heavy smoking and heavy drinking, and can auto-oxidize to form free radicals. Aldehydes are formed by automobile exhaust, cigarette smoke, smog, urban pollution, and are formed by the liver from alcohol.

These free radicals are associated with adverse cardiovascular, respiratory, and nervous system effects. Chains of Cysteine link up to form insulin, vasopressin, and somatostatin. It is also needed for proper structure of sulfur-containing protein hormones, neuropeptides, and enzymes.

Cystine is indispensable for formation of the skin. Both Cystine and Cysteine promote healing from surgical operations and burns, while also stimulating white blood cell activity in the immune system, necessary for resistance to disease.

L-GLUTAMIC ACID:

Glutamic acid is a non-essential amino acid. Glutamic acid serves as an acceptor and donor of ammonia. When coupled with ammonia, it becomes Glutamine and can safely transport ammonia to the liver where it becomes urea, and is excreted by the kidneys.

About 90% of the dry weight of the brain consists of protein. Approximately half of the amino acid composition in the brain is represented by Glutamic acid and its derivatives, which include L-Glutamine.

Glutamic acid has a function as a neurotransmitter in the central nervous system. Glutamic acid is called a "Brain Food" because it plays a special role in brain metabolism, essential to improve and maintain the functions of the brain.

Glutamic acid can pick up ammonia throughout the body. Glutamic acid is then converted to L-Glutamine which serves as a buffer against excessive ammonia in the brain.

Glutamic acid can also be converted and degraded to carbon dioxide and water and be transformed into sugar for the Krebs Cycle of energy. Glutamic acid also increases the water solubility of a protein.

Deficiency Symptoms:

A lack of Glutamic acid can be a contributing cause of Epilepsy, Hepatic Coma, Muscular Dystrophy, and Mental Retardation.

A lack of Glutamic acid could cause mood swings, brain upset, increased urination, brown out, loss of energy ignition, and a slow death.

Food Sources:

Wheat Gluten.

Glutamic acid is the most prominent amino acid in wheat protein. Glands and organs affected by Glutamic acid:

Adrenals
Pancreas
Solar Plexus
Spine

Complementary Vitamins:

Vitamin B-5 (Pantothenic Acid)
Vitamin C
Vitamin B Complex
Vitamin B-6
Niacin (Vitamin B-3)

Complementary Minerals:

Potassium
Sodium
Chromium
Zinc

L-GLUTAMINE:

L-Glutamine is a non-essential amino acid for it is an amide form of L-Glutamic acid. It is formed when a Glutamic acid attaches to an ammonia molecule. Therefore, L-Glutamine is primarily an ammonia carrier. L-Glutamic acid picks up ammonia in the central nervous system and delivers it to the kidneys for deamination.

L-Glutamine has improved intelligence. It is also reported to improve the I.Q. of the mentally retarded. L-Glutamine is presently being researched as a corrective and controlling nutrient to help alcoholics to recover by diminishing their desire and need for alcohol.

L-Glutamine has been used with other nutrients successfully against Petite Mal Epilepsy, Schizophrenia, and Senility. L-Glutamine has also helped ulcers to heal faster.

When amino acid concentrations are evaluated in blood plasma, L-Glutamine is the highest. Glutamine participates in creating urea (for excretion by the kidneys), and purines (genetic DNA material).

L-Glutamine is the antidote to the "Pepper, Pear, Peach, Plum," Nectoring Group.

Deficiency Symptoms:

A lack of L-Glutamine can cause breathing difficulties (as though caused by heart trouble) and cardiac dyspnea. A lack of L-Glutamine can also give flu symptoms.

Food Sources:

Beet Juice, and Wheat Protein
NOTE: L-Glutamine is the amino acid needed to neutralize peppers, peaches, pears, plums, and nectarines.
Glands and organs affected by L-Glutamine:

Lymph
Thymus
Heart

Complementary Vitamins:

Vitamin A
Niacin (Vitamin B-3)
Vitamin E

Complementary Minerals:

Chromium
Zinc
Calcium

Selenium
Magnesium
Sulfur

L-GLYCINE:

L-Glycine is a non-essential amino acid because the body can make it from other substances. L-Glycine is the simplest constructed amino acid. The nitrogen on the amino acid Glycine is exchanged readily with other amino acids. Glycine acts as a nitrogen pool for the synthesis of the other non-essential amino acids in the body by amination or transamination.

L-Glycine is needed for biosynthesis of heme (components of hemoglobin) and biosynthesis of serine, purines (DNA), and Glutathione. Glycine is also an inhibitory neurotransmitter in the central nervous system. Glycine has been effectively used to treat progressive muscular dystrophy.

Deficiency Symptoms:

A lack of Glycine can cause a disturbance in the oxygen carbon dioxide balance. A lack of Glycine can cause cardio/pulmonary disturbances causing heart trouble and difficult and labored breathing.

With a deficiency of Glycine (an inhibitory neurotransmitter), there is an over-excitability of certain portions of the brain leading to convulsions.

Glands and organs affected by Glycine:

Thyroid
Bones
Heart
Liver
Spleen

Complementary Vitamins:

Vitamin C
Vitamin A
Vitamin E
Niacin (Vitamin B-3)
Vitamin B-2
PABA
Vitamin B-Complex

Complementary Minerals:

Magnesium
Sulfur

L-HYDROXYPROLINE:

L-Hydroxyproline is a non-essential amino acid because it is manufactured in the body from other amino acids. Vitamin C also plays an important part in the manufacture of Hydroxyproline. Hydroxyproline is used in the manufacture of collagen (a substance of connective tissue), skin, ligaments, tendons, bone, and cartilage.

Deficiency Symptoms:

A lack of Hydroxyproline can be a cause of decaying bones, dizziness, hyperthyroid, overtaxed nerves, rickets, sciatica, and decaying of teeth. A lack of Hydroxyproline can cause a gradual deterioration of the spine making the electrical charge in the spine uncoordinated.

A lack of Hydroxyproline could also cause a mal-absorption of Vitamin D which would cause pains in the thighs and also a lack of Calcium absorption. Lack of Hydroxyproline can cause gradual hardening and loss of the functions of the vital organs.
Glands affected by Hydroxyproline:

Thyroid
Parathyroid

Complementary Vitamins:

Vitamin C
Niacin (Vitamin B-3)
Vitamin B-2
PABA
Vitamin A

Complementary Minerals:

Lithium
Fluorine
Sodium
Chlorine
Calcium
Selenium

Magnesium
Sulfur

Food Sources:

Gelatin

ORNITHINE

Ornithine is a non-essential amino acid which is manufactured in the kidney by Citrollin. Ornithine can also be a precursor of Citrulline and Arginine and when given orally has a very similar biological effect. Orally supplemented Ornithine can be converted by the body into Arginine, Glutathione or Proline.

Ornithine's primary end product is Arginine which is immediately converted back to Ornithine. Ornithine raises polymines which are usually high in cancer patients. Polymine's activity is associated with tissue growth. Ornithine releases growth hormone and is useful by athletes in training.

Toxic Effects:

An overdose of Ornithine over a long period of time can cause "gyrute atrophy", a very rare condition where the retina of the eye is affected and the visual field decreases. Cataracts, loss of visual sharpness and night blindness also occur. An overdose of Ornithine can also cause insomnia.

L-PROLINE:

L-Proline is a non-essential amino acid because it can be created in the body from Glutamic acid. L-Proline has a function in the joints and tendons of the body. Collagen, the main fibrous protein found in bone, cartilage, and other connective tissue, consists of 21% Proline.

Deficiency Symptoms:

Lack of Proline could cause joint and tendon dysfunction and swelling. A lack of Proline could also cause cardiac dysfunction and skin problems. Proline will also help to neutralize the "rice group" of allergies (Cinnamon, curry, blueberry, grapes, strawberry, watermelon, wine, pumpkin). A lack of Proline can cause a "ringing" in the left ear.

Glands and organs affected by Proline:

Bones
Duodenum
Stomach
Heart
Liver
Spleen
Thyroid

Complementary Vitamins:

Vitamin A   Trypsin
Vitamin E   Chymotrypsin
Vitamin B Complex   Vitamin B-2
Vitamin C   Vitamin B-12
Niacin   Folic Acid

Complementary Minerals:

Magnesium
Sulfur
Aluminum
Phosphorus
Calcium
Selenium
Chromium
Zinc

Food Sources:

Beet Sugar Molasses or Glucose, Casein (milk protein).

L-SERINE:

L-Serine is a non-essential amino acid because it can be synthesized in the body from other metabolites such as Glycine. L-Serine is very reactive in the body and plays an important role in the catalytic function of enzymes. L-Serine participates in Purine and Pyrimidine biosynthesis (utilized in the construction of RNA and DNA), Creatine (present in muscle, brain, and blood as a factor of muscle contraction), and Porphyrin (constituent of Heme in hemoglobin). It is also added as a natural skin moisturizing factor in cosmetics.

NOTE: The nerve gasses and insecticides work by combining with a residue of Serine which then inhibits proper enzyme activity and causes the neurotransmitter - Acetycholine to quickly reach dangerously high levels, resulting in convulsions and death.

Deficiency Symptoms:

A lack of Serine could cause a common cough, nervousness, hypersensing, and electric hypermotion.
Glands and organs affected by Serine:

Brain	Spine
Stomach	Hypothalamus
Pancreas	Eyes
Solar Plexus	Pineal

Complementary Vitamins:

Vitamin B Complex
Vitamin C
Pantothenic Acid (Vitamin B-5)
Niacin (Vitamin B-3)
Vitamin B-2
Vitamin B-12
Folic acid
Vitamin B-6
Vitamin A
Vitamin B-15
Vitamin E

Complementary Minerals:

Calcium
Selenium
Magnesium
Sulfur
Chromium
Zinc

L-TAURINE:

L-Taurine is a non-essential amino acid because it can be biosynthesized in the body from Methionine and Cysteine (two sulfur amino acids). Therefore, Taurine is a sulfur amino acid derivative. L-Taurine is found only in animal products (ox bile), and not in vegetable protein sources.

L-Taurine conjugates chemically with bile acids in the liver. This seems to be very important for the maintenance of proper bile composition, and for keeping cholesterol soluble. The liver is the only tissue where Taurine is metabolized, although there have been high levels found in the retina, brain, and heart.

Taurine in the body is conjugated to bile salts which makes bile less lithogenic and thus prevents gall stones. Taurine has been found to be concentrated in high quantities in the Pineal and Pituitary glands when an individual has been exposed to sunlight.

Stress has caused urinary spills of Taurine. L-Taurine works to spare the loss of Potassium from the heart muscle. Recent evidence indicates that Taurine may be the critical substance in the osmotic regulation of both Calcium and Potassium concentrations within the heart muscle, and also prevents Potassium or Calcium wasting, particularly during times of stress or weight loss and dieting.

L-Taurine is known to be an inhibitory neurotransmitter in the central nervous system. The brain is in subtle balance between the messages coming from the neuro-excitatory transmitters such as the Serotonin and Dopamine family, and the neuroinhibitory transmitters such as Gaba and Taurine. When there is a deficiency of neuroinhibitory transmitters, there is an over-excitation of certain portions of the brain which may lead to convulsions.

Taurine has been found to influence the movement of Calcium ions in the brain. Therefore, the observed anticonvulsant affects of Taurine may be a result of this biochemical effect. Taurine has been successfully used in the treatment of epilepsy. Taurine undoubtedly serves both as a neurotransmitter and a neuromodulator substance in the management of the central nervous system function.

Taurine has also been found to resemble the effect of insulin on blood sugar. It seems to promote regulation of blood sugar in the individual who may be insulin deficient.

Taurine is the second most abundant amino acid found in human milk, and infants may need more Taurine than the amount that is found in regular cows' milk and soy formula.

Deficiency Symptoms:

A lack of Taurine can cause epileptic seizures and heart problems due to the heart muscle being unable to retain Potassium. A lack of Taurine can also cause blindness. Taurine works with Zinc in the eyes, and deficiencies of Taurine have led to functional impairment of vision well before there was an actual structural alteration of the eye. Depletion of Taurine occurs slowly, but eventually leads to blindness.

Lack of Taurine can be caused by certain estrogenic hormone substances when given to women, who may then require more Taurine. A lack of Taurine can also cause memory loss and an allergy to fats. Complementary Vitamins:

Vitamin B-6
Vitamin B Complex
Vitamin C
Vitamin E

Complementary Minerals:

Zinc
Calcium
Potassium
Sodium
Chromium

Glands and Organs affected By Taurine:

Pineal
Pituitary
Thyroid
Parathyroid
Heart
Bones
Liver
Duodenum

NOTE: Excessive alcohol consumption will deplete the body of Taurine and Methionine.

Taurine is believed to be an "anti-aging" amino acid.

L-TYROSINE:

L-Tyrosine is a non-essential amino acid because it is formed from the amino acid L-Phenylalanine. L-Tyrosine plays an intermediary role in the synthesis of the neurotransmitter Norepinephrin from the amino acid Phenylalanine.

A neurotransmitter is a chemical that transmits signals between neurons and allows them to communicate. Since Norepinephrin is an appetite inhibitory neurotransmitter, Tyrosine will suppress the appetite.

Tyrosine is a useful agent in treating mental disorders. Tyrosine is an anti-depressant and plays a role in controlling anxiety. Tyrosine in combination with Tryptophane is a better sleep aid than Tryptophane by itself. Tyrosine also stimulates the release of growth hormones which causes muscular growth and reduces fat.

Tyrosine is a precursor to the adrenal hormone Epinephrin, Pituitary hormone Norepinephrin, and Thyroid hormone Thyroxin. Tyrosine also produces melanin, the pigment of the skin and hair.

Tyrosine is an anti-oxidant which bonds free radicals. Therefore, Tyrosine can be classified as an anti-aging amino acid.

Deficiency Symptoms:

A lack of Tyrosine can cause anxiety and depression which would also be caused by a deficiency of the neurotransmitter Norepinephrin at a specific site in the brain; this, in turn, relates to mood problems such as depression.

A lack of Tyrosine would make a person feel tired from the lack of formation of Thyroxin (Thyroid hormone). A lack of Tyrosine can also cause impotence and reduced flow of semen from the male.

Too much Tyrosine can cause an overload product-Tyramine, causing migraine headaches. Tyramine, when ingested in combination with anti-depressants of the class known as Monoamine Oxidase Inhibitors (MAOI), can cause an increase in blood pressure.

Food Sources:

Aged cheese, beer, wine, yeast, ripe bananas, avocado, pickled herring, and chicken livers.
Glands and Organs Affected By Tyrosine:

Anterior Pituitary
Thymus
Lymph
Tonsils
Appendix
Adrenal
Peyer's Patches

Skin

Complementary Vitamins:

Vitamin A
Vitamin C
Vitamin E
Vitamin B-5 (Pantothenic Acid)

Complementary Minerals:

Calcium
Selenium
Magnesium

I am enclosing a series of charts showing the Amino Acid acupuncture points.

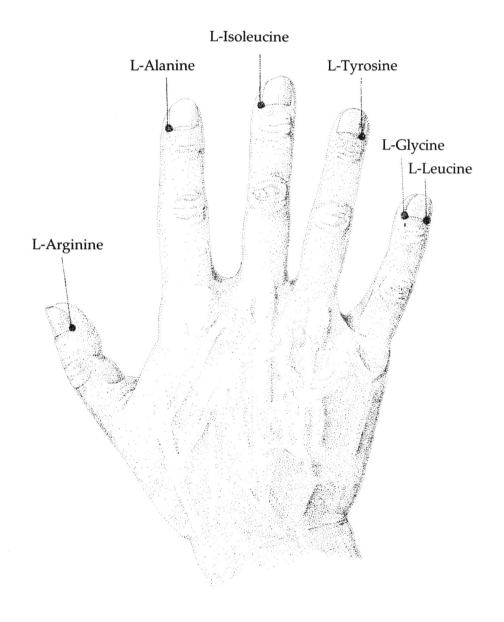

Figure 48

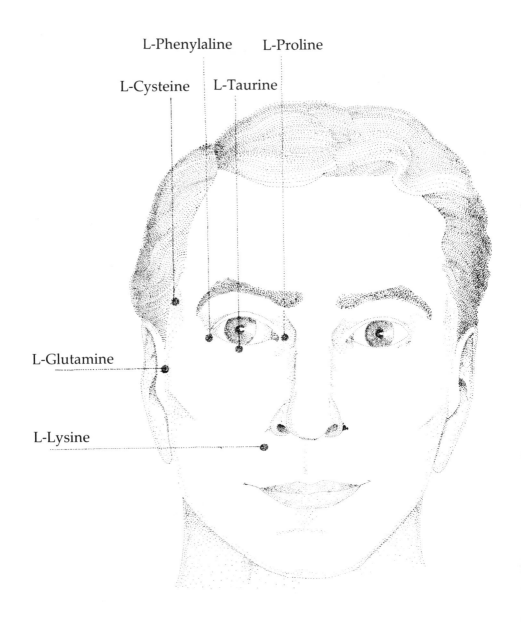

Figure 49

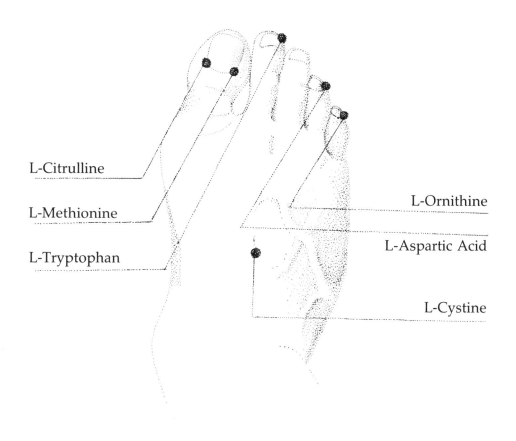

L-Citrulline

L-Methionine

L-Tryptophan

L-Ornithine

L-Aspartic Acid

L-Cystine

Figure 50

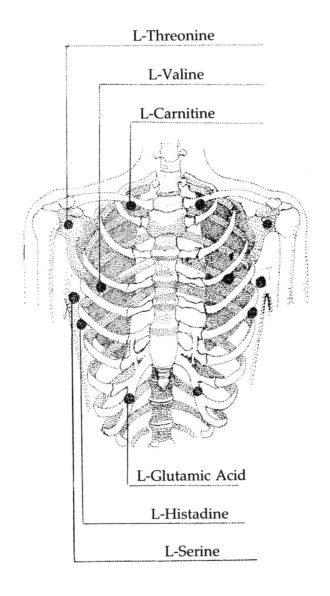

L-Threonine

L-Valine

L-Carnitine

L-Glutamic Acid

L-Histadine

L-Serine

Figure 51

CHAPTER 6

MISCELLANEOUS POINTS OF INTEREST

DIGESTIVE ENZYMES

The M.R.T. acupuncture point for the digestive enzymes is found one to one and a half inches to the right of the center seam line on the lower border of the rib cage.

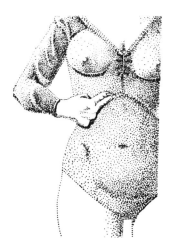

Figure 52

Function:

Pancreatic enzymes (Pancreatin components) are the body's most powerful digestive enzymes, having the ability to digest protein, starch, and fat. They are produced by the pancreas and delivered to the small intestines where they digest most of the food consumed. Pancreatic enzymes are Amylase, Protease, and Lipase.

Pepsin is the stomach's protein splitting enzyme, having the ability to reduce protein into Peptides and Polypeptides. Rennin, an enzyme formed only in infancy, causes coagulation of milk, changing its protein - Casein - into a usable form in the body.

Rennin releases the valuable minerals from milk, such as Calcium, Phosphorus, Potassium, and Iron that are used by the body to stabilize the fluid balance, strengthen the nervous system, and produce strong teeth and bones.

Lipase splits fats, which are then utilized to nourish the skin cells, protect the body against bruises, and ward off allergic conditions.

Enzymes are best available from uncooked vegetables and fruits. Each enzyme acts upon a specific food; one cannot substitute for the other. A deficiency, shortage, or even the absence of one single enzyme can mean the difference between illness and wellness.

Enzymes that end in "ase" are named by the food substance they act upon; for Phosphorus, the enzyme is called Phosphatase; for sugar (sucrose), the enzyme would be called Sucrase.

Bile is produced by the liver and aids in the digestion of fats.

The digestive aids that are available are: Acidophilus, Bromelain (from pineapple), Papain (Papaya), and comfrey.

NOTE: The Acidophilus Point is 1 inch lower than the collar bone on the right breast opposite the Vitamin "P" point. If there is a need for Acidophilus, sometimes the acupuncture point will hurt. Women sometimes mistake it for breast lumps or heart or thymus problems. If Acidophilus is administered it will stop hurting.

EPA: (Eicosapentaenoic Acid, "Max EPA")

The Muscle Response Testing (M.R.T.) method that I prefer is to hold the capsule in the hand while placing over the Solar Plexus and extending the opposite arm to be "pumped". See Figure 29, page 56.

EPA is a fatty acid found almost exclusively in fish and seafood. This Lipid (fatty acid) is distinctive because unlike other fats which have 18 or less carbons in their molecular make up, it can have 20 or more carbons per molecule. This means that the body can use EPA as a needed precursor (building block) to form anti-aggretory (tending not to clot or be overly adhesive) prostaglandins. Prostaglandins are chemical substances that can prevent and even reduce cholesterol build up, plaque, and arterial blockage.

Coronary health has also been improved when EPA is increased in the diet. Dr. William E. Connor, head of the Clinical Nutrition and Lipid Arteriosclerosis Laboratory at the University of Oregon Health Services Center, reports that after only ten days on a diet high in Salmon and Salmon Oil(EPA), normal test subjects (human) experienced an average of an 11% decrease in their cholesterol levels and a 33% reduction in their Triglyceride level (another form of fat found in the blood).

Test subjects with high blood fat levels showed a 32% reduction in cholesterol and a 66% drop in Triglycerides after the ten day Salmon diet! We find that heart disease is easier to prevent and reverse with Max EPA than we previously thought.

Ongoing research certainly points in that direction. Max EPA oil is prepared using natural processes that remove all Vitamin D and most Vitamin A from the oil. Max EPA oil is uniformly 18% EPA. If I find that a person needs Max EPA, and shows through testing that he needs as much as 4 capsules, I usually recommend that they take only 2 capsules at bedtime. I do this because I have found that if given their maximum amount needed, the person may "overdose" before his next visit, causing him to feel tired because as the Max EPA burns up Triglycerides and Cholesterol and other lipids, the body's fuel supply gets depleted. So by taking the Max EPA at night, the person will not experience this feeling of tiredness.

If the Max EPA is taken during the day, it may make a person feel sluggish and subconsciously feel the need to replace these fats by eating chocolate, hamburgers, french fries, milk shakes, bacon, sausage, or any other high fat-content foods.

HYDROCHLORIC ACID

The M.R.T. acupuncture point for hydrochloric acid is found one to one and a half inches to the left of the center seam line on the lower border of the rib cage.

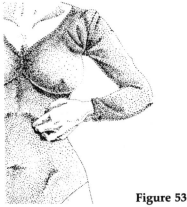

Figure 53

RDA: Not known

Function:

Hydrochloric Acid improves the digestion and assimilation of vitamins and minerals, especially Iron.

Because stress causes a "burn up" of Pantothenic Acid, which feeds the Adrenal glands which help to manufacture Hydrochloric Acid, most of us are low in Hydrochloric Acid. Most people think they have an over-acidity problem, so they take an antacid such as Maalox, Digel, Tums, Rolaids, or Alka-Seltzer, not realizing that it is the worst possible thing to do because the symptoms of not having enough acid are exactly the same as those of having too much!!

Most people don't have enough Hydrochloric Acid, and by taking an antacid they are dissolving the little acid they do have. This might relieve the gas pain, but the person will not assimilate any nourishment from the food he eats, and the food will probably pass into the colon undigested, sometimes causing constipation.

Also, most of the antacids contain Aluminum Hydroxide which is poisonous. Aluminum was not meant to be eaten!! One of the safest antacids to use (if you need the sodium) is Alka-Seltzer, which contains 500 mg. of Sodium. The use of antacids containing Aluminum Hydroxide can cause a loss of bone Phosphorus, causing tooth decay and bone deterioration (Arthritis).

A person who uses Tagamet will tend to produce too much Hydrochloric Acid. I have found that too much Hydrochloric Acid in the body can be neutralized by the Cell Salt Natrum Phos.

Deficiency Symptoms:

A lack of Hydrochloric acid can cause Pernicious Anemia, burning sensation in the stomach, systemic alkalosis, and allergies because of starvation caused by *non*-absorption of vitamins and minerals from foods.

Food Sources:

Apple Cider Vinegar, Betaine Hydrochloric (usually manufactured from Beet molasses).

NOTE: Apple Cider Vinegar contains Malic Acid (C_4, H_6, O_5) which is a natural organic constituent of apples and is an element involved in the digestive processes. It combines with alkaline elements and minerals in the body to produce energy that can be stored in the system as Glycogen for future use.

LECITHIN

The M.R.T. acupuncture point for Lecithin is located two to two and a half inches to the right of the center seam.

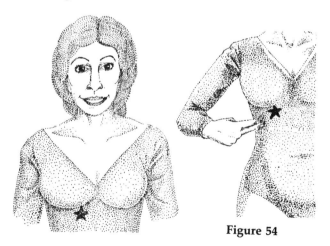

Figure 54

RDA: None established

Function:

Lecithin is found in all living cells of the human body. Lecithin helps in the digestion and absorption of fats and important oil-soluble vitamins by emulsifying them into tiny droplets that are utilized by every cell.

Lecithin is manufactured in the body by Choline and Inositol. Lecithin is high in Phosphorus and unites with Iron, Iodine, and Calcium to give power and vigor to the brain.

Phosphatidyl Choline (Super Lecithin) has been found useful in arresting Alzheimer's disease. Lecithin can help to restore the memory banks which we have found to be weakened by coffee. Coffee creates an Inositol deficiency. Inositol is needed to manufacture Lecithin in the body.

Lecithin breaks up cholesterol and allows it to pass through the arterial walls, helping to prevent Arteriosclerosis. Lecithin plays an important part in maintaining a healthy nervous system and is found naturally in the Myelin sheath, a fatty protective covering for the nerves.

Lecithin can prevent the formation of gallstones, and has also been found useful in weight control by helping to redistribute the fat of the body. Lecithin can also lower blood pressure.

Deficiency Symptoms:

A lack of Lecithin can cause forgetfulness, digestive problems such as intolerence to fat, nausea, and hypertension. A deficiency in Lecithin can cause joint and muscle problems such as bursitis, cramps, and soreness.

Food Sources:

Lecithin is found in Egg yolk, soybeans, corn, wheat, and nuts.

Lecithin as a supplement in capsules, liquid, or granule form is usually taken from a Soy source.

NOTE: If a Lecithin supplement is used in large dosages over a long period of time, please be sure to retest Calcium, as the Phosphorus in Lecithin can become out of balance to Calcium.

RIBONUCLEIC ACID (RNA)

The M.R.T. acupuncture point for RNA is found on the bridge of the nose, just between the eyebrows.

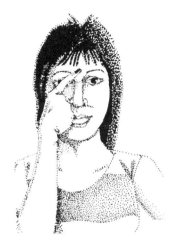

Figure 55

RDA: 30 to 100 mg.
 As much as 300 mg. is sometimes advised by Physicians.

Function:

RNA improves memory. The administration of RNA is regarded as valuable in recovery from neurological disorders. It sometimes helps to restore normal Thyroid functions.

Deficiency Symptoms:

A lack of RNA in the body could cause coldness of the hands and feet, coarse hair, a low resistance to stress, and/or a loss of weight. It should be noted that Zinc will help manufacture RNA in the body.

RNA may possibly be useful in reversing the degenerative effects of aging.

Food Sources:

Fish and shellfish, sardines, onions, and brewers yeast.

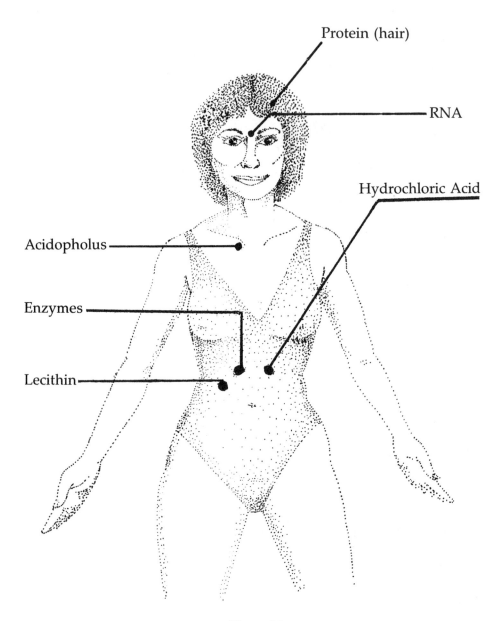

Figure 56

CHAPTER 7

HERB LAND

Herbs are Nature's Pharmacy. Every vitamin, mineral and amino acid is available to one from an herbal source, if you know where to look and for what.

This is what I will attempt to do in this chapter of this book.

First of all, Herbs are available to us from the Health Food Industry in many forms: (a) bulk teas; (b) bagged teas; (c) herbal capsules; (d) Herb pills; and in (e) Homeopathic tinctures.

The manufacturers of the tea forms argue that a tea of the herb can be more readily absorbed through the walls of the stomach. Herb capsule and pill manufacturers argue that there are non-water soluble substances that would remain in the tea bag or tea strainer that could dissolve in the stomach if taken in a pill or capsule form. The Homeopathy tinctures bypass all this by dropping the herbal extract under the tongue to bypass the stomach, thereby going directly to the blood stream, and are absorbed in minutes, if not seconds.

My personal preference is to use the capsule form because it is easier to measure by the M.R.T. system and it is tasteless.

With all the other systems, if the herb tastes or smells bad, your client will not take it anyway. (Have you ever smelled valerian root?) The capsule system insures that the client will not be "turned off" by his/her senses, which could discourage him/her and cause him/her to not take the amount of herbs you might suggest.

The way to ascertain the amount of capsules that should be taken would be to place the capsule in the client's left hand. Close the hand and place it over the solar plexus (mid section) while extending the other arm to be pumped. See figure 29, page 56.

If the arm that is extended seems to be weak, add a capsule at a time until the extended arm feels rigid. If the arm starts to get weak again, you may have added too many herbal capsules. Cut back on them until the extended arm tests strong.

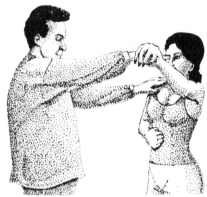

Figure 57

The way I use Herbs in my work is to use them wherever I can instead of specific vitamins, minerals, or amino acid capsules because they are in the organic form. For example, when I need to use Iron, I use a 500 mg. cap of Yellow Dock for every 60 mgs. of Iron needed. An Iron pill is basically an inorganic mineral pill but when I use Yellow Dock I'm using an organic source of Iron. Iron is mined from the earth as a mineral, but a plant like Yellow Dock goes into the ground and pulls out the inorganic Iron and converts it into its leaves as an organic source of Iron. Animals eat leaves, they don't eat dirt!! Now it is obvious that if the need for Iron is less than 40 mgs., then a Yellow Dock capsule may be an overdose.

Here are the vitamin, mineral and amino acid contents of herbs. It should be realized that the soil in which the herb is grown will determine its potency!!

VITAMIN	HERBS
A	Marshmallow, dandelion, alfalfa, chamomile, celery, blackberry, bee pollen, burdock, capsicum, catnip, chicory, comfrey, echinacea, eyebright, fenugreek, garlic, ginger, ginseng, golden seal, nettles, peppermint, red clover, red raspberry, rosehips, rosemary, sarsaparilla, saw palmetto, spearmint, strawberries, violet,

watercress, yarrow, yellow dock, yucca, dong quai, gotu kola, horehound, iceland and irish moss, saffron, sage.

B-COMPLEX   Bee pollen, royal jelly, blue cohosh, cascara sagrada, catnip, celery, eyebright, ginger, golden seal, hawthorn berries, kelp, parsley, rose hips, sarsaparilla, lady's slipper, licorice, anise, blessed thistle, burdock, caraway, hops, jojoba, strawberry, thyme, wormwood, yucca.

B12   Mistletoe, angelica, dong quai, ephedra (brigham tea), ginseng, mustard, saffron, white oak bark, coltsfoot.

B15   Black walnut.

PABA   Cornsilk, horsetail.

C   Chickweed, celery, burdock, blue vervain, blackberry, bee pollen, bayberry, barberry, capsicum, catnip, chicory, comfrey, echinacea, eyebright, garlic, ginger, golden seal, hawthorn berries, juniper berries, nettles, peppermint, pokeweed, queen of the meadow, rose hips, red raspberry, rhubarb, rosemary, sage, sarsaparilla, scullcap, shepherd's purse, spearmint, strawberry, thyme, violet, watercress, white pine bark, witch hazel, wormwood, yarrow, yellow dock, yucca, dandelion.

D   Alfalfa, basil, bee pollen, chickweed, eyebright, fenugreek, mullein, papaya, queen of the meadow, red raspberry, rose hips, sarsaparilla, thyme, watercress.

E   Angelica, bee pollen, birch, blue cohosh, blue vervain, burdock, dandelion, dong quai, ginseng, golden seal, gotu kola, horsetail, irish moss, jojoba, kelp, licorice, nettle, oatstraw, papaya, red raspberry, rose hips, scullcap, shepherd's purse, slippery elm, watercress, witch hazel, yarrow.

F   Gentian, golden seal, horseradish, irish moss,

nettle, red clover, red raspberry, safflower, slippery elm, yarrow.

K	Alfalfa, chicory , cornsilk, irish moss, cramp bark, gotu kola, kelp, papaya, plantain, safflower, shepherd's purse, slippery elm.
RUTIN (VITAMIN P)	Rue, burdock, chicory, colts foot, horseradish, nettle, red clover, rose hips, slippery elm, witch hazel.
MINERAL	**HERBS**
CALCIUM	Alfalfa, aloe vera, angelica, anise, basil, birch, blackberry, black cohosh, black walnut, blessed thistle, blue cohosh, blue vervain, cayenne, caraway, cascara sagrada, celery, chamomile, cloves, colts foot, comfrey, couch grass, dandelion, elecampane, flaxseed, garlic, ginger, ginseng, golden seal, horseradish, iceland moss, kelp, marshmallow, mistletoe, nettle, oatstraw, papaya, parsley, plantain, pokeweed, red clover, red raspberry, rhubarb, rose hips, rosemary, saffron, sage, scullcap, shepherd's purse, slippery elm.
COBALT	Caraway, ephedra (brigham tea), horsetail, juniper berries, kelp, lobelia, mistletoe, mustard, parsley, red clover, rhubarb, white oak bark, wormwood.
CHROMIUM	Jojoba, kelp, licorice, nettle.
COPPER	Birch, burdock, caraway, coltsfoot, comfrey, dandelion, echinacea, ephedra (brigham tea), eyebright, garlic, goldenseal, hops, horsetail, jojoba, juniper, kelp, lobelia, mistletoe, nettle, parsley, peppermint, valerian, watercress, white pine bark, witch hazel, yarrow, yucca.
FLUORINE	Hops, garlic, alfalfa, birch.
IODINE	Burdock, caraway, echinacea, eyebright (trace of Iodine), hops (trace of Iodine), horsetail, iceland moss, jojoba, kelp, licorice, mistletoe, mustard, peppermint.

IRON   Alfalfa, aloe vera, anise, barberry, basil, birch, blackberry, black cohosh, black walnut, blessed thistle, cayenne, caraway, chamomile, comfrey, dandelion, echinacea, eyebright, fenugreek, garlic, gentian, ginger, ginseng, golden seal, hawthorn berries, hops, horehound, horseradish, horsetail, jojoba, kelp, lobelia, mistletoe, mullein, mustard, nettle, papaya, parsley, peppermint, pokeweed, red raspberry, rhubarb, rose hips, rosemary, sarsaparilla, scullcap, shepherd's purse, slippery elm, yellow dock.

LEAD   Caraway, cascara sagrada, celery, gentian, hops, lobelia, valerian, white oak bark.

MAGNESIUM   Aloe vera, anise, basil, birch, black cohosh, black walnut, blue cohosh, cayenne, caraway, catnip, celery, chamomile, cloves, comfrey, couch grass, evening primrose, ginger, ginseng, hops, kelp, mistletoe, mullein, papaya, peppermint, spearmint, valerian, wood betony.

MANGANESE   Aloe vera, barberry, black walnut, blessed thistle, blue vervain, cascara sagrada, catnip, chamomile, chickweed, colts foot, garlic, gentian, ginseng, golden seal, hops, horsetail, kelp, licorice, mustard (trace of manganese), nettle, red clover, red raspberry, sarsaparilla, watercress, white pine bark, witch hazel, wood betony, wormwood, yarrow, yellow dock, yucca.

NICKEL   Dandelion, ephedra (brigham tea), hawthorne berries, kelp, white pine bark, yellow dock.

POTASSIUM   Alfalfa, aloe vera, birch, black cohosh, black walnut, blessed thistle, blue cohosh, burdock, cayenne, caraway, cascara sagrada, celery, chamomile, chaparral, cloves, colts foot, comfrey, couch grass, dandelion, echinacea, evening primrose, fennel, flaxseed, garlic, ginger, ginseng, golden seal, horehound, horseradish, iceland moss, irish moss, kelp, mistletoe, mullein, nettle, papaya, parsley, peppermint, plantain, rhubarb, rosehips, rosemary, saffron, sage, scull cap, shepherd's purse, slippery elm, spearmint, strawberry, valerian, white oak bark, wormwood, yarrow, yucca.

PHOSPHORUS   Alfalfa, barberry, basil, birch, black cohosh, black walnut, blessed thistle, blue cohosh, cayenne, catnip, celery, chickweed, cloves, comfrey, dandelion, ginger, ginseng, golden seal, hawthorn berries, horseradish, iceland moss, irish moss, kelp, licorice, marigold, oatstraw, papaya, pokeweed, red raspberry, rhubarb, rosemary, saffron, sage, slippery elm, strawberry, white oak bark, wood betony, yucca.

SELENIUM   Garlic, horsetail, lobelia, red clover, slippery elm, witch hazel, alfalfa, kelp.

SILICON   Birch, black cohosh, black walnut, burdock, caraway, celery, chaparral, cornsilk, couch grass, eyebright, gentian, ginseng, hawthorn berries, horsetail, jojoba, kelp, nettle, oatstraw, parsley, peppermint, thyme.

SODIUM   Alfalfa, aloe vera, birch, catnip, celery, chaparral, cloves, couch grass, dandelion, elecampane, fennel, ginger, ginseng, golden seal, hawthorn berries, hops, horseradish, horsetail, kelp, lobelia, mistletoe, nettle, papaya, parsley, pennyroyal, red clover, rhubarb, rose hips, rosemary, saffron, sage, sarsaparilla, shepherd's purse, slippery elm, thyme, white oak bark, white pine bark, wormwood.

SULFUR   Burdock, cayenne, catnip (trace of sulfur), celery, chaparral, comfrey, echinacea, fennel, garlic, gentian, ginseng, hawthorn berries, horehound, irish moss, juniper berries, kelp, lobelia, mullein, mustard, nettle, parsley, peppermint, plantain, rhubarb, rose hips, sage, sarsaparilla, shepherd's purse, spearmint, thyme, watercress, white oak bark.

TIN	Cascara sagrada, chaparral, dandelion, gentian, ginseng, hawthorn berries, juniper berries, red clover, rhubarb, shepherd's purse, white oak bark, wormwood.
TRACE MINERALS	Alfalfa, dandelion, lobelia, plantain, kelp, irish moss.
ZINC	Aloe vera, burdock, chamomile, chickweed, comfrey, dandelion, eyebright, garlic, gentian, golden seal, hops, hawthorn, jojoba, kelp, licorice, marshmallow, nettle, rosemary, sarsaparilla, scullcap, shepherd's purse, slippery elm, taheebo, valerian, witch hazel.

ENZYMES	**HERBS**
Eight Essential	Alfalfa
	Bee Pollen

AMINO ACIDS	**HERBS**
	Bee Pollen (35% protein), Comfrey (18 amino acids, especially lysine), Dandelion (rich in Protein), Ginger, Nettle.

Now that we have discussed the vitamin and mineral contents of herbs, we should not use them for this purpose only, for each herb has a personality and therefore a unique individuality. So that you might familiarize yourself with each herb, I am listing the ones that are easily obtainable, and those which I have successfully used over the years.

Here they are alphabetically:

ALFALFA:

Alfalfa is very rich in the vitamins A, E, K, D, B6 and U. Alfalfa contains a tremendous amount of minerals such as Calcium, Phosphorus, Iron, Magnesium, Silicon, Sodium and Potassium. Alfalfa also contains trace minerals. I have found that dried alfalfa juice concentrate is a very rich source of Potassium and Sodium with a ratio of 2 (Potassium) units to 1 (Sodium) unit. Alfalfa has eight digestive enzymes which help with nutritional assimilation.

I have found that alfalfa is one of the best herbs to combat and cure allergies. Because of its Potassium and Sodium content, it is one of the best herbs to use when Rheumatoid Arthritis is present. It is almost a miracle herb. It is the most important source of electrolytes and will give the body's muscles strength when one seems exhausted.

I have used alfalfa juice concentrate capsules with excellent results to arrest lupus, A.L.S. (Lou Gehrig's disease), and other strength debilitating diseases. The ratio of Potassium to Sodium in a normal alfalfa pill is 2:1. In the alfalfa juice concentrate the capsule is triple the strength of the pill. It is also a heart strengthener.

Time of Administration:

Before meals, or upon rising in the morning, at noon, and at supper time, because of its anti-allergic affect upon foods.

ALOE VERA:

Part used:

Gel from inside of leaves.

Aloe Vera contains Calcium, Potassium, Sodium, Manganese, Iron, Lecithin and Zinc.

Aloe Vera applied externally will heal, disinfect and soothe abscesses, burns, wounds, insect bites and all skin irritations.

Aloe Vera Juice taken internally can correct chronic constipation, gastritis, hyperacidity, and stomach ulcers. Aloe Vera taken internally acts like a chelating agent to detoxify the body of heavy, poisonous metals. Aloe Vera contains substances which promote the removal of dead skin, and promote the normal growth of living cells.

It has been discovered that liquid aloe vera taken internally will help to heal and mend tissues that have been damaged by Cobalt Radiation used in the treatment of cancer in Nuclear Medicine. Aloe Vera applied externally will heal X-ray burns and will also prevent scar tissue from forming inside the body of the site of a surgical incision. If Aloe Vera gel is frequently applied after surgery, the incision will heal rapidly and leave practically no scar.

Time of Administration:

I prefer late evening for oral consumption, so that the resultant Bowel Movement should occur in the A.M. upon arising!

For external use any time is okay.

ANISE (Pimpinella Anisum):

Known also as "sweet cummin".

Parts used:

Oil and seed.

Anise contains B Vitamins, Choline, Calcium, Iron, Potassium and Magnesium, 1.5 - 3.5%. Volatile oil (Anethole) is used clinically as an intestinal stimulant for colic.

Anise is believed to be high in estrogen content.

Anise is used for colic, indigestion, intestinal gas, halitosis (bad breath). Anise has also been used as an expectorant for mucus congestion in the lungs and for whooping cough.

Anise will also increase the flow of milk from a lactating mother.

Time of Administration:

When needed to alleviate a condition.

BARBERRY (Berberis Vulgaris):

Part used:

Root Bark

Barberry is high in Vitamin C. Barberry also contains Iron, Manganese and Phosphorus.

Barberry will normalize the bowels. Barberry will stimulate the flow of bile from the liver. Barberry is effective in almost all liver problems, especially Jaundice.

Barberry dilates the blood vessels, and therefore will lower blood pressure. Barberry is sometimes used as a mouthwash and a gargle because it has antiseptic qualities. A gall bladder condition can also be soothed by Barberry.

Time of Administration:

Morning and all day.

BASIL (Ocimum Basilicum)

Part used:

Leaves

Basil contains Vitamins A, D, and B2 as well as Calcium, Phosphorus, Iron and Magnesium.

Basil when taken internally can help stop stomach cramps because it is an antispasmodic. Basil will also alleviate constipation. Basil will help in digestion. Basil when applied externally can draw out insect, bee, wasp or snake venom when so bitten.

Time of Administration:

Afternoon or when needed.

BAYBERRY (Myrica Cerifera):

Parts used:

Bark, Root

Bayberry contains Vitamin C.

Bayberry is a blood tonic. Bayberry will help to rejuvenate the adrenal gland, and help to clear the sinus on both sides of the nose. Bayberry will aid digestion and circulation. Bayberry can ward off cold-like symptoms if taken at the first sign of the symptoms.

Bayberry when combined with Ginger has successfully combatted Cholera. A douche made with Bayberry tea can be used to treat excessive menstrual bleeding, vaginal infections, and prolapsed uterus. Bayberry tea gargle can soothe a sore and infected throat. A bayberry tea mouthwash can arrest bleeding gums.

Time of Administration:

Evenings.

BEE POLLEN:

Please see description in the "Miracle Food" section.

BIRCH (Betula Alba):

Parts used:

Bark and Leaves
Birch contains Vitamins A, C, E, B1, B2, Calcium, Chloride, Copper, Iron, Magnesium, Phosphorus, Potassium, Sodium, Silicon and is high in Fluoride.
Birch is a blood purifier and is used to treat bladder problems. Birch can be used externally for treating Eczema.
Powdered Birch can be used to brush teeth.

Time of Administration:

Anytime.

BLACKBERRY (Rubus Fructicosus):

Parts used:

Leaves, root bark, berries
Blackberry contains Vitamins A, B1, B2, B3, and C, and the minerals Iron and Calcium.
Blackberry (Blackberry tea or brandy) has the ability to stop diarrhea and dysentery.
Blackberry tea has the ability to dry up one's sinus.

Time of Administration:

When the body's condition needs it.

BLACK COHOSH (Cimicifuga Racemosa):

Part used:

Root

Black Cohosh contains impressive amounts of Calcium, Potassium, Magnesium and Iron. It also contains minimal amounts of Vitamin A, Inositol, B5, Silicon and Phosphorus.

Black Cohosh is a sedative. Black Cohosh contains natural estrogen, the female hormone. Black Cohosh was used by the American Indian women for all pelvic conditions, female complaints, and uterine troubles. Black Cohosh relieves pains associated with childbirth and menstrual cycles. Black Cohosh also neutralizes toxins in the blood-stream and helps to dispel uric acid out of the body. Black Cohosh can normalize blood pressure. It should be noted that an overdose will produce nausea and vomiting.

Time of Administration:

Because of Black Cohosh's sedative effect, I recommend taking it before bedtime.

BLACK WALNUT (Juglans Nigra):

Parts used:

Hulls and leaves

Black Walnut is rich in organic Iodine, B15 and Manganese. Black Walnut also contains Potassium, Silica, Magnesium, Calcium, Phosphorus, Iron and Protein.

Black Walnut oxygenates the blood to destroy parasites. It also contains juglone, ellagic acid, and a barium alkaloid. Ellagic acid in the Black Walnut affords an ideal protective antidote to electrical shock, accidental electrocution and lightning mishaps.

Black Walnut can be used externally also as an antiseptic and is very useful for poison oak, ringworm and skin problems. Black Walnut can be used to restore tooth enamel.

NOTE: Black Walnut should not be taken internally by lactating mothers because it can dry up the milk flow.

Time of Administration:

Morning - external; midday - internal.

BLESSED THISTLE (Cerbenia Benedicta):

Part used:

The Herb

Blessed Thistle contains B-complex, Manganese, Calcium, Iron, Phosphorus and Potassium.

Blessed Thistle is a general tonic. It improves digestion and circulation, and strengthens the heart, liver, lung and kidneys. Blessed Thistle acts as a brain food and stimulates memory, by bringing oxygen to the brain. Blessed Thistle increases Mother's milk and balances hormones. Blessed Thistle helps with cramps and headaches caused by female problems and menopause problems.

Blessed Thistle has also been used for treating internal Cancer.

Time of Administration:

Morning to evening; (afternoon - peak strength).

BLUE COHOSH (Caulophyllum Thalictroides):

Parts Used:

Root

Blue Cohosh contains Vitamins E and the B-complex and minerals Calcium, Magnesium, Phosphorus, Iron, Silicon and Potassium.

Blue Cohosh can ease childbirth and relieve pain associated with childbirth. This is done by Blue Cohosh aiding the elasticity of the neck of the uterus if given hours before delivery. Blue Cohosh is a strong anti-spasmodic.

Blue Cohosh will relieve muscle cramps and spasms, thereby relieving painful menstruation. Blue Cohosh is a blood alkaliner. Blue Cohosh can help aid epileptics.

NOTE: Blue Cohosh should not be used by pregnant women except during the last weeks of pregnancy.

Time of Administration:

Evening.

BLUE VERVAIN (Verbena Hastata):

Part used:

The Herb

Blue Vervain contains Vitamins C and E and minerals Calcium and Manganese. Blue Vervain contains an important glycoside called Verbenalin. Verbenalin works on the sensory nerves leading to the brain, and is tranquilizing to the mind so that calm and order will prevail instead of restlessness and agitation. Verbenalin induces restfulness and sleep in those suffering from insomnia.

Blue Vervain can expel worms from the intestines. Blue Vervain can induce sweating, allay fevers, and it can settle the stomach.

Blue Vervain can help alleviate asthma, bronchitis and other upper respiratory inflammation which would be aggravated by nervousness.

Time of Administration:

Preferably evening.

BRIGHAM TEA (Malvang) (Ephedra Species) (Mormon Tea, Squaw Tea):

Parts used:

The Herb (leaves)

Brigham Tea contains Vitamin B12, Cobalt, Strontium, Nickel, Copper and Ephedrine.

The Chinese Herb name for Brigham Tea is Ma Huang. Ma Huang is a "natural high". Ma Huang's most active ingredient is Ephedrine which is similar to adrenalin. Ephedrine excites the Pituitary Gland which activates all of the other glands. Ephedrine stimulates the heart and central nervous system, and has a slight local anaesthetic action on all of the body's muscle and mucous membranes so that physical ability is enhanced. I have found that my work day is easier because I have the energy to perform. But when the Ma Huang wears off there is usually a "crashing feeling". This is caused by the Potassium and Sodium depletion that occurs when the endocrine system is activated. So in conjunction with Ma Huang, I suggest ALFALFA and Spirulina be consumed as well as a few glasses of carrot and celery juice in order to replace the burned up electrolytes.

Do not use Ma Huang as an everyday herb but as a casual "up", if you wish. In the Soviet Union, Brigham Tea is used for treating Rheumatism and Syphilis. Brigham Tea is considered a bronchial dilator and decongestant. Brigham Tea increases blood pressure so it should not be used by persons who have high blood pressure.

Time of Administration:

Morning to late afternoon.

BUCHU (Barosma Betulina)

Parts used:

Leaves

Buchu is a strong antiseptic for the urinary tract, one of the best herbs for any infection of the urinary organs. Buchu neutralizes uric acid so as to reduce urine burning in the bladder. Buchu will help to dissolve kidney stones. Buchu will neutralize gas and aid digestion. Buchu leaves can help stabilize the blood sugar level at the early stages of diabetes.

Buchu leaves contain mucilage resin, calcium oxalate and a volatile oil containing diosphenol. The odor of the oil is caused by its high Sulfur content.

Diosphenol acts as a mild antiseptic, also as a cardiac and circulation stimulant. Diosphenol also stops diarrhea.

Time of Administration:

Late afternoon.

BURDOCK (Arctium Lappa):

Parts used:

Root

Burdock root contains inulin, mucilage, sugar, lappin resin, fixed and volatile oil, and some tannic acid. Burdock contains good amounts of Vitamin C (ascorbic acid) and Iron. It also contains some amounts of A, P, B-complex, E, PABA, Sulfur, Silicon, Potassium, Copper, Iodine and Zinc.

Burdock stimulates and nourishes the hypothalamus and pituitary glands to help adjust the hormone balance in the body.

Burdock is one of the best blood purifiers for chronic infection, arthritis, rheumatism, skin diseases and sciatica. Burdock can reduce swelling around joints and break down calcification deposits. It clears the kidney of excess wastes and uric acid by increasing the flow of urine. Burdock is excellent for Gout. Burdock, like most blood purifiers, will heal eczema and most skin conditions.

Time of Administration:

Morning and afternoon.

CACTUS (Cactoceae):

Parts used:

Cactus is helpful to persons who have diabetes, infection, hemorrhaging and arthritis.

Cactus is an internal cleanser. The pulp from the slashed leaf, applied as a poultice to painful Tarantula Bites will cause the immense swelling to disappear rapidly. Juice from the cactus neutralize internal poisoning and act as an efficient antidote.

The Nopal pads of the Prickly Pear also contain natural, organic insulin which will strengthen the pancreas and help overcome Diabetes.

Time of Administration:

Afternoon.

CAPSICUM OR CAYENNE (Capsicum Frutescens):

Part used:

Fruit

Capsicum is high in Vitamins A, B-complex, C, Iron and Calcium. Capsicum also has Magnesium, Phosphorus, Sulfur and Potassium.

Capsicum is a "catalyst" herb as it carries all the nutrients in the other herbs to the sites in the body where they are most needed, and increases their effectiveness.

Many folk healers claim Cayenne can help to heal stomach ulcers.

I have found the opposite to be true. When Cayenne was *continually* ingested on a daily basis, ulcers either developed or were further agitated. Some researchers have observed that the intestines can adapt themselves within a short period of time to Cayenne and form a protective coating of mucous inside. This is why some people who ingest Cayenne capsules daily often find that their stools are full of mucous. Erroneously, they think that they are actually cleaning "bad wastes" out of their bodies, when in fact they are only stimulating further secretions of mucous in order to protect their intestines and colon from the presence of Cayenne.

Capsicum will stop bleeding both internally and externally by sprinkling powdered Cayenne on bleeding cuts. The bleeding stops immediately.

Capsicum can help strengthen the heart and improve blood circulation.

Time of Administration:

Morning to afternoon (Afternoon peak chemical activity).

CASCARA SAGRADA (Rhamnus Purshiana):

Part used:

Bark

Cascara Sagrada contains B-complex, Calcium, Potassium, Manganese, traces of Tin, Lead, Strontium and Aluminum.

Cascara Sagrada is man's best "Roto-Rooter". It will normalize severe cases of constipation. Cascara Sagrada contains Chrysophanic Acid. This acid gives Cascara Sagrada its laxative properties by stimulating the muscle walls of the lower bowel into eliminative action.

Cascara Sagrada also contains emodin, which creates a tightening mood. The checkmate presence of amodin keeps control on the Chrysophanic acid's strong laxative abilities, so that extreme diarrhea will not occur.

Cascara Sagrada is not habit-forming and, through its use over a period of time, the colon will actually become normalized.

Cascara Sagrada will also help the gall bladder duct to discharge any gall stones.

Time of Administration:

At bedtime.

CATNIP (Nepata Cataria):

Part used:

Tops

Catnip is high in Vitamins A, B-complex and C. Catnip contains Magnesium, Manganese, Phosphorus, Sodium and a trace of Sulfur.

Catnip tea is wonderful for children and infants, when stomach cramps, spasms, colic, gas, or nervousness are present. Catnip tea can be used internally to alleviate the symptoms from chicken pox, small pox and mumps. Use Catnip tea as an enema to expel worms, release gas, or to treat fevers and hysterical headaches. The enema will also increase urination.

An external fomentation of Catnip can be used to place on mumps or a swollen part of the body to bring down the swelling. Catnip Tea has been used to stop diarrhea and lung congestion. Catnip is said to help to prevent miscarriage and premature births.

NOTE: Clinical Psychologists report hallucinogenic properties are less severe than marijuana attached with its use in cigarettes by young patients desiring to get "high".

Time of Administration:

Morning and evening.

CELERY (Apium Graveolens):

Parts used:

Root and Seed

Celery contains Vitamins A, B and C and has much Calcium, Potassium, Phosphorus, Sodium and Iron. Celery has lesser amounts of Sulfur, Silicon and Magnesium.

Celery's Sodium and Potassium content make it an excellent Alkaline source to neutralize the body's Acidity. Celery is useful to counter incontinence of urine, arthritis, gout, lumbago, neuralgia and dropsy. The whole plant can be used to treat kidney ailments and rheumatism.

Time of Administration:

A.M. and noon.

CHAMOMILE (Matricaria Chamomilla):

Part used:

Flower

Chamomile contains Vitamin A, Calcium, Magnesium, Potassium, Iron, Manganese and Zinc. Chamomile also contains the amino acid Tryptophan, which works like a sedative to the body and will induce sleep. Chamomile also contains chamazulene, which has recognized anti-allergenic and anti-inflammatory properties. Chamomile is one of the best herbs for soothing an upset stomach, releasing gas and colic conditions in babies and inducing sleep. Chamomile is a sedative without any harmful side effects. Chamomile can be applied externally as a fomentation to sore muscles, swelling and painful joints.

Chamomile tea can also be used as an eyewash, and a wash for open sores and eczema. Chamomile can alleviate menstrual cramps and cramps caused by drug withdrawal.

Time of Administration:

When needed, preferably morning to evening (in stormy weather); Morning (in fair weather).

CHAPARRAL (Larrea Divaricata)

Part used:

Leaves

Chaparral is high in Potassium and Sodium. Chaparral also contains Silicon, Tin, Aluminum, Sulfur, Molybdenum, Chlorine and Barium.

Chaparral is "Herb Land's" best antibiotic used both internally and externally. Chaparral can successfully treat bacterial, viral and parasitic infections. Chaparral contains an anti-tumor substance called NDGA (NORDIHYDRO- GUARARETIC ACID) which has anti-cancer properties. Chaparral has been known to treat cancer melanomas, leukemia, venereal disease and L.S.D. toxic residue successfully.

As a fomentation it can be used topically for herpes, eczema, skin diseases and arthritic pains. Chaparral has the ability to strengthen the eyes as well as dissolve Cataracts. Chaparral has also been used to heal hemorrhoids.

Chaparral's saponins seem to act as kind of a natural "detergent" in scrubbing the human body clean of toxic impurities.

Time of Administration:

Afternoon.

CHICKWEED (Stellaria Media)

Parts used:

Tops

Chickweed is rich in Vitamins A, B-complex, C and D. Chickweed contains Iron, Copper, Calcium, Sodium and a trace amount of Manganese, Phosphorus, Zinc and Molybdenum in its flowers, leaves and stalk.

Chickweed's leaves contain a resin and assorted glycosides which yield wonderfully peculiar antiseptic properties when exposed to the blood. These glycosides are antidotes to minor blood poisoning. Chickweed's mucilage qualities are helpful in healing stomach ulcers and inflamed bowels. Chickweed has been called an effective anti-cancer agent. It has been used as a poultice for burns, boils, skin problems, swollen testes and sore eyes. Chickweed is said to be an appetite depressant and therefore an aid in obesity control.

Time of Administration:

Internal - morning and late evening.
External - early morning and early evenings.

COMFREY (Symphytum Officinale)

Parts used:

Leaves and root

Comfrey contains Vitamins A and C, and minerals Calcium, Potassium, Phosphorus, Iron, Magnesium, Sulfur, Copper, and Zinc. Comfrey also contains 18 amino acids of which the amino acid Lysine is predominant. Comfrey Root contains a mucilage property that coats the intestinal lining acting like a demulcent and a lubricant. Such a coating would soothe ulcerations in the digestive tract and also would destroy any amoebic-like bacteria that might be existing, thus aiding digestion. Comfrey Root also contains Allantoin, which is a "cell proliferant agent" which stimulates healthy tissue formation. The allantoin present in the Comfrey Root helps deal with acne, scalp problems and infected or slow-healing wounds. Comfrey taken internally can help remedy cough, catarrh, ulcerated bowels, stomach and lungs. It stops dysentery and regulates blood sugar. Comfrey Tea can stop bleeding internally and externally and builds new flesh during wasting diseases.

Externally as a poultice, apply bruised leaves to burns, wounds, open sores, gangrene and moist ulcers.

NOTE: A recent scientific study indicates that Comfrey Root and leaves may be carcinogenic to the liver if frequently ingested over a long period of time. For further information read Rodale Press' *Organic Garden*, October, 1979, p. 100.

With our M.R.T. Testing system there is no danger because when the body cannot tolerate any more Comfrey, the extended arm will be unable to sustain a pull.

Doctor Norman R. Farnsworth, of Illinois School of Pharmacy and Pharmacology, University of Illinois School of Medicine, Chicago, believes that making a tea of the root and leaves solves the problem altogether.

In my own research, I suggest using Comfrey for the first week of the Program because it permits the ultilization of a multi amount of different nutrients in therapeutic amounts.

Comfrey feeds the Pituitary with its natural hormone to accelerate growth of the body's skeleton flesh. Comfrey is an over-all tonic.

Time of Administration:

(Fresh) Blossoms - morning
Leaves - afternoon
Root - evening
Dried - mid-morning to mid-afternoon

CORNSILK (Stigmata Maidis):

Part used:

Silk
Cornsilk contains Vitamin B, PABA, K, Silicon, Maizenic acid, fixed oils, resin, and mucilage.
Cornsilk has the ability to remove gravel from the kidneys, urethra, bladder, and prostate gland. Cornsilk is valuable in the treatment of renal and cystic inflammation. Cornsilk will help when the urinary tract needs opening up or when there is mucus in the urine. Cornsilk has a cleansing effect on urea and will neutralize scalding urine and solve bed-wetting problems.

Time of Administration:

Late evening.

CRAMP BARK (Viburum Opulus):

Parts used:

Bark and Berries
Cramp Bark contains C, K, Potassium, Calcium and Magnesium. Cramp Bark also contains viburnin, bitter resins, tannin, sugar and various acids which are citric, malic, oxalic and valeric. The presence of Valeric acid gives it that "Valerian-like" smell.
Cramp Bark is used as an antidote to muscular spasms of any kind, epileptic seizures, all types of nervous disorders, severe menstrual pain during periods or labor pain during birth. Cramp Bark is an excellent uterine sedative and is the best relaxant for the ovaries and uterus.

Cramp Bark Berries are used fresh or dried to normalize high blood pressure and normalize heart problems.

Externally, a decoction of Cramp Bark Flowers has been used for eczema and other skin problems.

Time of Administration:

Unknown

DAMIANA (Turnera Aphrodisiaca):

Parts used:

Leaves

Damiana contains volatile oils from which Thymol, a copaene o-cadinene and calaminene have been isolated, damianin, resins, and gum. Thymol has been used as an agent against fungus, intestinal worms, parasites, jaw and lung tumors, and athlete's foot.

Damiana is a rejuvenator of the sexual organs. Damiana will increase sperm count in males, and Damiana will also balance the hormones in women as well as strengthen their eggs. Damiana in small doses will aid in correcting nervousness, weakness and exhaustion.

Damiana has the reputation of having the ability to restore natural sexual functions of females and also males. It can help combat frigidity, hot flashes, and menopause problems in women, and prostate problems in males.

Damiana has also been used in cases of bronchitis, emphysema and Parkinson's Disease where exhaustion is a factor in the causation.

Time of Administration:

Afternoon.

DANDELION (Taraxacum Officinale):

Parts used: Leaves and Roots

Dandelion contains Vitamins A, B, C and E, Potassium, Calcium, Sodium, Phosphorus, Iron, Nickel, Cobalt, Tin, Copper, and Zinc.

Dandelion also contains taraxerol, choline, levulin, inulin, and pectin. Dandelion Root is well known for its liver-strengthening, water-removing, and detoxifying properties. The inuline content in Dandelion Root is up to 25% which makes Dandelion very helpful to the kidney and the pancreas.

Dandelion has been used where jaundice and gallstones are present.

Dandelion can be considered a survival food, because it contains all the nutritive salts that are required for the body to purify the blood.

Dandelion juice from a broken stem can be applied to warts and allowed to dry. If done four times a day for two or three days, the Dandelion juice will dry up the wart. It can also be used on corns, acne, and blisters.

In my own nutritional practice, I use Dandelion as an organic multi-mineral source, and a Vitamin A source.

The phosphorus content in Dandelion will help improve the enamel of the teeth. Dandelion will also lower blood pressure.

Time of Administration:

Morning to evening.

DEVIL'S CLAW (Harpagophytum Procumbens):

Parts used:

Devil's Claw has the ability to cleanse deep into muscles and tissue walls.

Devil's Claw is a natural cleaning agent which will clean the blood, cells, and joints of toxins, and especially remove uric acid from the systems. For these reasons, Devil's Claw is very useful to combat gout, rheumatism, arthritis, arteriosclerosis, gallstones, and liver diseases.

Time of Administration:

Morning and evening.

DONG QUAI (Anglica Sinensis):

Part used:

Root
Dong Quai contains Vitamins A, B12, and E. Dong Quai is the

"Queen" of all Female Herbs. Dong Quai can rejuvenate and normalize the female's ovaries, and strengthen the womb. Dong Quai stimulates the female hormone production so as to stop hot flashes and growth of ovarian cysts. Dong Quai has a sedative affect on the central nervous system. Dong Quai helps to rebuild the blood by purifying and cleansing. Dong Quai increases circulation and nourishes the brain cells.

Time of Administration:

Late afternoon and evenings.

ECHINACEA (Echinacea Augusti Folia):

Part used:

Root

Echinacea contains Vitamins A, C and E, and minerals Iron, Iodine, Copper, Sulfur and Potassium.

Echinacea is called the "King of the Blood Purifiers", Echinacea Root contains inulin, sucrose, betain, echinacein, myristic acid, echina coside (a caffeic acid glycoside), resins, and various fatty acids.

Betaine has antiseptic properties. Betaine and caffeic acid glycoside in echinacea root rearrange and reorganize enzyme pattern systems within the body. This removes viral formations that might be hostile to the organism. Both betaine and caffeic acid glycoside in Echinacea Root are cell manipulators and can help to heal certain forms of cancer. Inulin is a tasteless, white, semi-crystal carbohydrate sugar found in echinacea root. Inulin is rapidly absorbed into the kidneys where it cleanses and strengthens that organ as well as the spleen, pancreas and liver.

Echinacea will raise the white blood cell count in the body considerably through stimulation of the lymphatic system. This improves lymphatic filtration and drainage, and it helps remove toxins from the blood. Echinacea does wonders for raising the immunity level of the body. Echinacea contains myristic acid, which causes a catabolic effect on fatty adipose tissue and it causes a disintegration of serum cholesterol.

Echinacea has proved helpful to persons with prostate gland enlargement and weakness. Echinacea is also good for arresting carbuncles, all pus diseases, gangrene, lymph swelling, and snake and spider bites.

Externally a fomentation (tea) can help open wounds to clean out and painful swelling tissue to normalize.

Time of Administration:

Evening; also when needed.

ELECAMPANE (Inula Helenium):

Parts used:

Root
Elecampane contains Calcium, Potassium and Sodium.
Elecampane is one of the richest sources of natural insulin and can be helpful to Diabetics. Elecampane has antiseptic properties and therefore is helpful in treating rabies and worms, and is a poison antidote. Elecampane is helpful in all respiratory problems. Elecampane promotes expectoration, and is therefore useful in catarrhal conditions, especially whooping cough and bronchitis. Elecampane aids in digestion and can stop diarrhea.
Elecampane reduces tooth decay and tightens the gums.
Elecampane used externally as a wash can help cure skin diseases.

Time of Administration:

Evenings.

EVENING PRIMROSE (Oenothera Biennis):

Parts used:

Bark, Leaf oil, Flower seeds oil
Evening Primrose contains Vitamin F, Potassium and Magnesium. The oil from the seed of the flower is rich in polyunsaturated fatty acids, as much as 9% gamma-linolenic acid and 72% linoleic acid. Polyunsaturated fatty acids are essential nutrients. We have found them to be an antidote to wheat and corn allergies. Evening Primrose can be useful in many ways. There is a suggestion that it could be helpful in many Multiple Sclerosis (M.S.) cases.

Research showed that brain tissue and blood cells from some M.S. patients had reduced levels of linoleic acid.

In my own research, I have found Evening Primrose to help regenerate skin when taken orally. Evening Primrose's polyunsaturated fatty acids have been effective in lowering cholesterol levels, thereby inhibiting the formation of clots and plaque which will then lower blood pressure in those with mild to moderate hypertension. It also cleans out the liver and spleen.

Evening Primrose has been an asset in obesity control also.

Time of Administration:

Small amounts from early morning to late evening.

NOTE: If the person has a "fat allergy", do not administer evening primrose till the "fat allergy" is corrected. (See chapter on allergy and antidotes.) (Also see chapter on Sulfur, Methionine, Cystein, Taurine, Carnitine and Threonine. Please read the chapter on Vitamin F).

EYEBRIGHT (Euphrasia Officinalis):

Parts used:

The Herb

Eyebright contains Vitamins A, B-complex, C, D, and E. Eyebright also contains Sulfur, Potassium, Iron, Silicon, a trace of Iodine, Copper and Zinc.

Eyebright also contains tannic acid, euphrastic acid, mannite, glucose, volatile oil, and possibly a saponin.

Eyebright strengthens all of the eye's tissues. Eyebright provides an elasticity and resiliency to the nerves and optic mechanics which permit us to see. If there is a weakness in any of the parts, Eyebright will help normalize them. Eyebright regulates the tensile strength of all fibrous mass in the eyes, by normalizing them. Eyebright is cooling to the blood and will help the liver to detoxify. This also helps clear vision, and thought.

Externally Eyebright, when used as an eyewash with powdered Yucca Root, has helped to reverse cataract formation in the eye. When the Eyebright eyewash is applied to the eyes, the eyebright's volatile properties are activated by sunlight to saturate the conjunctiva, cornea, sclera, choroid, ciliary muscle and process, iris, suspensory ligaments, both posterior and anterior fluid chambers, lens, retina, optic nerve, and other miscellaneous tissue membranes connected in the eye.

Eyebright has antiseptic properties that fight infection such as conjunctivitis, ophthalmia and all other eye problems.

Eyebright is also helpful in measles, mumps, and chicken pox. A warm oil or tincture of Eyebright applied with a cotton swab to a tooth will help a toothache, and applied to an ear will help an earache.

Time of Administration:

Internally, mid-morning to early evening.
Externally, when there is sufficient sunlight.

FENNEL (Foeniculum Valgarg):

Parts used:

Seeds

Fennel contains Vitamin E, Potassium, Sodium, and Sulfur. Fennel seeds contain one to four percent (1-4%) volatile oil. The active constituents of the oil are a Phenolic ether, anethole, and fenchone. The Phenolic ether has antiseptic qualities, Anethole serves as an intestinal stimulant, and the Fenchone acts as an internal anesthetic. These activities take place in the bowels.

Fennel is used to settle acid stomach, colic, cramps, and for treating intestinal gas.

Fennel seed is also used as an appetite suppressant. Fennel will increase the flow of urine, menstrual blood, and mother's milk.

Fennel seed has an anticonvulsive and pain-relieving property. Fennel is recommended as a sedative for small children. Fennel has a diuretic effect because of its Potassium content.

Time of Administration:

Taken before each meal.

FENUGREEK (Trigonella Foenum-Graecum):

Parts used:

Seeds

Fenugreek contains Vitamins A, B1, B2, B3 (nicotinic acid), cholines, Vitamin D, Lecithin, Iron, Trigonelling, and Trimethylamine.

Fenugreek seeds are a strong, mucilaginous antiseptic and kill infection of any kind in the lungs.

The alkaloids Trigonelling and Choline work as Antiseptic agents.

Fenugreek can soften and dissolve hardened masses of accumulated mucus. Fenugreek expels mucus and phlegm from the bronchial tubes.

Fenugreek contains Choline and Lecithin which dissolve cholesterol and fat deposits in the blood stream, expelling toxic waste through the lymphatic system. The major antiviral activity in the Fenugreek seed is found in the 3 mgs. of nicotinic acid that each seed contains.

The Nicotinic acid is able to destroy parasites and make Fenugreek useful to treat smallpox.

Oil of Fenugreek is an ideal insect repellant.

Fenugreek seeds are sometimes used to deter bugs from going into grain storage bins.

Some authorities consider Fenugreek seeds as an aphrodisiac.

Time of Administration:

When needed.

FIGS (Ficus Carila):

Parts used:

Fruit, stem, and leaves

Figs are excellent to relieve constipation, heal boils and carbuncles, and for lung inflammation.

Externally, by using the stem and leaves, to cover and heal warts.

Some authorities claim Figs have helped lymphatic cancer.

Time of Administration:

Morning and evening (generally when cool).

FO-TI (Polygonum Multiflorum):

Part used:

Root

FO-TI is a Chinese herb that is known as an "Elixer of Life" herb. The Chinese name for the herb is Ho-Shou-Wu.

FO-TI stimulates the kidneys and acts as a diuretic. FO-TI also helps the liver to detoxify the blood. FO-TI is a tonic for the endocrine glands, and will rejuvenate them.

FO-TI increases stamina and resistance to disease.

FO-TI is very helpful in taking away the pain of a Sciatica condition, as well as knee joint pain.

FO-TI is helpful in reversing premature graying hair.

FO-TI is an excellent digestive tonic. It also is a safe aphrodisiac.

GARLIC (Allium Satiuum):

Parts used:

Bulb

Garlic contains Vitamins A, B1 and C and Selenium, Sulfur, Calcium, Manganese, Copper, Iron, Potassium, and Zinc.

Garlic contains volatile oils, which are composed of allicin and many sulfur-related compounds, plus citral, geraniol, linalool, A-phellandrene, and B phellandrene. Garlic also contains the enzymes allinase, peroxidaze, and myrosinase.

Garlic also contains approximately seventeen percent (17%) protein and lipids.

Garlic is nature's antibiotic. It is sometimes called Russian Penicillin.

Garlic can dissolve cholesterol in the blood stream and is therefore useful in lowering and normalizing blood pressure. Garlic also reduces symptoms of dizziness, angina, headaches, and backaches. Garlic, because of its sulfur content, is useful in correcting a "fat allergic" condition. Garlic has a rejuvenative affect on all body functions, and therefore is helpful in combatting cancer.

Garlic also kills parasites if taken internally.

Externally, oil of garlic can be applied to heal ringworm, skin parasites, tumors, and warts.

Garlic oil used as an enema can correct bowel infections and parasites.

Garlic as a douche (using small amounts of tincture or juice, oil or powder) can correct Yeast infections.

Garlic oil can be prepared by peeling fresh garlic (4 to 8 ounces), mincing it, and putting it into a wide mouth jar. Pour cold-pressed Olive Oil over it until all the garlic is covered. Close tightly and allow it to set for three to seven days. Shake it daily. Strain. Put it in a dark bottle and store in a cool place.

In the event that Garlic Oil is needed immediately, purchase garlic oil pearls (caps). Break open and mix the garlic contents with Olive Oil.

For earaches put two or three drops twice daily in the ear that aches.

Garlic's sulfur can detoxify the blood of toxic metals such as lead, mercury and cadmium.

Time of Administration:

Late evening til early morning.

GENTIAN (Gentiana Lu Tea):

Parts used:

Root

Gentian contains B-complex, Inositol, Niacin, F, Manganese, Silicon, Sulfur, Tin, Lead, and Zinc.

Gentian Root is rich in natural plant sugars, including sucrose. These sugars help the breakdown and proper assimilation of food into the system. Gentian's chief action is upon the liver and stomach. Gentian improves appetite, increases digestion, and increases circulation. Gentian Root is used to strengthen female organs and to combat gout.

Gentian promotes the secretion of bile from the Gallbladder and exhibits strong anti-inflammatory properties in case of Rheumatoid Arthritis.

Gentian has been known to reduce cancerous tumors.

Gentian stimulates the glands to produce more hormones for the body.

For all cases of debility caused by great illness, Gentian can be used.

Time of Administration:

Anytime.

GINGER (Zingibar Officinale):

Parts used:

Root

Ginger Root contains Vitamins A, B-complex and C and minerals Calcium, Phosphorus, Iron, Sodium, Potassium and Magnesium.

Ginger contains protein and an oil called Ginerol. This oil is an oleo-resin which "binds" or "holds together" the other herbs administered and delivers them as a unit to the colon. Because of this, Ginger Root acts as a transporter of the other herbs to organs they are designed to heal. If Ginger Root is grouped with Hawthorne Berries (a cardiac herb), then Hawthorne Berries will definitely reach the heart.

Ginger Root will stop nausea, morning sickness and motion sickness, e.g., car or air.

Ginger Root aids in digestion, and alleviates stomach and colon spasms and constipation.

Ginger Root is an excellent herb to help fight off the symptoms of colds and flu, because of its detoxification personality.

Ginger Root sometimes relieves headaches, and aches and pains caused by poisons. Ginger Root is a helpful herb for the respiratory system. Ginger Root will raise the body temperature when taken in frequent doses.

Ginger is very good to stop intestinal gas. Ginger Root lowers serum cholesterol levels. Ginger Root can kill vaginal trichomonads, (parasitic protozoan) that inhabit the vagina and urethra of women, if used as a douche. Ginger Root contains the amino acid Tryptophane, which gives it the ability to be tranquilizing to the central nervous system. Ginger Root also contains Lecithin.

Time of Administration:

When needed.

GINSENG (Korean: Panax Schin-Seng, Siberian: Eleutherococcus, Wild American: Panax Quinque Folium)

Parts used:

Root

Ginseng is considered king of all the Herbs.

There are 3 different species of Ginseng on the Herbal Market. They are American (Panax Quinque Folium—considered the same as the Chinese species), Siberian (Eleutherococcus), and Korean (Panax Shin-Seng).

I have found in my research that the American variety is the most potent, the Siberian less in potency, and the Korean the weakest. Ironically, the Korean is the most popular because it is the cheapest on the wholesale market and is being sold at the retail level at almost the same price of the other varieties to the uninformed consumers. The higher profit margin permits the distributor of the Korean variety some extra funds for promotion!

Ginseng contains B1 (Thiamin), B2 (Riboflavin). Biotin, B3 (Niacin), and B5 (Pantothenic Acid), Vitamin A, E, Rutin (Vitamin P-Bioflavonoid) and also the minerals Calcium, Iron, Phosphorus, Sodium, Silicon, Potassium, Manganese, Magnesium, Sulfur, Tin and Germanium. Germanium oxide is a mineral salt which stimulates the formation of red blood cells on account of its influence upon the bone marrow. Germanium enables the blood's malignant cells to attract oxygen and so normalize themselves and thus be effective in curing cancers.

The Korean variety Ginseng does have the greatest amount of Germanium because of the great amount of Germanium in Korean soil.

Ginseng contains an anti-diabetic substance which lowers blood sugar. Ginseng contains panaxin which stimulates the brain, improves muscle tone, and acts as a tonic for the cardiovascular system.

These vitamin and mineral substances and panquilon (a glycoside) activate the endocrine system to increase the hormonal level in the blood, so that rejuvenation can occur.

Ginseng is a tonic which stimulates the body's resistance to adverse influences, stress, and mental and physical fatigue. Ginseng can reduce blood cholesterol and prevent Arteriosclerosis.

Ginseng, because of its endocrine system revitalization, is said to be an anti-aging herb. In the Orient it is considered a cure-all herb. It is a neutralizer of drugs, toxic chemicals, and radiation. Some say it improves vision, hearing, and work performance. Ginseng can give one more poise and composure by checking irritability.

Ginseng does promote the appetite and increases one's sex drive.

Ginseng is also said to remove age spots and alleviate depression as well as stop hemorrhaging.

Time of Administration:

In morning and mid-day.

GOLDEN SEAL (Hydrasic Canadensis):

Parts used:

Rhizume and Roots.

Golden Seal contains Vitamins A, B-complex, C, E and F. Golden Seal also contains minerals Calcium, Copper, Potassium, Phosphorus, Manganese, Iron, Zinc and Sodium.

Golden Seal Root has anti-viral, antibiotic properties which have been useful in fighting infections from conjunctivitis to gangrene, and even to cancer.

The alkaloid derivative, Hydrastine, is what gives Golden Seal Root its ability.

Golden Seal can be used externally as well as internally to stop infection and kill poisons.

As a fomentation, Golden Seal can be used externally on open sores, inflammations, eczema, ringworm, or other itchy skin afflictions.

Internally, Golden Seal is recommended for all problems of the mucous membranes. As a douche, Golden Seal is excellent for vaginal infection. As an eyewash, Golden Seal can safely be used. Golden Seal is an excellent antiseptic mouthwash for pyorrhea, and a gargle for tonsillitis.

Golden Seal has the ability to lower blood sugar and should be used by diabetics but not by hypoglycemics. Golden Seal has the ability to soften the bowel stools, enabling relief from constipation. As a retention enema, it will reduce swollen hemorrhoids. Golden Seal has the ability, upon entering the bloodstream, to regulate liver functions, thereby being the best general medicinal herb in the Herbal Kingdom.

GOTU KOLA (Hydrocotyle Asiatica):

Parts used:

Herbs
GOTU KOLA contains Vitamins A, B, E, G and K. Gotu Kola is rich in Magnesium.

Gotu Kola does NOT contain any caffeine!! The other Kola Nut contains caffeine. Gotu Kola does contain Vallerine, an oil which is a pale yellowish color with a pungent and persistant taste and a marked odor. Gotu Kola's Vallerine has been effective in treating eye lesions and cataracts before the posterior chamber becomes involved.

Gotu Kola is also called "food for the brain", because it increases mental and physical power. Gotu Kola has an energizing effect on the cells of the brain. Gotu Kola neutralizes blood acids and will lower body temperature as well as lower blood pressure.

Gotu Kola has rejuvenating properties and will regenerate the brain to prevent senility, depression, and mental fatigue. Gotu Kola is used in the treatment of Leprosy.

We have found that it also strengthens the Pituitary Gland to hold on to the body's needed electrolytes Potassium and Sodium.

Time of Administration:

Morning, noon, supper, and bedtime.

HOPS (Humulus Lupulus):

Part used:

Flower.

Hops is rich in the Vitamin B-complex. Hops also contains Magnesium, Zinc, Copper, traces of Iodine, Manganese, Iron, Sodium, Lead, Fluorine and Chlorine. Hops contains Lupulin, which constitutes ⅐ of Hops' major ingredients. Lupulin is a sedative and will induce sleep where insomnia is present.

Hops is the Herb Kingdom's best nervine for it is strong but safe. Hops increases the flow of bile and relaxes the liver and gall duct.

Hops is good for a nervous stomach, poor appetite, gas, and intestinal cramps. Hops taken before meals will increase digestion. Hops will reduce sexual desire and provoke urination.

Hops also will help the bowels move. Hops used externally as a poultice or fomentation will be effective in treating boils, tumors, painful swelling, and skin inflammations. Some authors say Hops placed inside a pillow case will induce sleep.

Time of Administration:

Evenings.

HOREHOUND (Marrubium Vulgare):

Horehound contains Vitamins A, B-complex, C, E and F. Horehound also contains the minerals Iron, Potassium, and Sulfur. Horehound contains a substance called Marrubiin (*Merck Index*, p. 645.) which gives Horehound its expectorant properties. Horehound has been used in "cough drops" to loosen phlegm, bronchial catarrh, and will relieve sore throats and pulmonary problems.

Horehound will act as a tonic to the respiratory organs and to the stomach, but in large doses Horehound will act as a laxative.

Externally the dried Horehound applied topically has been used for Herpes Simplex, eczema and shingles.

Time of Administration:

Morning.

HORSERADISH (Ammor Acia Lapathi Folia):

Part used:

Root.

Horseradish contains rich amounts of Vitamins B1 and C and minerals Sulfur and Potassium. Horseradish also contains Vitamins A, B-complex, P, and minerals Calcium, Phosphorus, Iron and Sodium. Horseradish contains a lot of ascorbic acid (Vitamin C) and Sinigrin.

Horseradish will promote stomach secretion to stimulate digestion. Horseradish will also clear up sinus congestion and clear the nasal passage of infection. Horseradish will activate the kidneys to promote urination. Horseradish is sometimes helpful in expelling worms from the body. Horseradish does have antibiotic action.

NOTE: Horseradish left in contact with the skin can cause blistering. Avoid contact with the eyes.

Time of Administration:

Morning to late afternoon.

HORSETAIL or SHAVEGRASS (Equise Tum Arvense):

Part used:

The Herb.

Horsetail is rich in Silicon, Selenium, and Calcium. It also contains Vitamin E, Pantothenic acid, PABA, Copper, Manganese and Sodium; and some Cobalt, Iron and Iodine.

Horsetail is high in Silica, so herbalists use it for skin, hair, and eye conditions. Horsetail is used to alleviate glandular swelling and pus discharges. Horsetail aids circulation and blood coagulation and is helpful in decreasing bleeding and menstruation. Fractured bones will heal much faster when Horsetail with Comfrey is taken.

Horsetail strengthens the heart and lungs and will remove gravel from the bladder and kidneys.

Horsetail applied externally will stop bleeding of wounds and heal them.

Time of Administration:

Morning and evening.

NOTE: Horsetail can be irritating to the kidneys when used for
prolonged periods, e.g., daily for more than one month. It
works best in small frequent doses.

HAWTHORN (Crataegus Oxycantha):

Part used:

Fruit (berries).

Hawthorn Berries contain the Vitamin B-complex and Vitamin C.

Hawthorn also contains Potassium and Sodium in a 1:1 ratio; it also
contains Silicon, Phosphorus, Iron, Zinc, Sulfur, Nickel, Tin, and
Beryllium. Hawthorn Berries have an abundance of Choline which is
the basic constituent of Lecithin which helps control cholesterol by
breaking up fat into tiny particles which can then pass very easily into
the tissues of the body.

Hawthorn Berries prevent hardening of the arteries and is excellent
for feeble heart action, vascular insufficiency, and irregular pulse.
Hawthorn Berries are a cardiac tonic with antispasmodic properties and
are valuable in angina pectoris.

Hawthorn Berries will normalize blood pressure, inflammation of the
heart muscle and arteriosclerosis. Hawthorn has the ability to neutralize
acid conditions of the blood. Hawthorn can also be used for
nervousness and in preventing miscarriage.

Time of Administration:

Morning, noon, supper.

HYDRANGEA (Hydrangea Arborescens):

Parts used:

Leaves and root

Hydrangea contains Calcium, Potassium, Sodium, Sulfur,
Phosphorus, Iron, and Magnesium.

Hydrangea is an aquatic plant of the swamps and marshes.

Hydrangea is similar to Yucca and Chaparral in its action on arthritis, gout, and rheumatism.

Hydrangea possesses alkaloids within its complex root system that behave similarly to cortisone and clean with the same kind of "detergent" power that Chaparral does.

Hydrangea prevents gravel from forming in the kidney. Hydrangea helps alleviate pain when gravel passes through the ureters from the kidney to the bladder.

Hydrangea is also useful for bladder infections, gallstones, gout, kidney stones, gonorrhea, and backaches.

Time of Administration:

Throughout the day.

IRISH MOSS OR CARRAGEEN (Chondrus Crispus):

Parts used:

The whole plant.

Irish Moss contains Vitamins A, D, E, F, and K. Irish Moss contains Iodine, Calcium and Sodium in high amounts. Irish Moss also contains some Phosphorus, Potassium and Sulfur. Irish Moss contains 15 different elements needed by the human body. Irish Moss is high in mucilage which makes it soothing to inflamed tissue, especially of the lungs, intestines, and kidney.

Externally, Irish Moss can be used as a fomentation to be used on dry and burning skin diseases. It will also soften the skin and prevent wrinkles.

The Iodine obtained from Irish Moss is converted to Iodide in the gastrointestinal tract. Its absorption is rapid and complete. Once Iodide enters the blood, it is distributed throughout the body fluids. The thyroid gland uses the Iodide to manufacture the thyroid hormones, giving the body's glandular system an energizing effect.

Irish Moss could be used to reduce and heal a goiter condition.

Time of Administration:

Morning and noon.

JOJOBA (Simmondsia Chinensis):

Part used:

Oil.

Jojoba contains B-complex, Vitamin E, Silicon, Chromium, Copper and Zinc, and is very high in Iodine (81.7% of the total contents.).

The iodine content helps Jojoba to heal acne, athlete's foot, cuts, mouth sores, pimples, and warts. The Jojoba Oil, which also contains Vitamin E removes the sebum which tend to collect around hair follicles, causing dandruff, hair loss, and dry scalp.

Jojoba is used in some hair shampoos and hair conditioners because it is believed that Jojoba will promote hair growth and relieve scalp problems.

Time of Administration:

Anytime.

JUNIPER (Juniperis Species):

Parts used:

Berries.

Juniper Berries are high in Vitamin C, Sulfur, and Copper, and have a high content of Cobalt and a trace of Tin.

Juniper Berries contain a volatile oil which gives the characteristic flavor. Oil of Juniper has certain terpenes (turpentine-like compounds) which give it an antiseptic quality. Juniper Berries afford a natural immunity in the system against contagious diseases.

Juniper Berries activate the kidneys to throw out uric acid. Juniper Berries will help to heal Diabetes, Gonorrhea, Insect Bites (Poisonous), Snake Bites, Tuberculosis, Typhoid Fever, and Catarrhal inflammation.

Juniper Berries will stop water retention.

Juniper Berries will help restore the function of the Pancreas which malfunctions and will cause Diabetes.

Time of Administration:

Throughout the day.

KELP (Fucus Visiculosis):

Part used:

Whole plant.

Kelp is one of the most nutritional herbs as it contains Vitamins A, B-complex, C, E, and K. Kelp contains over 30 minerals, being richest in Iodine, Calcium, Sulfur and Silicon. Kelp also contains Phosphorus, Iron, Sodium, Potassium, Magnesium, Chlorine, Copper, Zinc, and Manganese. Kelp contains trace amounts of Barrium, Boron, Chromium, Lithium, Nickel, Silver, Titanium, Vanadium, Aluminum, Strontium, Bismuth, Chlorine, Cobalt, Gallium, Tin, and Zirconium.

The vast assortment of trace elements, vitamins and minerals in this nutritional seaweed presents an all-around balance of those nutrients the body requires. The Iodine helps to rejuvenate the endocrine system, specifically the Pineal, Pituitary, Thyroid, Hypothalamus, and Lymph glands.

Kelp contains alginic acid which absorbs toxins in the system so that they can be more easily eliminated later on. Kelp has a protective reaction against radiation and heavy metals toxicity.

When Kelp stimulates the thyroid, it will normalize the metabolism of the body.

In Kelp there is a factor called Sodium Alginate which binds with radioactive Strontium-90 in the intestines and carries it out of the body.

Time of Administration:

In the morning and at noon.

LADY'S SLIPPER (Cypripedium Pubescens):

Parts used:

Root.

Lady's Slipper contains B-complex. Lady's Slipper contains volatile oil in fresh (non-dried) plants which can cause severe dermatitis, on contact with the skin, much like Poison Ivy, Oak, or Sumac. Certain compounds within the herb itself act quite profoundly on the central nervous system. Lady's Slipper has a calming affect on body and mind.

Lady's Slipper can alleviate pain, hysteria, neuralgia, tremors, and shakes.

Lady's Slipper acts primarily on the medulla, helping to regulate breathing, sweating, saliva, and heart functions. If Lady's Slipper is taken in large enough quantities, it can induce hallucinations similar to those caused by Marijuana.

Lady's Slipper acts as a tonic to rebuild the exhausted Nervous system.

Time of Administration:

Throughout the day.

LICORICE (Glycyrrhiza Glabra):

Parts used:

Root.

Licorice contains Vitamin B-complex, Pantothenic acid, Niacin, Biotin, Vitamin E, Phosphorus, Lecithin, Manganese, Iodine, Chromium, and Zinc.

Licorice Root also contains Glycoside Glycyrrhizin also known as Glycyrrhizinic Acid or Glycyrrhizic.

Glycyrrhizinic Acid deals with all kinds of ulcers by stimulating the adrenal and lymph glands and aids in the production of white blood cells, thereby raising the body's immune levels. The anti-septic constituents of Thujone (found also in Western Red Cedar) and Fenchone (present in Fennel and Lavender) inhibit the growth of harmful viruses that might be present in one's system. Licorice Root has activity similar to those of Cortisone and Estrogen.

Licorice Root is a mild laxative. Licorice Root has been used medically to treat Rheumatoid Arthritis, Addison's Disease, and Hypoglycemia.

Licorice Root has a high content of sugar which means that Diabetics should use it cautiously only since it could also raise the blood sugar. That is why it is excellent for hypoglycemics. Licorice Root also tends to stimulate the endocrine system to the effect that Potassium and Sodium, the body's electrolytes, are consumed at a faster rate leading to a depletion. So test Potassium and Sodium levels daily when using Licorice Root, to avoid a depletion. Tell-tale signs are swollen ankles, pain in the heart area and an increase in blood pressure.

Time of Adminstration:

Evening.

LOBELIA (Lobelia Inflata):

Parts used:

The herb and seeds.

Lobelia contains Sulfur, Iron, Cobalt, Selenium, Sodium, Copper, and Lead.

Lobelia contains Alkaloids, the most important of which is Lobeline. Lobeline has been used in places like Sweden as an oral deterrent to smoking, and internally as a respiratory stimulant for the lungs.

Taken orally, Lobelia is both a relaxant and a stimulant. Small doses of Lobelia will act as a tonic and a stimulant. Large doses of Lobelia will act as a sedative.

Externally, Lobelia is used to wash infected or itchy skin diseases.

Too much Lobelia can cause nausea, vomiting, and *convulsions*.

Time of Administration:

Throughout the day.

MANDRAKE (American) (Podophyllum Peltatum)

Part used:

Root

Mandrake effects the liver, gall bladder, intestines, skin, and all the glands.

Mandrake is one of the antidotes of mercurial poisoning. Mandrake has an anti-tumor effect in destroying many different kinds of cancer cells in the body. It is presently being used in Cancer Chemotherapy in some hospitals. But it does possess some side effects like nausea, vomiting, diarrhea, and fever when over used. Mandrake has been successful in clearing up human Condyloma Acuminata. This is a condition of soft warts (venereal warts) which usually accumulate near the Rectum and Genital Organs of men and women alike.

Mandrake is also known to destroy intestinal worms as well as being a rejuvenator for sterile women.

Time of Administration:

Evenings.

MARIJUANA (Cannabis Sativa)

I personally feel Marijuana should not be legalized because of its side effects!! Every user of Marijuana whom I have tested, showed two distinctive problems. They are:

1.) The displacement from the brain of L-Glutamine (a protein which is food for the thinking brain). This causes a confusion in the thinking ability of the Marijuana User, causing illogical decisions. This can be checked by placing the pointer finger of the person to be tested on the left side of the head about 1½" above the ear and then extending the other arm to be pumped. It will always test weak!! Now place the predetermined amount of L-Glutamine in the test palm and place it on the left side of the head 1½" above the ear. Now pump the extended arm, it should test strong!!

After, place the L-Glutamine which just tested strong, and a couple of (2) joints of Marijuana together in the same palm, place both again on the thinking brain point (1½" above the ear) and pump the other arm which is extended. It will *always* go down!! (Testing Weak) Marijuana does weaken the thinking brain!! And if not controlled, because it is ADDICTIVE, can eventually destroy a person's ability to make decisions, accept responsibility, and can endorse bizzare illogical behavior.

2.) Marijuana also weakens the adrenal glands. Every Marijuana user had weak adrenals causing them to behave explosively. They were unable to cope with every day problems, which appeared to them to be growing more complex daily. The years I've spent as a professional musician enabled me to observe my fellow performers, who, by smoking "POT", etc., thought they sounded better than ever because of the use of the Marijuana. In reality they sounded 10 times worse but they didn't realize it!! Their performance was not enhanced but they really thought it was, because of the euphoric effect marijuana had on their minds. As far as I'm concerned Marijuana should not be used for any MEDICINAL purposes and therefore should not be legalized.

MARIGOLD (Calendola Officinalis)

Part used:

The Herb (Flower)
Marigold is High in Phosphorus, and Vitamins A and C.
Marigold has the marvelous ability to cause cells to heal. Marigold as a salve or fomentation can heal sores, burns, and wounds. A strong tea used as a sitz bath can heal bleeding hemorrhoids. A salve used as a suppository in the rectum also can help to heal hemorrhoids.

The Marigold Tea can also be used as a vaginal douche and the Marigold salve as a vaginal suppository to heal infections, ulcers, pruritus, and bleeding. Marigold can be used as a "SNUFF" to discharge mucus from the nose. Also, the nose can be irrigated with Marigold tea as a nasal wash for sinus problems.

Marigold oil can be placed in the ear and left overnight to help alleviate earaches.

Marigold Tea taken as a warm infusion can normalize body temperature, help heal ulcers, and help stop cramps. Marigold is excellent as a healing salve on burns or wounds.

Time of Administration:

When Needed

MARSHMALLOW

Parts Used:

Root, Flowers and Leaves
Marshmallow contains about 18,000 IU per ounce of Vitamin A. Marshmallow is high in Calcium, Zinc, Iron, Sodium, Iodine, B-Complex, and Pantothenic Acid.

Marshmallow is high in mucilage which helps aid the expectoration of phlegm and helps relax the bronchial tubes while soothing and healing. Marshmallow is good for all lung ailments. It can be very useful for asthma because it helps to remove mucus from the lung.

Marshmallow is also helpful in Emphysema, Diabetes, Whooping Cough and Breast Problem.

Marshmallow used as a poultice externally is excellent to treat gangrene, burns, wounds, bruising, or blood poisoning.

Marshmallow encourages the body to manufacture the necessary material for new tissue production.

Marshmallow Tea is excellent as a douche for vaginal infections as well as for use as an eyewash.

Marshmallow can be used with other Herbs to release stones and gravel from the kidney. Marshmallow can combat dysentery and diarrhea.

The leaves of Marshmallow have been used as a poultice for Bee Stings.

Marshmallow Root triggers muscle reflexes in the mammary gland which produce milk, increasing the flow of milk of lactating mothers.

Marshmallow is also used internally to treat inflammation and Mucosal affliction of the genito-urinary tract, including cystitis, incontinence, painful urination, gonorrhea, enteritis and cholera.

Time of Administration:

Throughout the Day

MISTLETOE (Viscum Flavescens)

Part Used:

The Tops

Mistletoe contains B-12, Calcium, Sodium, Magnesium, Potassium, Iron, Cobalt, Iodine, Copper, and Cadmium.

Mistletoe is a Vasoconstrictor and should not be used by people that have hypertension.

Mistletoe is a natural tranquilizer and is good to arrest dizziness, vertigo, and headaches.

Mistletoe effects the uterus. It will increase uterine contraction and lessens bleeding. Mistletoe can be used early in labor to give tone to contractions and make the contractions much more regular as opposed to spasmodic contractions.

It should be noted that Mistletoe can be toxic and should be used cautiously.

Time of Administration:

Anytime, Taken as needed

MULLEIN (Verbascum Tapsus)

Part Used:

Leaf

Mullein contains Vitamins A, D and B-Complex. Mullein is also high in Iron, Magnesium, Potassium, and Sulfur.

Mullein loosens mucus and expels it out of the body. Mullein is used for all lung problems because it nourishes as well as strengthens the lungs. The oil of Mullein is considered one of the best remedies for an ear infection. Place two or three drops of warm oil in the ear overnight and/or two to three times daily.

Mullein contains a glycoside called Verabascose which has a healing effect, when applied externally to skin conditions, open wounds, and sores. The strong antiseptic properties of the Verbascose explains the use of Mullein in the treatment of tuberculosis in India. The Mullein flower and leaves contain Saponins which act as strong disinfectants to the lungs when smoked. Smoking Mullein Leaves is recommended for asthmatics and those who have bronchitis. A syrup made of the leaves and/or seeds of Mullein is great to stop chronic coughing (i.e. smoker's cough, whooping cough, consumption).

Mullein leaves can be used to dress open wounds and sores, and to alleviate leprosy, shingles, hives, and hemorrhoids. If a poultice of fresh Mullein Leaves is placed on swollen lymph glands, the glands will reduce to normal. A poultice of Mullein Leaves has been used to remove warts.

Mullein is a pain killer and helps induce sleep. Mullein Tea is useful in treating dropsy, sinusitis, swollen joints, and to sooth inflamed kidneys.

Time of Administration:

Afternoon to Evening

MUSTARD (Sinapis Olba)

Part Used:

Seeds

Mustard contains Calcium, Phosphorus, Potassium, Sulfur, Iron, Cobalt, and Traces of Manganese and Iodine. Mustard also contains Vitamins A, B-1, B-2, B-12, and C.

Mustard Seeds help digestion because the Sulfur content counteracts a "Fat Allergy" or "Fat Sensitivity". This is why Mustard is used on "Hot Dogs."

An infusion of Mustard Seed Tea will stimulate urination and possibly bring on a woman's menstrual period if it is late.

Mustard Seed Tea can be used as an emetic (vomit inducing) for narcotic poisoning.

Externally Mustard Seed can be used as a warm plaster or poultice to help treat Muscular Problems. Mustard Seed plaster will detoxify the area so as to loosen up the muscles which are sore.

Time of Administration:

Anytime - when Needed

MYRRH (Balsamodendron Myrrha)

Part Used:

Resin

Myrrh is a Bacteriostatic inhibitor which stops the production of staph and E. Coli Viruses.

Myrrh is useful as a vaginal douche for it helps treat uterus and vaginal infections.

Myrrh taken orally is a healing agent to the stomach and colon.

Myrrh has been used to treat chronic bronchitis and heavy mucus accumulations in the lungs. Myrrh is considered a useful dental aid. Powdered Myrrh has been used to strengthen gums and whiten teeth. Gingivitis, bleeding gums, loose teeth, gum inflamation, and plaque build up have all been treated sucessfully with Myrrh.

Myrrh mixed with Red Raspberry leaves makes an excellent mouthwash and gargle for relief of sore throats.

Myrrh has the antiseptic property to alleviate skin rash through topical applications. Myrrh taken internally can also clean out the colon and heal Hemorrhoids.

Time of Administration:

Late Evening to Early Morning

NETTLE (Urtica Dioica)

Part Used:

Leaves

Nettles contain Iron, Silican, Calcium, Sulfur, Sodium, Copper, Manganese, Chromium, and Zinc. Nettles also contain the Vitamins A, C, D, E, F and P. Nettles are also rich in Chlorophyll.

Nettle leaves used externally as a poultice draw uric acid out of the body offering relief from Rheumatic pains.

Fresh Nettle juice, taken one teaspoon every hour, can stop intestinal bleeding. Nettle Tea will expel phlegm from the lungs and can also be used to stop diarrhea and dysentery. A poultice of Nettles and Slippery Elm will arrest bleeding when applied to the skin and is therefore helpful in healing piles and hemorrhoids.

Nettle Tea if used as a hair rinse will help restore the hair to its NATURAL color. Nettles will also lower blood pressure. Nettles is useful in relieving hayfever.

Time of Administration:

Morning and Evening

OAT STRAW (Avena Sativa)

Part Used:

Stem

Oat Straw is rich in Silicon, Calcium, Manganese, and Phosphorus. Oat Straw is also high Vitamins A, B-1, B-2 and E.

Oat Straw applied externally as a hot compress on a kidney area during a kidney stone attack, has brought relief.

Adding one gallon of Oat Straw Tea to a warm bath, can bring relief for gout, rheumatic problems, lumbago, sore kidneys, and itchy skin.

Oat Straw Tea can be used internally to alleviate kidney and chest ailments. Bedwetting by children can be curtailed by drinking Oat Straw Tea.

A Tincture made from the fresh flowering plant can be used to treat arthritis, rheumatism, paralysis, liver infection and skin diseases.

Time of Administration:

When Needed

PAPAYA (Carica Papaya)

Parts Used:

Fruit and Leaves

Papaya contains Vitamins A, B, D, E, G, K, and C. Papaya also contains the minerals Calcium, Iron, Phosphorus, Potassium, Sodium, and Magnesium.

Papaya fruit has as its chief constituent a natural digestive enzyme, Papain, as well as Carpain and Carposide (a glucoside).

Papain is capable of enzymatic action in either acid, neutral or alkaline states. The protein digesting enzyme of the Papaya, Papain enables Papaya juice to dissolve corns, warts, and pimples. Papain can digest dead tissue without affecting the surrounding live tissue. Medicinally, Doctors have used it to prevent adhesions from occuring and in treating infected wounds. Papaya has been called a "Biologicalpel". In Africa, natives place strips of the Papaya fruit over open infected sores and wounds with excellent results.

Papaya has been used internally to heal ulcers and other internal bleeding.

Carpain is used as a depressant for the central nervous system.

Papaya is used by the food industry as a meat tenderizer.

The digestive enzyme, Papain, administered internally is also a powerful abortive agent and can induce abortion in a developing fetus as well as change the cellular structure of the surrounding placenta.

Papaya seed is administered with honey to expel worms. Papaya seed paste can be applied to skin diseases like ringworm with good results.

Papaya will normalize the colon and stop constipation or chronic diarrhea. Papaya fruit is best taken after the meal to aid digestion.

Time of Administration:

Morning to Evening

PARSLEY (Petroselinum Sativum)

Part Used:

Leaves

Parsley contains the Vitamins A, B-1, B-2, B-3, and C, Folic Acid, and the minerals Iron, Potassium, Sodium, Copper, Silicon, Sulfur, Calcium, and Cobalt.

Parsley can be used to treat kidney inflammation and bladder infections because the Parsley increases bladder release activity.

Parsley herb (leaf) oil contains as much as 85% Myristicin which corrects infection and inflammation in the prostate.

Parsley is an excellent tonic for the urinary system.

Parsley also contains Volatile Oil Apiol which effects the body three ways: (a) it lowers blood pressure, (b) relaxes uterine tissue, and (c) stimulates the lymphatic glands. Because of this, menstruation is normalized in some women. Parsley should not be used during pregnancy, it could bring on labor pains.

Fresh Parsley juice has helped in conjunctivitis and blepharitis (inflammation of the eyelid).

Parsley has been used as a cancer preventative, because it is said to contain a substance in which cancerous cells cannot multiply.

Parsley can be used to dry up mother's milk after birth.

Time of Administration:

Morning to Early Evening

PASSION FLOWER (Passiflora Incarnata)

Part Used:

The Herb

Passion Flower contains an indole alkaloid called Harman. Passion Flower also contains flavonoids like Apiqenin, Saponaretin and Saponarin which all have a tranquilizing effect on the sympathetic nervous system. Passion Flower has been used as a sedative in treating neuralgia, insomnia, restlessness, headache, hysteria, twitching, epilepsy, and convulsions especially in young children.

In older people, it can help to alleviate sciatica and nerve debility.

Passion Flower can lower blood pressure, slow the pulse rate and stimulate respiration. Passion Flower can be used for inflamed eyes and dimness of vision.

Time of Administration:

When Needed, Probably Late Evening

PENNYROYAL (Hedeoma Pulegioides)

Parts Used:

Flowers and tops

The dried flowers and tops of the Pennyroyal plant contain the volatile oil Ketone Pulegone. The pulegone is a yellow or greenish-yellow oil and yields a strong aromatic odor and taste. When applied externally, the Pennyroyal oil will provide great relief from mosquito, chigger, gnats, and other insect bites.

Pennyroyal taken orally will have an opening effect on the pores of the skin, cause sweating and a release of toxic poisons. The reaction to the ingestion of Pennyroyal will cause the stomach to remove gas. It will also stimulate menstruation in females.

Pennyroyal can be used as a tea and a foot bath to induce abortions. Pregnant women should not use Pennyroyal for the first three months of a pregnancy if they do not wish to abort.

Pennyroyal Tea can be used for an external wash for skin eruptions, rashes, and itching. Pennyroyal can be of help in treating leprosy.

Pennyroyal's oil, Pulegone, also works on the central nervous system and produces a mild, tranquil effect.

Time of Administration:

Anytime

PEPPERMINT (Mentha Piperita)

Part Used:

Leaves

Peppermint contains Vitamins A, C, and E. Peppermint also contains the minerals Magnesium, Potassium, Inositol, Niacin, Choline, Copper, Iodine, Silicon, Iron, and Sulfur.

Peppermint Leaves contain a volatile oil that is composed of Menthol, Menthone, Menthyl Aletate, Menthofuran, and Limonene. Other constituents in the oil include Viridfioral (an antibiotic), Pulegone (also in oil of Pennyroyal), Piperitone, Bicycloelemene (another antibiotic), Tocopherols that are part of the Vitamin E complex, Carotenoids (Provitamin A), Betaine, Azulenes, Rosmarinic Acid, and Tannin.

Peppermint is excellent for cleaning and strengthening the entire system, including the nerves. Peppermint's menthol in the oil of the leaves has an exhilarating effect on the brain by sending oxygen into the blood stream.

Peppermint oil (5 to 10 drops poured into 2 quarts of hot water) breathed in through the mouth and nostrils will open the sinuses. To do this, boil the water, add the oil, turn off the stove, place a towel over your head and lean over the pot. Try to keep the steam from leaking out under the towel. This also is good for a facial steam bath.

Peppermint enemas are excellent for colon problems.

The natural-occuring Tannin in peppermint suppressed the activity of influenza virus, Type A.

Peppermint aids in digestion by stimulating the salivary glands. Peppermint can be used to alleviate colic, constipation, stomach cramps, gas, heartburn, morning sickness, sea sickness, and vomiting.

Peppermint can be used as a refreshing mouthwash also.

Time of Administration:

Morning and Evening

PERIWINKLE (Vinca Major/Vinca Minor)

Parts Used:

Herb, Leaves

Periwinkle has two alkaloids, vinblastine and vincristine, which act as a liquid "sponge" causing the blood to absorb oxygen, thereby nourishing the brain.

Periwinkle has been used to treat Leukemia in children. Verblastine sulphate, which is in Periwinkle, has shown promising results for choriocarcinoma and Hodgkin's disease. Periwinkle use is being researched in lung cancer.

Periwinkle will stop internal hemorrhaging, bloody noses and bleeding piles.

Periwinkle Tea, if used as a hair rinse will remove dandruff. If used as a body wash it will heal skin sores and other skin diseases.

Periwinkle taken internally will reduce nervousness, nightmares, hysteria, and fits.

Periwinkle also counteracts chronic constipation.

Time of Administration:

When Needed

PLANTAIN (Plantago Major)

Parts Used:

Leaves and Seeds

Plantain is rich in Vitamins C, K, and T. Plantain is rich in minerals Calcium, Potassium, Sulfur, and Trace Minerals.

Plantain contains a glucoside, Aucubin, which tends to medicate bladder infections and stomach ulcers.

Plantain also contains Potassium salts, citric acid, the enzymes invertin and emulsin, olionic acid, fats, and rubber.

Plantain can be used for uterine, kidney, and bladder infection. Plantain can be used to expel intestinal worms.

Plaintain Tea can be used as an enema to heal hemorrhoids and also as a vaginal douche.

Plantain Leaves ground up can be applied to snake and insect bites.

A salve or fomentation on the skin can clear up eczema, boils, and carbuncles. Fresh Plantain Juice applied to the skin stops itching.

Plantain will neutralize poisons and stomach acid, and normalize all stomach secretions.

Plantain seeds work similarly to psyllium seeds and can be used as a colon cleanser (laxative).

Time of Administration:

Morning to Evening

PLEURISY ROOT (Asclepias Tuberosa)

Part Used:

Root

Pleurisy Root contains Asclepiadin, Resins, and a volatile oil. Pleurisy Root is an excellent expectorant for colds, flu, bronchitis, and other lung problems. Pleurisy Root is considered to be one of the finest herbs to combat tuberculosis and emphysema.

Pleurisy Root can be used to treat dysentery.

Pleurisy Root Tea can be used as an enema for bowel complaints and for asthma and pneumonia. Pleurisy Root Tea will bring on sweating to help detoxify the body and lower fevers.

Time of Administration:

Afternoon to Late Afternoon

POKE ROOT (Phytolacca Americana)

Parts Used:

Root, Young Shoots, and Berries

Poke Root contains Vitamins A, and C, and minerals Calcium, Iron, and Phosphorus.

Poke Root is helpful in treating rheumatism, tonsillitis, mumps, lymphatic swelling, laryngitis, thyroid glands, spleen, and liver enlargment. Poke Root is very potent. It should not be taken more than one teaspoon, three times a day. An overdose will cause vomiting and diarrhea. Externally, Poke Root can be added to salves for skin diseases such as scabies, eczema, and infections. The decoction can also be used as a fomentation for these conditions.

Poke Root makes a good poultice for breast tumors and caked breasts. The poultice should be made by grinding the root into a powder and mixing it with slippery elm and water. Apply to the swellings and remoisten it when it drys. Keep the poultice on all day and change it every 3 days.

Poke Root consists of resins, tannin, about 10% natural plant sugar, phytolactic acid, and the non-essential amino acid asparagine. Poke Root has been used medically as an internal agent for parasitic infection.

Poke Root contains steroids resembling cortisone making it useful in treating psoriasis. A powdered root poultice has been used for skin cancer.

Time of Administration:

Early to Late Morning

PSYLLIUM (Plantago Ovata)

Part Used:

Seeds

Psyllium seeds are like a "Roto-Rooter" for the colon and intestines. Psyllium will clean and lubricate as well as heal the intestine and colon, by strengthening the tissues and restoring tone. Psyllium Powder or the soaked seed will assist easy evacuation by increasing water content in the colon.

Externally a poultice of psyllium seed powder can draw out pus from boils, carbuncles, and sores, because it is a drawing agent.

The way to make an effective external poultice would be to stir together Psyllium Seed Powder, pieces of unleaven bread, and water until the mixture becomes thick like paste.

To move the bowels take a teaspoon of Psyllium Seed Powder in a cup of warm water or juice, and drink it down three times a day until results are obvious.

Time of Administration:

When Needed

QUEEN OF THE MEADOW or GRAVEL ROOT (Eupatorium Purpurem)

Parts Used:

Leaves and Root

Queen of the Meadow contains Vitamins C, D and P. Queen of the Meadow contains eupatorin and resin, both of which exert a contracting influence on the bladder to permit increased fluid elimination. Queen of the Meadow also contains quercetin. Queen of the Meadow (Gravel Root) will dissolve kidney or bladder stones if used with considerable frequency with Juniper Berries. Queen of the Meadow (Gravel Root) will also eliminate gallstones.

Queen of the Meadow will neutralize uric acid deposits in the joints, relieving pain and the gout.

Queen of the Meadow is also a nerve tonic as well as a diuretic.

Time of Administration:

Morning to Late Afternoon

RASPBERRY (Rubus Idaeus)

Part Used:

Leaf

Red Raspberry contains Vitamins A, B, C, D, E, and F and the minerals Phosphorus, Magnesium and Calcium.

Red Raspberry Leaves are high in Iron, enriching early colostrum found in breast milk. Red Raspberry prepares the mother's breast for a pure milk supply for her nursing infant. Red Raspberry Leaf is one of the best herbs for women. The tannic acid in the leaves alleviates female abdominal cramps, morning sickness, false labor pains, and will reduce labor pains and ease childbirth. Drinking Red Raspberry will strengthen the uterus wall, relieve painful menstruation, and aid in normalizing menstrual flow.

Red Raspberry leaves have been used to treat hyperglycemia (high blood sugar) and mild high blood pressure.

Red Raspberry aids the eyes to reduce mucus, as well as stopping any cataracts that may be forming.

Too much Red Raspberry Leaf Tea can cause loose bowels.

Time of Administration:

Morning to evening

RED CLOVER (Trifolium Pratense)

Part Used:

Flowers

Red Clover contains Vitamins A, B-Complex, C, F, and P. Red Clover also contains the minerals Iron, Phosphorus, Magnesium, Calcium, Copper, Selenium, Cobalt, Nickel, Manganese, Sodium, Molybdenum and Tin.

Red Clover is exceedingly good for all kinds of cancer throughout the body. It is especially useful for esophageal and mammary cancer. Red Clover affects the mammary glands in a positive way by helping to increase lactation in nursing mothers.

Red Clover is a blood purifier that can be used to treat spasms, lung congestion, bronchitis, and whooping cough. Red Clover can be used externally as a wash (tea) or a salve for healing burns, psoriasis, shingles, acne, and any other skin condition.

Red Clover tea can be used as a gargle for all throat swelling and infections, and as an enema or a douche.

Red Clover has been shown to possess antibiotic properties against several bacteria especially against the pathogen that causes tuberculosis.

Red Clover contains the plant-estrogen Coumerol which explains its estrogenic activity.

Time of Administration:

Early Morning to Late Morning

ROSE HIPS (Rosa Species)

Parts Used:

Fruit, Petals, Buds

Rose Hips has Vitamins A, B-Complex, C, D, E, P and Rutin. Rose Hips also contains the minerals Iron, Calcium, Sodium, Potassium, Sulfur, and Silica.

A tea of fresh Rose Petals can help purify the blood, and alleviate headaches, cramps, and dizziness. Five to ten flowers or buds steeped in hot water for twenty minutes can alleviate diarrhea. One cup of this tea has more vitamins than 10 or 12 dozen oranges.

Time of Administration:

Early Morning, Afternoon to late Afternoon

ROSEMARY (Rosamarinus Oficinalis)

Part Used:

Leaves

Rosemary contains Vitamins A and C. Rosemary also contains the minerals Iron, Calcium, Magnesium, Phosphorus, Potassium, Sodium, and Zinc.

Rosemary possesses a large amount of Magnesium which causes a tranquilizing effect on frayed nerves.

Rosemary Tea taken internally will alleviate gas, colic, indigestion, nausea, and fever. Rosemary Tea will also relieve hysterical depression and strengthen the nervous system.

Rosemary Tea used as a hair rinse will help to alleviate baldness by stimulating the hair bulbs. Rosemary, because of its nutrient value, will also stimulate the cardiovascular system. Rosemary helps liver function, the production of bile, and improves circulation.

Rosemary normalizes blood pressure. Rosemary is excellent when used for all women's ailments. It helps regulate menses and should be used when there are pains from the uterus followed by hemorrhage. Rosemary is a good tonic for the reproductive organs. Rosemary oil when added to liniments and salves is good for rheumatism, eczema, stings, sores, arthritis, and wounds.

Rosemary Tea is a good mouthwash to treat halitosis.

An herbalist warns against drinking too much Rosemary Tea. Three cups per day should be the limit.

Time of Administration:

When Needed

RUE (Ruta Graveolens)

Part Used:

The Herb

Rue contains large amounts of Rutin (Vitamin P), which will strengthen capillaries, and veins, and harden bones and teeth.

Rue Tea is an excellent remedy for stomach problems, cramps in the bowel, nervousness, hysteria, spasms, dizziness, and congestion in the female organs. Rue Tea should not be taken by pregnant women.

Rue Tea has been found to be very effective in preserving sight by strengthening the ocular muscles.

Rue has helped to remove deposits that formed in the tendons and joints, especially the joints of the wrist.

Rue applied externally as a poultice (with fresh leaves only) has been able to relieve headache and sciatica pain. Rue has the ability to expel poisons from the body and has also been used for snake bite, scorpion, spider, or jellyfish bites.

When a poultice of fresh Rue leaves is to be used, it is suggested to first rub a vegetable oil on the body part where the poultice is to be placed.

Time of Administration:

As Needed

SAFFLOWER (Carthamus Tinctorius)

Part Used:

Flowers
Safflower contains Vitamins F and K.

Safflower Tea will produce perspiration which will detoxify the body of uric acids and is useful in alleviating the flu and fever.

Safflower has the ability to remove hard phlegm from the lungs, therefore being valuable in all respiratory conditions. When Safflower Flowers are dried and stored for any length of time, oxygen in the air unites with the volatile properties of Safflower to create a form of natural sugarlike compounds which induce the adrenal gland to produce more adrenalin and the pancreas to produce more insulin, although this herb is not for diabetes. Safflower has been used as a remedy for jaundice, sluggish liver, and gall bladder problems.

Safflower oil is a polyunsaturated oil that is being used to lower the cholesterol level in the blood stream. Safflower oil also contains Vitamin F which is an essential fatty acid needed to regenerate the skin and combat a wheat, corn, dust, feather, or wool allergy.

Time of Administration:

Afternoon

SAGE (Salvia Officinalis)

Part Used:

Leaves

Sage contains Vitamins A, B-Complex, and C. Sage contains the minerals Calcium, Potassium, Sulfur, Silicon, Phosphorus and Sodium.

Sage is helpful in alleviating mental exhaustion. Sage has improved the memory and strengthens the ability to concentrate. Sage has been used to treat some types of insanity. Sage Tea is an excellent gargle when combined with freshly squeezed lemon juice and honey for all mouth disease. Sage Tea can be taken to help normalize stomach troubles, diarrhea, gas, dysentery, colds, and flu.

Sage Tea or Enema will expel worms in children and adults. Externally, Sage Tea used as a hair rinse will stimulate hair growth and remove dandruff.

Sage Tea is an excellent wash for wounds that heal slowly and for other skin eruptions.

Lactating mothers should not drink cold sage tea for it will dry up the milk in the breasts.

Sage tea will stop "Night Sweats" and perspiration. Sage will decrease secretions, and excessive mucus discharges of the lungs, sinuses, throat, and all mucous membranes.

Sage has also been used internally and as a douche to alleviate yeast infections.

Time of Administration:

Late Morning to Late Afternoon

SARSAPARILLA (Smilax-Ornata)

Parts Used:

Root

Sarsaparilla contains Vitamins A, B-Complex, C and D.

Sarsaparilla also contains the minerals Iron, Manganese, Sodium,

Silicon, Sulfur, Copper, Zinc and Iodine. Sarsaparilla contains the amino acids Methionine and Cystein. Sarsaparilla contains a sapogen called Diosgenin which contains the female hormone progesterone and the male hormone testosterone. The dried roots of Sarsaparilla contain Sarsaponin, Smilacin, Paroaparic Acid, Resin, and Volatile Oil.

The Saponins in the Sarsaparilla root help the body to better absorb other nutrients taken along with it.

Sarsaparilla helps strengthen the nerve fibers and tissues of the brain, spinal cord, lungs, and throat. Sarsaparilla has been accepted as an effective deterrent to venereal disease. The saponins in Sarsaparilla Root act as cleaning agents removing the accumulated toxic waste and calcification from around the joints and also from the system itself, thereby having anti-inflammatory properties. Sarsaparilla is useful in treating mercury poisoning, and is especially good for removing heavy metallic contaminants from the blood, which are received through the nostrils in the foul, smog filled air of urban areas. Sarsaparilla influences the genes within the human organism to various extents. Sarsaparilla exerts a considerable force upon the RNA and DNA factors within the body, virtually guaranteeing a normal behavior pattern for the genes to follow.

Sarsaparilla Root, which contains testosterone, will help hair to regrow.

Sarsaparilla Tea used externally is useful as a fomentation or wash for skin eruptions, pustules, sores, wounds, and ringworm. Sarsaparilla Tea is also a good eyewash. Sarsaparilla Tea taken internally will increase urine, break up gas, and increase sweating to break up fevers.

Time of Administration:

Late Morning to Late Afternoon

SAW PALMETTO (Sereno Serru Lata)

Part Used:

Fruit

Saw Palmetto contains Vitamin A, Alkaloids, Resin, Dextrin, Glucose, Volatile Oil, and Fixed Oil (12%).

Saw Palmetto Berries help rebuild the body by feeding the endocrine system to rebuild atrophied flesh. Saw Palmetto Berries can help rebuild sexual reproductive organs, such as atrophied testicles in elderly men. Saw Palmetto Berries work well for female organs also. Saw Palmetto Berries have been known to increase the size of small breasts.

Certain unidentified alkaloids in the volatile and fixed oils of Saw Palmetto Berries act as a sedative on mucus membranes and muscles in the body, being very helpful in the reduction of such spasms as in whooping cough and croup. The Saw Palmetto Berries act as an anti-inflammatory agent on the mucous tissue of the lungs, throat and colon. Saw Palmetto is useful in treating gonorrhea in the advanced stages. Saw Palmetto Berries, because of nutritional effect on the glandular system, can be effectively used to combat diabetes in the early stages.

One remarkable characteristic of Saw Palmetto Berries is the great nutritional value it has on any kind of wasting disease. The Saw Palmetto Berries will increase flesh strength and weight.

Time of Administration:

Anytime as Needed

SCULLCAP (Scutellaria lateriflora)

Part Used:

The Herb

Scullcap contains the Vitamin C and E. Scullcap also contains the minerals Calcium, Potassium, Magnesium, Iron, and Zinc.

Scullcap contains Scutellarin, Volatile Oil, Tannin, and bitter Principles.

Scullcap's Scutellarin acts on the central nervous system and exerts most of its influence in the spinal column and brain as a sedative. Scullcap is valuable in any kind of deliriums produced by raging fever or rabies. Scullcap is sometimes useful in epilepsy and in twitching problems.

Scullcap's scutellarin produces natural endorphins in the body to act on the brain to aid in headaches and act as a tranquilizing opiate on the body.

Scullcap has been used as an aid in weaning individuals from barbiturate addiction and excessive use of Valium. Scullcap Tea mixed

2:1 with American Ginseng Tea has been used as treatment for alcoholics.

Scullcap Tea combined with Pennyroyal and Crampbark Teas has been known to cure Nymphomania. It seems to work by quieting the Cerebrospinal Centers and by calming the heart and hysterical excitement.

NOTE: Scullcap top should be used as fresh as possible since much of its activity is lost with prolonged storage.

Time of Administration:

Evenings

SENNA (Cassia Acutifolia)

Parts Used:

Leaves and Pods

Senna contains Chrysophanol, Aloe-emodin, Rhein, and other Glucosides and Glycosides.

Senna is an effective laxative and should be combined with Ginger, or Anise, or Fennel to avoid stomach griping or cramping. Senna pods are milder than the leaves. Senna Tea should be drunk cold, so that there will be less griping.

To make a tea, use one ounce of Senna, 1/10 ounce Ginger, Anise or Fennel. Steep the combination for 20 minutes. Then drink this Tea *cold*. Only drink 2 oz. three times a day.

Senna does not agree with Peruvian Bark, limes and mineral acids. In my own practice I refrain from using Senna for the reason it seems to displace or burn up Magnesium which is essential for good bowel movements.

Senna should not be used when there is inflammation anywhere in the intestinal tract or rectum, or if there are piles, or prolapsed intestines or rectum. Senna should not be used during pregnancy.

Senna does expel parasites and worms.

Time of Administration:

When Needed

SHEPHERD'S PURSE (Capsella Bursa-Pastoris)

Part Used:

The Whole Plant

Shepherd's Purse is high in Vitamins C, E and K. Shepherd's Purse contains the minerals Iron, Magnesium, Calcium, Potassium, Tin, Zinc, Sodium, and Sulfur.

Shepherd's Purse also contains Acetylcholine which plays an important role in the transmission of nerve impulses. Acetylcholine has a stimulating action on the uterine muscle.

Shepherd's Purse can be used after childbirth to arrest excessive bleeding.

Shepherd's Purse is helpful to stop all internal hemorrhaging, especially bleeding of the lungs, colon, bladder, kidneys and hemorrhoids, because it contains Vitamin K. The tops should be used fresh for this. Shepherd's Purse will stop diarrhea when all else fails.

Externally Shepherd's Purse has been found to be useful as a poultice on Rheumatic Joint Pain and as a salve on wounds. It helps to close the wounds.

Culpepper recommends "The Juice of Shepherd's Purse being dropped into the ear, heals the pains, noise and muttering".

Shepherd's Purse normalizes blood pressure and heart action.

Time of Administration:

Morning to Evening

SLIPPERY ELM (Ulmus Fulva)

Part Used:

Inner Bark

Slippery Elm contains the Vitamins C, E, F, K, and P. Slippery Elm also contains Iron, Sodium, Calcium, Selenium, Iodine, Copper, Manganese, Zinc, Potassium, and Phosphorus.

Slippery Elm is helpful in alleviating inflammation of the mucus surfaces of the mouth, throat and lungs. Slippery Elm Bark is useful for sore throats and pleurisy.

Slippery Elm is nourishing for children or the elderly with weak stomachs or ulcers. Slippery Elm has the ability to neutralize stomach acidity and to absorb foul gases. Slippery Elm will relieve constipation or diarrhea.

Externally Slippery Elm can be used as a poultice to heal sores, wounds, burns, open sores, poison ivy, and infected skin. Externally Slippery Elm can be used as a douche or an enema when there is inflammation and burning.

Slippery Elm is a mucilaginous herb. Make sure it does not plug the apparatus.

Slippery Elm aids in boosting the adrenal glands' output of cortin hormone, which helps send a stream of blood-building substances through the body. Slippery Elm has been used in the treatment of Cancer and Asthma.

Time of Administration:

Morning to Evening (Especially at meals)

SPEARMINT (Mentha Viridis)

Part Used:

Leaves

Spearmint contains Vitamins A, B-Complex, and C. Spearmint also contains the minerals Calcium, Sulfur, Iron, Iodine, Magnesium, and Potassium.

Spearmint activates the production of saliva and digestive enzymes in the mouth to aid in the start of the digestive processes. Spearmint helps to alleviate nausea and vomiting, especially in pregnancy.

Spearmint will alleviate gas, cramps, and slight spasms.

Externally, Spearmint can be used as an enema to stop restlessness.

Time of Administration:

Morning and Evening

SQUAWVINE (Mitchella Repens)

Part Used:

The Herb

Squawvine contains Alkaloids, Bitter Glycosides, Tannin, and Saponin. Squawvine also contains the amino acid Tryptophan.

The Saponins in Squawvine help to regulate and stimulate the amount of contractions which help to facilitate childbirth. The bitter alkaloids and tannins, being natural antiseptics, help alleviate vaginal infections. Squawvine will alleviate "Morning Sickness". Squawvine taken during pregnancy will also insure milk production for successful lactation.

Squawvine is a uterine tonic and will relieve congestion of the uterus and ovaries. Squawvine is excellent to alleviate P.M.S. and absent menstruation.

Squawvine is also a diuretic that can aid in removing gravel from kidneys and bladders.

Time of Administration:

Late Evenings

TA HEEBO (Tabebuia Avellanedae)
(Pau D'Arco or Ipe Roxo)

Part Used:

Inner Bark

Ta Heebo (Pau D'Arco) contains the minerals Iron and Zinc.

Ta Heebo is found in South America, where it is being used in some hospitals in cancer therapy.

Ta Heebo contains antibiotic properties with virus-killing ability. Ta Heebo from Brazil is presently of questionable quality for the Brazilians are using Agent Orange to defoliate its jungles.

Ta Heebo Tea is one of the ingredients of Jonathan Winters' Miracle Cancer Cure Tea.

Time of Administration:

When Needed

THYME (Thymus Vulgaris)

Part Used:

The Herb

Thyme contains the Vitamins B-Complex, C, and D. Thyme also contains Iodine, Sodium, Silicon, and Sulfur.

Thyme contains a powerful germicide, Thymol, which is an antiseptic as well as a parasiticide. Thymol has been used to treat Hookworms. Thymol can cause mental excitement and has been used as "Smelling Salts". Thyme is useful as a tincture to treat all throat and bronchial problems, especially bronchitis, laryngitis, and whooping cough. Thyme is good for all stomach and intestinal problems such as diarrhea, gastritis, lack of appetite, gas, and colic.

Externally, an oil of Thyme added to vegetable oil can be used as an antiseptic for ringworm, athlete's foot, scabies, crabs, and lice. For a bath add thyme to the water and soak for at least 45 minutes and itchiness will stop.

A fomentation of Thyme can help heal wounds, warts, and varicose veins.

Thyme can be used as a douche to help alleviate leucorrhea.

Thyme Tea can also take away headaches.

Time of Administration:

Evenings

UVA URSI (Arctostaphylos Uva Ursi)
(bar berry)

Part Used:

Leaves

Uva Ursi leaves contain Arbutin, Allantion, and Tannins.

The Arbutin found in Uva-Ursi has strong disinfectant properties. Therefore Uva Ursi will work as an effective urinary antiseptic, killing any types of viral infection that may occur. The Allantoin that occurs in Uva Ursi will relieve the pain of and help to heal kidney inflammation. Uva Ursi has been recommended for nephritis, cystitis, urethitis, or kidney and bladder stones. Uva Ursi increases the flow of urine but has a sedative and tonic effect to the bladder wall.

Uva Ursi is best known as the diabetic remedy to decrease excessive sugar in the system.

Uva Ursi should not be used in large quantities during pregnancy because it is a vasoconstrictor to the uterus which will cut down the circulation to the fetus.

Externally, a bath with one cup of Uva Ursi Leaves submerged in a sock, is beneficial for skin infections, hemorrhoids, inflammations and can also be used after childbirth.

Tincture of Uva Ursi taken internally can help to restore the womb to normal size after child birth.

Externally a tea of Uva Ursi is an excellent douche for vaginal infection.

Time of Administration:

As Needed

VALERIAN (Valeriana Officinalis)

Part Used:

Root

Valerian is rich in Magnesium, Potassium, Copper, and some Lead and Zinc.

Valerian Root contains a volatile oil, alkaloids, Valeric Acid, Formic Acid, Malic Acid, Tannins, Gums, Resin, and iridoid compounds.

The iridoid compounds, called Valpotriates, infiltrate brain tissue, blood cells, and the central nervous system where they produce a strong sedative effect on the entire body.

Valerian Root is useful in pain-relieving remedies because it relaxes muscle spasms.

The Valepotriates in Valerian Root help to heal Erysipelas, an acute inflammation of the skin due to a disturbance in the red blood cells caused by strep virus infection.

Valerian Root also can treat hives, shingles, backache, and certain eye inflammations.

Valerian Root should be recommended for short-term use. Prolonged or excessive use can cause mental depression.

Valerian Root is sometimes used as a substitute for the synthetic drug, Valium. The difference between the two is (a) the Smell!! and (b) one is natural and the other is synthetic. Also an overdose of Valerian will bring on a headache while an overdose of Valium can lead to coma and death.

Time of Administration:

Late Evening & Early Morning

VERVAIN (Verbena Officinalis)

Part Used:

Tops

Vervain is helpful in pneumonia, asthma, and all other congestive chest diseases, especially upper respiratory inflammations.

Vervain Tea will settle a nervous stomach and help combat insomnia. Vervain Tea drunk warm will alleviate pains or cramps in the stomach and bowels. Too much Vervain can induce vomiting!

Time of Administration:

Evenings

VIOLET (Viola Odorata)

Parts Used:

Flower and Leaves

Violet contains Vitamins A and C.

Violet can be helpful in alleviating sore throats, asthma, difficult breathing, bronchitis, coughs, especially whooping cough, and head or sinus congestion.

The characteristic of Violet leaves and flowers is that it is able to saturate the blood stream and lymphatic systems so that they are carried to the body where needed.

Externally, a poultice or fomentation of Violet flowers or leaves can treat tumors, boils, abscesses, pimples, swollen glands, and cancerous growths. It's now being researched for its cancer-treating ability. Violet is very effective in treating internal ulcers.

Time of Administration:

When Needed

WATERCRESS (Nasturium Officinale)

Part Used:

The Whole Plant

Watercress contains an abundance of Vitamins A, B, C, D, and G. Watercress also contains the Minerals Iron, Iodine, Calcium, Copper, Sulfur, and Manganese.

Watercress is a blood purifier and tonic. It stimulates the flow of bile. Watercress has been used as a blood tonic where anemia or other blood disorders are present.

Watercress can be used internally and externally to treat skin disorders such as acne, eczema, and age spots. Watercress helps to heal internal tumors, and uterine cysts. Kidney problems and stones have been helped by Watercress. Watercress will increase the amount of milk production by a lactating mother.

Time of Administration:

When Needed

WHITE OAK BARK (Quercus Alba)

Part Used:

Bark

White Oak Bark contains B-12, Calcium, Phosphorus, Potassium, Iodine, Sulfur, Iron, Sodium, Cobalt, Lead, Strontium, and Tin.

White Oak Bark tea is recommended for bleeding of the stomach, lungs, and rectum. White Oak Bark tea will stop diarrhea. White Oak Bark tea used as a douche will correct vaginal infections and used as an enema will heal piles and hemorrhoids.

White Oak Bark tea taken internally will help gallstones and kidney stones pass out of the body. White Oak Bark tea also increases the flow of urine and cleans the stomach of mucus.

Externally, White Oak Bark tea is an antiseptic and is good for bathing scabs, wounds, sores, poison oak, and insect bites. White Oak bark tea used externally as a fomentation will reduce tumors, swollen glands, goiter, and lymphatic swelling.

White Oak Bark tea is also a good mouthwash and gargle, and is also a good treatment for sore gums, pyorrhea, and gingivitis.

Time of Administration:

When needed.

WILD YAM (Diocorea Villosa):

Part Used:

Root.

Wild Yam roots contain two steroidal saponins; dioscin and diosgenin, which provide antiseptic strength to the liver, spleen, pancreas, and gallbladder.

The steroid diosgenin is a precursor of the sex hormone progesterone. Wild Yam Roots contain true estrogen. Wild Yam root can yield as much as 40% diosgenin.

Wild Yam roots were used by the American Indians as a "birth control pill". They claim that if wild yam roots are eaten every day for over 2 months, conception will not occur as long as the wild yam roots are consumed. Ovulation and the menstrual cycle will not be interrupted, but the woman's eggs are resistant to fertilization during the period that the wild yam is ingested. When the Indians decided to become pregnant they merely stopped the wild yam ingestion and within one month the female would then become fertile again.

Time of Administration:

When desired.

WHITE WILLOW (Salix)

Part Used:

Bark.

White willow bark is a natural alternative to aspirin. The major active ingredient in white willow bark is salicin. White willow bark can alleviate headaches, fevers, neuralgia, and pains in the joints.

White willow bark tea taken internally can soothe kidney, urethra, and bladder irritations. White willow bark tea taken internally is a helpful remedy for gout, rheumatism and arthritic pains. White willow tea is an excellent gargle for throat and tonsil infections.

Used externally, white willow bark tea is a strong antiseptic and an excellent wash for infected wounds, ulcerations, eczema, and all other skin inflammations. White willow tea can also be used as an eye wash.

WITCH HAZEL (Hamamelis Virginiana)

Part Used:

Bark.

Witch hazel contains the Vitamins C, E, K, and P. Witch hazel also contains the minerals Iodine, Manganese, Zinc, Copper, and Selenium. The most active ingredient in witch hazel is Hamamelitannin.

Taken internally witch hazel bark tea will stop excessive menstruation and hemorrhages from the lungs, stomach, uterus, and bowels. Witch hazel bark tea can be used as an enema to stop piles and hemorrhoids from bleeding. Witch hazel bark tea can also be used as a douche to stop vaginal discharges and infections.

Externally, witch hazel bark tea can be used as a wash for bed sores, wounds, oozing skin diseases (poison ivy), and inflamed eyes and insect bites.

Witch hazel bark tea makes an excellent mouth wash and gargle. It will also stop bleeding gums and aid an inflamed condition of the throat or mouth.

Time of Administration:

Evenings.

WOOD BETONY (Betonica Officinalis)

Part Used:

The Herb (tops)

Wood betony contains Magnesium, Manganese, and Phosphorus. Wood Betony is a valuable nervine. It soothes the Pineal gland area which is the "Crown Chakra".

Wood Betony is excellent for any headaches on the top of the skull. Wood Betony can also stop migraine headaches if it is used daily over a period of time. Wood Betony will also nourish the Pineal gland and protect it from degeneration. Degeneration of the Pineal gland can cause insanity and Vitiligo (a disorder of the skin marked by a loss of natural pigment resulting in patches of white on the skin).

In using Wood Betony to correct a Vitiligo condition it can take months before you finally see an improvement. The improvement is usually first noticed in the center of the patch where it will gradually fade to look like a doughnut until it finally disappears.

Wood Betony is useful in treating nerve twitching of the face and palsy. Wood Betony tea will successfully open up obstructions of the liver and gall bladder while soothing the spleen, thus being useful in treating jaundice.

Wood Betony tea taken 3 to 4 times a day in 3 ounce dosages will also kill worms.

Time of Administration:

Throughout the day. Morning to night.

YARROW (Achilea Millefolium)

Part Used:

Flower.

Yarrow contains Vitamins A, C, E, F, and K. Yarrow contains the minerals Manganese, Copper, Potassium, Iodine, and Iron.

Yarrow promotes perspiration and opens the pores of the skin, thereby permitting toxic impurities to leave the system, particularly uric acid and ammonia.

Yarrow helps the liver to produce bile and stops any kind of internal hemorrhaging and will strengthen the blood.

Yarrow tea is excellent for shrinking hemorrhoids and piles if used as an enema after each bowel movement. If there is much pain, use a warm tea (112 to 115 degrees Fahrenheit) and it will soothe and alleviate the pain. Yarrow tea can also be used as a douche to stop secretions and hemorrhage. A Yarrow tea douche is also helpful in arresting yeast infections.

It should be noted that because Yarrow causes perspiration, the user should have Sodium and Potassium levels checked in order to replace any that may have been lost through perspiration.

Time of Administration:

Early morning to late evening.

YELLOW DOCK (Rumex Crispus)

Part Used:

Root.

Yellow Dock root contains Vitamins A, B, and C. Yellow Dock root also contains the minerals Iron, Manganese, Nickel, Sulfur, and Calcium.

Yellow Dock root also contains Emodin, Chrysophanic acid, Lapathin, a Volatile Oil, Resin, Tannin, Rumicin, Starch, and various mineral salts. The Yellow Dock root is somewhat of an antibiotic and inhibits the growth of staph and E. coli bacteria.

Yellow Dock root is an astringent & blood purifier. Yellow Dock is valuable for skin diseases such as leprosy, eczema, psoriasis, ringworm of the scalp, cradle cap, and hives. Yellow Dock root stimulates the flow of bile and acts like a laxative.

We use Yellow Dock root capsules in our program instead of inorganic Iron pills. One 500 mg. capsule of Yellow Dock root contains approximately 60 mg. of organic Iron. However, not everyone is able to tolerate Yellow Dock because of its nickel content so this should always be checked by using Muscle Response Testing.

Time of Administration:

Morning to evening.

YUCCA (Yucca Glauca)

Part Used:

Root.

Yucca root contains Vitamins A, B-Complex, and C. Yucca also contains the minerals Calcium, Potassium, Phosphorus, Iron, Manganese, and Copper.

Yucca root contains special steroid saponins which are able to strengthen the flora of the intestines, thereby breaking down organic wastes in the body like uric acid. The Yucca root saponins are also cleansing agents of mineral and salt deposits which might exist in the joints of the body. Yucca root saponins possess cortisone-like properties, thereby making it greatly useful for arthritic joint problems.

The highly absorbable organic Manganese content of Yucca makes it useful in restoring the connective tissue of the body to alleviate stiffness in the joints and back. Yucca root can also be useful in reconstructing deteriorated or damaged discs of the spinal column.

Dr. Asplund, of the chemistry and biochemistry department of the University of Wyoming at Laramie discovered that the Yucca flower has anti-cancer properties.

Time of Administration:

Afternoon

HERBAL BOOKS FOR FURTHER STUDY:

1.) *Science of Herbal Medicine*, by John Heinerman, published by Woodland Books.
2.) *Today's Herbal Health*, by Louise Tenney, published by Woodland Books.
3.) *Natural Healing with Herbs*, by Humbart Santillo, B.S., M.H., published by Hohm Press.
4.) *The Encyclopedia of Herbs and Herbalism*, edited by Malcolm Stuart, published by Crescent Books, N.Y., distributed by Crown Publishers.
5.) *Herbal Medication*, a Clinical and Dispensary Handbook, A.W. Priest & L.R. Priest, published by L.N. Fowler & Co., LTD, London England.

6.) *The Herbal Connection*, by Ethan Nebelkopf, M.A., M.F.C.C., published by Bi-World publishers, Utah.

7.) *Herb Walk*, by Learta Moulton, published by Gluten Co., P.O. Box 482, Provo, Utah.

8.) *Advanced Treatise in Herbology*, by Dr. Edward E. Shook, published by Trinity Center Press, P.O. Box 335, Beaumont Ca. 92223.

9.) *Secrets of Chinese Herbalists*, by Richard Lucas, published by Parker Pub. Co., West Nyack, N.Y.

10.) *Chinese Herbal Medicine*, by Richard Hyatt, published by Thorson Publishing Co., Inc.

11.) *Back to Basics with Herbs*, by James D. Jenks, H.M.D., published by Woodland Books.

12.) *Kneipp Herbs*, by Dr. B. Lust, published by Benedict Lust Publications, P.O. Box 404, N.Y., N.Y. 10016.

13.) *The Herb Book*, by John Lust, published by Benedict Lust Publications.

14.) *The Way of Herbs*, by Michael Tierra, C.A., N.D.

15.) *Common & Uncommon uses of Herbs for Healthful Living*, by Richard Lucas, published by Arco Publishing Co.

16.) *Using Plants for Healing*, by Nelson Coon, published by Rodale Press.

17.) *The Rodale Herb Book*, edited by William H. Hylton, published by Rodale Press.

18.) *Herbal Medicine*, by Dian Dincin Buchman, published by Gramercy Publishing Co.

19.) *Growing & Using Healing Herbs*, by Gaea & Shandor Weiss, published by Rodale Press.

20.) *Health Through God's Pharmacy*, by Maria Treben, published by Wilhelm Ennsthaler, Steyr, Australia.

21.) *The Little Herb Encyclopedia*, by Jack Ritchason, published by Woodland Books.

22.) *School of Natural Healing*, by Dr. John R. Christopher, available from Woodland Books.

CHAPTER 8

FLOWER REMEDIES

THE FLOWER REMEDIES

In my research, I have found the flower remedies to be a valid form of treatment for certain problems. I have found that they modify behavior problems gradually and are especially helpful to people who have personality problems and psychological "hang ups". How they work God only knows, but they do work!!

Many noted psychologists and psychiatrists use the flower remedies in their practices, but in order to use them most effectively they take the time to analyze their patients to find out which remedy is best suited for that particular person.

I have discovered a simple way to determine the proper flower remedy by using the "Lepore Technique". Place a list of the 39 different flower remedies on a flat firm surface. The person who is being tested should then place their index finger over the first flower remedy name while extending the opposite arm to the side to be "pumped". You should also "think" the remedy name as you pull down on the person's extended arm.

If the arm goes down when it is "pumped" by the other person, it shows that the person does not need that specific flower remedy. You would then move the finger onto the second flower remedy while extending the opposite arm to again be "pumped" by the other person (also think the name of the remedy). If the arm is now strong when it is "pumped" it is one of the remedies that may help the person. You should then proceed to check the rest of the flower remedies the same way to find out which ones are negative and positive to that person.

However, it is not advisable to prescribe 6 different remedies at the same time.

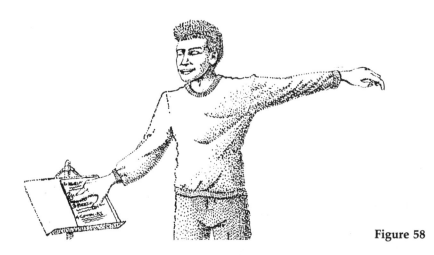

Figure 58

After you have found the appropriate remedies for the person on the list sheet, double check it by using the Muscle Response Testing method with the bottle which actually contains the remedy. Have the person being tested place the bottle containing the remedy in the hand while it is held to the Solar Plexus and extend the opposite arm to be "pumped". You should now pull down on (or "Pump") client's arm to determine whether the remedy is positive or negative. If the arm goes down or tests weak, you should then add a second or third bottle of the remedies which originally tested strong on the list until the pumped arm feels strong and rigid. When you have found the remedies which finally make the arm strong and rigid, this means that this specific remedy is very much needed, so the intake should be doubled. If the arm was strong when the first bottle was tested, it means that the remedy is needed, but in an average dose. It should be noted that one cannot "overdose" on the flower remedies, and there are no adverse side effects.

An average dose of the flower remedies is 4 drops under the tongue 4 times a day. The liquid should be held in the mouth so that it can enter the bloodstream through the saliva glands. The flower remedies are prepared from highly potent, vital seedbearing, non-poisonous, flowers. The remedies are simple to prepare using pure water, sunlight, fresh blossoms, & a clean glass bowl.

The following is a list of the different flower remedies:

1.) **Agrimony:** This remedy is especially used for those who suffer considerable inner torture which they try to dissemble behind a facade of cheerfulness.
2. **Aspen:** Useful for feelings of anxiety and apprehension.
3. **Beech:** Good for those who are critical and intolerant of others. Also good for those who are arrogant.
4. **Centaury:** Useful for those with a weakness of will and for those who let themselves be exploited or imposed upon by others.
5. **Cerato:** For those who lack confidence in their own judgment and are constantly seeking the advice of others, often being misguided.
6. **Cherry Plum:** For those with a fear of mental collapse and of doing something desperate. Also for the uncontrolled temper.
7. **Chestnut Bud:** For those who refuse to learn from experience, and constantly repeat the same mistakes.
8. **Chicory:** For those who are over-possessive and are constantly trying to put others right, usually demanding the attention of those close to them. Full of self pity, martyrs.
9. **Clematis:** For the dreamy sort of person who doesn't pay much attention to what's going on around them.
10. **Crab Apple:** For those who feel unclean or ashamed of their ailments. A cleanser for those feelings of self disgust and condemnation.
11. **Elm:** Good for temporary feelings of inadequacy and those overwhelmed by responsibilities.
12. **Gentian:** Good for feelings of discouragement and resultant self-doubt.
13. **Gorse:** For those with feelings of despair, hopelessness, and utter despondency.
14. **Heather:** For those who are obsessed with their own problems and experiences and constantly relate these to others. These types drain the vitality of others and are poor listeners.
15. **Holly:** Use for those who are jealous, revengeful, envious, and suspicious. For those who are hateful.
16. **Honeysuckle:** For those who are nostalgic and constantly dwell in the past. Also for feelings of homesickness.
17. **Hornbeam:** This remedy is good for those who need strength to deal with their daily duties (though they usually succeed in fulfilling their task). For that "Monday morning" feeling.
18. **Impatiens:** Good for those who are impatient and irritable.
19. **Larch:** For those with feelings of despondency because they lack

self-confidence, always expecting failure so they never make an attempt. Also for feelings of inferiority.

20. **Mimulus:** For those who are shy and timid and those with a fear of known things.
21. **Mustard:** For those with feelings of deep gloom which come and go quite suddenly for no apparent reason.
22. **Oak:** For those in despair, but not willing to give up. This type is brave and struggles on despite feelings of despondency. Plodders.
23. **Olive:** For exhaustion and weariness. Good for mental and physical exhaustion.
24. **Pine:** For feelings of guilt and self-reproachfulness. The feeling that one should do (or has done) better. Good for those who blame themselves for the mistakes of others.
25. **Red Chestnut:** For those with excessive fear or anxiety for others.
26. **Rock Rose:** For those with feelings of terror and extreme fear or panic.
27. **Rock Water:** For those who martyr themselves in their pursuit of an ideal. For the rigid minded and inflexible. Also for feelings of self denial.
28. **Scleranthus:** For feelings of uncertainty and indecision. For those who are one way one minute, and another the next.
29. **Star of Bethlehem:** This remedy is good for all kinds of shock and the after effects of trauma.
30. **Sweet Chestnut:** For those in despair, feeling that they have reached the limits of endurance.
31. **Vervain:** For those who are over-enthused, fanatical and highly strung. Those who are incensed by injustices.
32. **Vine:** For those who are dominating and inflexible, those who are ruthless and crave power (leaders).
33. **Walnut:** This remedy helps to give protection from outside influences and over sensitivity. This is the link-breaking remedy for transition and change, such as puberty, menopause, etc.
34. **Water Violet:** For those who are proud, aloof, superior, reserved. This type does not interfere in the affairs of others.
35. **White Chestnut:** For persistent unwanted thoughts. Also good for those pre-occupied with some worry or episode. Good for quieting "mental arguments".
36. **Wild Oat:** For those with feelings of dissatisfaction with not having found one's goal in life.

37. **Wild Rose:** For those with little desire to make an effort, and feelings of resignation. Good for those who are apathetic.
38. **Willow:** For those with feelings of resentment and bitterness. Those with a "not fair" attitude.
39. This is the "Rescue Remedy" which is a composite of Cherry Plum, Clematis, Impatiens, Rock Rose, and Star of Bethlehem.

CHAPTER 9

CELL SALT THERAPY

CELL SALT THERAPY
(Tissue Salt Therapy)

Dr. Schussler, a German Homeopathic Physician in 1873, amplified and expounded this therapeutic science of biochemistry. Schussler believed the 12 different cell salts were all that were necessary to maintain perfect health in the human body.

Should a deficiency occur in one or more of the cell salts, an abnormal condition arises. These are misdiagnosed as specific diseases.

By properly balancing the patient biochemically, the client will remove the cause of the symptoms and it will disappear. Therefore, the disease symptoms will also disappear, healing the patient!! The importance of cell salts in biochemical balancing is their speed of absorption by the body. Cell salts are available in two different forms: Miniature homeopathic type pills which are dissolved under the tongue, or a liquid form which is also deposited under the tongue. These do not enter the digestive track, but by-pass it by being absorbed by the blood stream via the saliva ducts. This gives the patient immediate absorption of the biochemical remedy!

What I have found in my own research, is that cell salts may be utilized with patients who cannot swallow pills. This may be a real physical problem. When a pill is not right for a person, the client will usually gag because of being allergic to the pill, or because the dosage is too high. When a person tries to swallow a pill which is not needed, the esophagus will actually try to close up to save the person from ingesting a pill that may be harmful. If a pill won't go down, I instruct my clients not to take it. Something is wrong with it. People who have had a bad social interaction in the past with pills, often give cell salt therapy a chance.

In my experience, I have found that there are two things wrong with the cell salts. One is that the homeopathic type pills have a milk lactose base. This type will dissolve readily under the tongue, and have a long "shelf life", but if a person has a milk allergy it will give them an allergic reaction. Usually it will form little white blisters on and under the tongue. The only cell salt that will not do this is Kali Phos, because the Potassium in that pill will antidote the milk allergy. Kali Mur will cause a reaction because if a milk allergy exists, so will the chlorine allergy since they are both governed by Potassium. So in a Kali Mur pill, the Potassium is weakened by the Chlorine, and therefore not strong enough to handle the milk lactose allergy.

The other form of cell salts is the liquid form, which has a distilled water and alcohol base. Originally, when they were first marketed, they did not have alcohol in them and I used them quite successfully. But I guess the alcohol was added as a disinfectant to the dropper mechanism. What the alcohol did do was affect the rubber end of the dropper and give the substance a "rubber taste".

These bottles should always be upright so as to avoid this problem. If your store stocks the bottles on their sides, this will cause rubber or plastic erosion into the bottle contents which could be toxic to you!!

If you find a source of these liquid cell salts that is good, you can rid the bottle of its alcohol content by placing the opened bottle in a sauce pan of water and boiling it for about 5 minutes (let stand before use). By doing this, the alcohol should be boiled out.

To biochemically balance the body we have used vitamins, minerals, amino acids, herbs, juice therapy, and cell salts. I have found cell salts to be useful in cases where a person has a phobia about taking pills, or with infants that need biochemic balancing.

For example, if an infant needs Iron and is not allergic to the milk lactose base, I will have the mother place the Ferrum Phosphoricum in the baby's formula or drinking water. If the baby is breast feeding, the thing to do in this case would be to bring up the mother's Iron level by giving Iron-rich sources such as the herb Yellow Dock, and Beet Powder (or beet juice). By doing this, the Iron level of the mother's milk will increase and the infant will receive the Iron through the mother's milk. If you wish to use the liquid type of cell salt, it should be de-alcoholized before it is given to the infant.

Explanation of cell salt potencies:

A 3× potency contains 1 part of the cell salt to 999 parts of lactose (milk sugar), or 1:1000 of the cell salt.

A 6× potency contains 1 part cell salt to 999,999 parts lactose, or 1:1,000,000.

12× potency would be 1:1,000,000,000,000.

In my practice, I use the 1× or 3× potency because I am more interested in the physical action of the cell salt rather than the etherical action. 6× is the most common on health food store shelves because it tastes sweeter than the 1× or 3×.

To determine what cell salts you need you must first learn the characteristic and function of every cell salt!! The next thing would be to use the mineral M.R.T. points to determine where the weakness may be. This can be done by placing the fingers of the right hand at a mineral point such as the Magnesium point (which is the navel) and have someone pump the extended left arm. If the arm goes down, this will indicate a need for Magnesium. You can now determine the amount needed by placing the cell salt Mag-Phos (which is Magnesium Phosphate) in the palm of the hand while still holding the finger in the navel. Pump down on the extended arm while holding the cell salts in the other hand with the finger in the navel. Try different amounts until the arm shows strong and rigid. When the arm is rigid, you have found the amount that is needed by that person.

Another way of testing the amount of cell salts needed would be to hold them in the palm to the solar plexus area and pump the other arm as previously described.

Please see figure 29, page 56.

To test for cell salts:

Place cell salts in hand while holding to specific mineral point you are testing, or hold to solar plexus area. Now pump extended opposite arm to determine the amount of cell salts needed.

According to Dr. Schussler, the body needs only 12 cell salts, they are:

1. Calcarea Fluorica
   (Calcium Fluoride)
2. Calcarea Phosphorica
   (Calcium Phosphate)
3. Calcarea Sulphurica
   (Calcium Sulphate)

4. Ferrum Phosphoricum
   (Iron Phosphate)
5. Kali Muriaticum
   (Potassium Chloride)
6. Kali Phosphoricum
   (Potassium Phosphate)
7. Kali Sulphuricum
   (Potassium Sulphate)
8. Magnesia Phosphorica
   (Magnesium Phosphate)
9. Natrum Muriaticum
   (Sodium Chloride)
10. Natrum Phosphoricum
    (Sodium Phosphate)
11. Natrum Sulphuricum
    (Sodium Sulphate)
12. Silicea
    (Silicon, Quartz)

Now, what happens if a person needs Zinc, Manganese, Sulfur, or Chromium? Some of these elements were introduced by Dr. Eric Graf Von Der Goltz, whose writings on biochemistry are of great assistance. They will be listed and explained after Schussler's 12 cell salts. Please try and memorize each cell salt, its properties, and the field of action of each so that when the symptoms crop up, you will know which one to use.

1.) Calc. Fluor. (Calcium Fluoride)

Calc. Fluor. gives to the tissues the quality of elasticity. It combines with the organic substance, albumin, to form organic elastic tissue and is found in the walls of the blood vessels, in muscular tissue, in connective tissue, in the surface of bones, and in the enamel of teeth. A deficiency of Calc. Fluor. results in a loss of elasticity and a consequently relaxed condition. Its main function is the preservation of the contractile power of elastic tissue.

Whenever symptoms are traceable to a relaxed condition this tissue salt is indicated, e.g. a relaxed condition of veins and arteries, piles, sluggish circulation, or a tendency to cracks in the skin, notably in the palms of the hands and between the toes. Calc. Fluor. is also useful in the treatment of diseases affecting the surface of the bones and joints and when the teeth become loose in their sockets and decay rapidly.

The elasticity of muscular tissue and supporting membranes becomes impaired when this tissue-salt is deficient, resulting in muscular weakness, bearing-down pains, etc. The symptoms are generally worse in humid conditions and are relieved by massage and warmth.

2.) Calc. Phos. (Calcium Phosphate)

Calc. Phos. is the tissue-salt concerned with nutrition. It combines with albumin and its need is indicated when there are albuminous discharges. Without Calc. Phos. there could be no blood coagulation. It will assist the action of a more directly indicated tissue-salt and thus produce more rapid results. It promotes healthy cellular activity and restores tone to weakened organs and tissues. This tissue-salt is concerned with the formation of bone and teeth and thus becomes an important remedy for children. It aids growth and normal development and should be given in cases of backwardness, more particularly where there is bone weakness or recurring tooth troubles.

Calc. Phos. is the biochemic remedy for rickets. It is a combination of saliva and gastric juice. It assists digestion and assimilation and favors the building up of a sturdy, robust constitution. This is the remedy for the period of convalescence. Its restorative power will speed recovery and replenish the body's reserves of strength. Calc. Phos. is the tissue-salt for blood poverty and conditions associated with imperfect circulation. In the anemic states often seen in young girls, this remedy should be given. Calc. Phos. pains can be severe and "fixing" and they tend to be worse at night. There may be a creeping sensation of the skin, also numbness and coldness of the limbs. Calc. Phos. has always been prized as a restorative.

3.) Calc. Sulph. (Calcium Sulphate)

Calc. Sulph. is a blood purifier and healer. It is found in the liver where it helps in the removal of waste products from the blood stream and it has a cleansing and purifying influence throughout the system. Calc. Sulph. cleans out the accumulation of non-functional, organic matter, so that it may not lie dormant or slowly decay and thus injure the surrounding tissues.

Calc. Sulph. is indicated in conditions arising from impurities in the blood stream. It supplements the action of Kali Mur. in the treatment of catarrh, acne, etc., and it should always be given when "pimples" occur in adolescence. It checks the weakening drain of suppuration too long continued, e.g. abscesses and wounds which will not heal readily and tend to become septic. If taken in the early stage, it will prevent a sore throat from developing and in the same way, it will often cut short a threatening cold. The symptoms are generally worse after getting wet and are better in a warm, dry atmosphere.

4.) Ferr. Phos. (Iron Phosphate)

Ferr. Phos. is the pre-eminent Biochemic First-Aid. It is the oxygen-carrier. It enters into the composition of hemoglobin, the red coloring matter of the blood. It takes up oxygen from the air inhaled by the lungs and carries it in the blood stream to all parts of the body, thus furnishing the vital force that sustains life. It gives strength and toughness to the circular walls of the blood vessels, especially the arteries. Freely circulating, oxygen-rich blood is essential to health and life and for this reason Ferr. Phos. should always be considered, as a supplementary remedy, no matter what other treatment may be indicated by the symptoms.

Congestion, inflammatory pain, high temperature, quickened pulse, all call for more oxygen, and it is Ferr. Phos. that is the medium through which oxygen is taken up by the blood stream and carried to the affected area. This tissue-salt can be given with advantage in the early stage of most acute disorders, and it should be administered at frequent intervals until the inflammatory symptoms subside. It is also indicated where there is a lack of red blood corpuscles, as in anemia, and as a first-aid remedy for hemorrhages. It would be difficult to find a case of illness where Ferr. Phos. could not be used to advantage, irrespective of any other treatment that may be given. It is an excellent remedy for ailments associated with advancing years and it is one of the most frequently needed remedies in the treatment of children's ailments. Bleeding from wounds, cuts, and abrasions, can be controlled with a little powdered Ferr. Phos., applied directly to the injured parts. A few tablets may be crushed for this purpose or the tablets may be dissolved and used as a lotion (see directions, external applications). Ferr. Phos. should also be thought of as a first-aid in cases of muscular strains, sprains, etc.

NOTE: Ferr. Phos. is in no sense an Iron tonic. Its action is entirely nutritional and without any side-effects.

5.) Kali Mur. (Potassium Chloride)

Kali Mur. is the remedy for sluggish conditions. It combines with the organic substance, fibrin. Thus a deficiency of this tissue-salt causes fibrin to become non-functional, and to be thrown off in the form of thick white discharges, giving rise to catarrhs and similar symptoms affecting the skin and mucus membranes. Its action is complementary to that of Calc. Sulph., as both remedies are concerned with cleansing and purifying the blood. In conditions calling for Kali Mur. the blood tends to thicken and to form clots. When alternated with Ferr. Phos. it is frequently needed for the treatment of children's ailments.

Kali Mur. is the remedy for thick, white fibrinous discharges. Other prominent symptoms are a white-coated tongue and light colored stools (lack of bile). Torpidity of the liver is another indication. When alternated with Ferr. Phos. it is frequently needed in the treatment of inflammatory diseases, particularly those affecting respiration—coughs, colds, sore throats, tonsillitis, bronchitis, etc.; also for children's ailments such as measles and chicken pox and where there are soft swellings, e.g. mumps, or croup. Kali Mur. is concerned with the production of saliva and is therefore important in the early stages of digestion. The symptoms may be worse after eating fatty or rich foods and there may be a lack of appetite. With Nat. Mur. it is utilized in the production of hydrochloric acid, and is thus an essential link in the process of digestion. This tissue-salt is useful as a first-aid for the treatment of burns.

6.) Kali Phos. (Potassium Phosphate)

Kali Phos. is a nerve nutrient. It is the remedy for ailments of a truly nervous character. School children often need this tissue-salt; it helps to maintain a happy, contented disposition and sharpens the mental faculties. Early symptoms may be very slight, scarcely noticeable in fact, except to a mother's watchful eye. There may be fretfulness, ill-humor, bashfulness, timidity, laziness, and similar indications; indeed, any display of what is sometimes described as "tantrums" may be regarded as a Kali Phos. symptom.

Kali Phos. is the remedy for nervous headaches, nervous dyspepsia, sleeplessness, depression, languid weariness, lowered vitality, grumpiness and many other conditions which may be summed up in the modern colloquial phrase, "lack of pep". But do not regard Kali Phos. as merely a pick-me-up. This tissue-salt is an important constituent of nervous tissue and consequently has a wide and powerful influence on the bodily functions. It covers those ailments comprehended by the term "nerves". Kali Phos. is also indicated in the treatment of irritating skin ailments, such as shingles, to correct the underlying nervous condition. It is helpful for breathing in nervous asthma. The symptoms are usually worse from mental and physical exertion and from cold. They are ameliorated by rest, warmth, and sometimes by eating.

7.) Kali Sulph. (Potassium Sulphate)

Kali Sulph. works in conjuction with Ferr. Phos as an oxygen-carrier. It assists in the exchange of oxygen from the blood stream to the tissue-cells, thereby completing the respiratory process initiated by Ferr. Phos. Internal breathing of the tissues depends upon Kali Sulph.; external breathing is the function of Ferr. Phos., if we designate the exchanges of gases in the lung in this way. Kali Sulph. has a beneficial effect on respiration and is indicated in those cases where there is a feeling of "stuffiness" or desire for cool air. It is also the anti-friction salt ensuring the smooth working of all parts, thus acting in the manner of a lubricant.

Kali Sulph. is indicated when there is a sticky, yellowish discharge from the skin or mucous membranes, as in certain forms of catarrh. Eruptions on the skin and scalp, with scaling, call for this remedy and it helps to maintain the hair in a healthy state. Other symptoms include chilliness and shifting, fleeting pains. It is useful in the treatment of intestinal disorders, stomach catarrh, and in inflammatory conditions to promote perspiration. The symptoms are generally worse in the evening, or in a closed, stuffy atmosphere, and are better in the fresh air.

8.) Mag. Phos. (Magnesium Phosphate)

Mag. Phos. is known as the anti-spasmodic tissue-salt. Its main function is in connection with the nervous system where it supplements the action of Kali Phos. When a deficiency of Mag. Phos. occurs, the white nerve fibers contract, causing spasms and cramps. This tissue-salt is of importance to muscular tissue ensuring rhythmic and coherent movement. Mag. Phos. is quick to relieve pain, especially cramping, shooting, darting, or spasmodic pains.

Mag. Phos. is indicated for nerve pains, such as neuralgia, neuritis, sciatica, and headaches accompanied by shooting, darting stabs of pain. It relieves muscular twitching, cramps, hiccups, convulsive fits of coughing and those sudden, sharp twinges of pain that are so distressing. It also relieves menstrual pains. Stomach cramps and flatulence respond to treatment with this tissue-salt. These symptoms may be aggravated by cold and by touching and are relieved by the application of heat, by pressure, and by bending double. The doses may be taken at frequent intervals until relief is obtained.

Because Magnesium has been assumed to be plentiful in the diet, some authorities have considered a deficiency unlikely. But this is not necessarily so, as recent research has proved that some diets provide insufficient Magnesium for the body's needs.

NOTE: Mag. Phos. will often act more rapidly when the tablets are taken with a sip of hot water.

9.) Nat. Mur. (Sodium Chloride)

Nat. Mur. is the water-distributing tissue-salt. It enters into the composition of every fluid and solid of the body. Because of its powerful affinity for water, it controls the ebb and flow of the bodily fluids; its prime function being to maintain a proper degree of moisture throughout the system. Without this tissue-salt, cell division and normal growth could not proceed. It is closely associated with nutrition, with glandular activity, and with the internal secretions which play such an important part in the physiological process. Excessive moisture or excessive dryness in any part of the system is a clear indication of a Nat. Mur. deficiency. The resulting symptoms are many and varied but always, underlying them, will be found this predominant condition of too much or too little water. Here are some typical symptoms:

Low spirits, with a feeling of hopelessness; headaches with constipation; blood thin and watery with pallor of the skin, which sometimes has a greasy appearance; difficult stools, with rawness and soreness of the anus; colds with discharge of watery mucus and sneezing; dry, painful nose and throat symptoms; heartburn (water brash) due to gastric fermentation with slow digestion (the food remains too long in the stomach); great thirst; tooth-ache and facial neuralgia with flow of tears and saliva; eyes weak, the wind causes them to water; hay fever, drowsiness with muscular weakness; chafing of the skin; hangnails; unrefreshing sleep - tired in the morning; after-effects of alcoholic stimulants; loss of taste and smell; craving for salt and salty foods. For stings and bites of insects apply locally as soon as possible.

An important function of Nat. Mur. is the production of Hydrochloric Acid. Too little acid means slow digestion, especially of Calcium rich foods.

Remember, approximately two-thirds of your body is composed of water; hence the vital role played by Nat. Mur., the water distributor, in all the life processes.

10.) Nat. Phos. (Sodium Phosphate)

Nat. Phos. is an acid neutralizer. It is the principal remedy for the wide group of ailments arising from an acid condition of the blood. This tissue-salt is also of importance for the proper functioning of the digestive organs. The assimilation of fats and other nutrients is dependent on the action of this remedy. A deficiency of Nat. Phos. allows uric acid to form salts which become deposited around the joints and tissues, giving rise to stiffness and swelling and other painful rheumatic symptoms.

Nat. Phos. is indicated whenever symptoms of acidity are present, such as acid dyspepsia, pain after eating, and similar digestive disorders. Other indications are highly colored urine, golden-yellow or creamy coating at the root of the tongue (the whole tongue may sometimes present the appearance of a piece of washleather), worms, or nervous irritability. Sleeplessness caused by indigestion can sometimes be remedied with a dose of Nat. Phos. kept handy by the bedside. This remedy is of importance in the treatment of rheumatism, lumbago, fibrositis and associated ailments. An acid state of the blood occurs when there is a deficiency of the soothing acid-neutralizing tissue-salt, Nat. Phos.

11.) Nat. Sulph. (Sodium Sulphate)

Nat. Sulph. regulates the density of the intercellular fluids (fluids which bathe the tissue-cells) by eliminating excess water. This tissue-salt largely controls the healthy functioning of the liver. It ensures an adequate supply of free-flowing, healthy bile, so necessary for the late stages of digestion. The removal of poison-charged fluids, which are the normal result of the chemical exchanges constantly taking place in the tissue-cells, is brought about by the action of Nat. Sulph. If conditions arise which allow these waste fluids to accumulate in the blood and tissues, autointoxication (self poisoning) is the result. Nat. Sulph. ensures the disposal of these poison-charged fluids and its importance in the treatment of rheumatic ailments is therefore self-evident.

Nat. Sulph. is indicated in the treatment of ailments affecting the liver, e.g. biliousness. Sandy deposits in the urine, watery infiltrations, a brownish-green coating of the tongue and a bitter taste in the mouth are some of the symptoms. It is the principal remedy in the treatment of influenza. Humid asthma, malaria, and other conditions associated with humidity need this remedy. A few doses of Nat. Sulph. will help to dispel that languid feeling so often experienced during a spell of humid, oppressive weather.

12.) Silica (Silicic Oxide)

Silica is a cleanser and an eliminator. It is a deep acting remedy which helps the body to throw off non-functional organic matter that may have arrived at a given point during Nature's effort to eliminate it from the system. It can often initiate the healing process by promoting suppuration and breaking up pathological accumulations, e.g. abscesses. Silica is a constituent of the hair, skin, nails, and surfaces of the bones. It also acts in the manner of an insulator for the nerves. In cases of checked perspiration, Silica restores the activity of the skin, thereby aiding this important cleansing process. It is the biochemic remedy for offensive perspiration of the feet and arm-pits.

Silica is indicated wherever there is pus formation or threatened suppuration, e.g. abscesses, boils, gumboils, styes, etc. It is useful in the treatment of tonsillitis when pus has begun to form. Brittle or crippled nails and diseases affecting the surfaces of the bones need this remedy. Silica is helpful as a supplementary remedy in cases of dyspepsia and pains in the region of the stomach. The symptoms are usually worse at night or in the morning and are relieved by the application of heat.

THE NEW REMEDIES

13.) Aurum Mur. (Chloride of Gold)

Gold is found in the brain, glands, and bones and for biochemic purposes, the Chloride is probably the best form. It is given for morbid mental conditions, sclerosis, female troubles, uterine tumors, some forms of paralysis, and also has some value in cases of high blood pressure. It seems to be well indicated in those persons who are inclined to produce growths of various kinds—the sycotic type.

We use this as an antidote to an Aluminum allergy.

14.) Argentum Nit. (Nitrate of Silver)

Silver acts mainly on the spinal cord and motor nerves. It is a powerful remedy for disorders associated with the motor nerves and for paralysis. In some respects it is similar to Kali Phos. Indeed, when the motor nerves are badly affected, Argentum Nit. probably takes first place as a dependable remedy. It may be administered from the $6\times$ potency upwards.

We use this as an antidote to Mercury poisoning.

15.) Antimonium Tart. (Tartrate of Antimony)

Antimonium Tart. has a profound action on the respiratory organs and mucous membranes. Given promptly it will often abort an attack of asthma, and is excellent for bronchitis, colds, coughs, and nasal catarrh. While the homeopaths employ this remedy over a wide field, the biochemist will use it mainly for the disorders mentioned in this book.

16.) Baryta Carb. (Carbonate of Baryta)

As with all other salts, this element is found in the blood and tissues.

It is helpful to backward and scrofulous children. Baryta Carb. is employed by biochemists mainly in the treatment of enlarged and septic tonsils, quinsy (for which it is a marvelous remedy), and for throat affections generally. It is helpful in paralysis, senile decay, and cysts.

Baryta Carb. has great value as a remedy for elderly people and may be taken in alternation with any indicated remedy.

17.) Calc. Iod. (Iodine of Lime)

The chemical laboratories of the body are the glands, and Iodine is one of the most important of the basic elements employed by the glandular system for the manufacture of its inimitable compounds. Iodine in the form of Calcium Iodide is, perhaps, the most important of the various Iodine combinations used in biochemistry.

When the endocrine glands are involved, Kali Iod. may be of greater value than Calc. Iod.

It is advised for emaciation with keen appetite, degeneration of the glandular tissues, weakness, malnutrition, toxemia, rheumatism, glandular disorders, chronic cough, night sweats, anemia, copious menses, movable nodules under the skin, atrophy of ovaries, dysentery, pustules and some skin diseases, painful discharges, deep-seated organic disease, etc.

Calc. Iod. works well with other indicated salts and is of profound importance in all wasting diseases. Cases calling for Iodine are usually "nervy" and restless. Dark, lean folk appear to require Iodine more than fair types, although it is often indicated for the latter.

18.) Cuprum (Copper)

This is found chiefly in the liver, also in the blood and nerve cells. Cuprum is used for anemia, especially when the liver is at fault, cramps, heavy sleep, hysteria, spasmodic affectations (similar to Mag. Phos., often producing effects when the salt fails), colic, dysmenorrhea, amenorrhea, and chlorosis. (Use the $6\times$ potency or higher)

19.) Cadmium Sulphate (Cadmic Sulphate)

This element surpasses Kali Phos. as a remedy for great depression. This remedy also kills the influenza virus, and the reader will note that influenza is always associated with mental depression. It is very doubtful if a better remedy exists for the above conditions. Cadmium also acts on the blood and nervous systems, so it is useful in cases of auto-toxemia and for some nervous complaints. For the treatment of influenza, the 30th potency should be given: five drops or five pills every two hours. Each dose may be taken with Ferr. Phos. and Kali Mur., also in the 30th potency. When the fever has gone, cease the Cadmium and take lower potency Schussler salts as indicated.

20.) Erbium (The metal)

This trace element is one of the new discoveries in medicine. Its action on the kidneys and nervous system is profound. Many serious kidney ailments and sclerosis have responded to Erbium, and for kidney trouble it appears to be superior to any other remedy. It may be administered from the 6th to the 30th potency. All the new trace elements are found in the human organism in very minute quantities, but are as vital as the smallest cog in an intricate machine.

21.) Graphites (Plumbago-Black Lead)

Strictly speaking this remedy does not come under the heading of biochemistry, but Carbon in this form plays such an important part in therapeutics that it has been included. It has a very wide range of action and is indicated in some nervous disorders, ear troubles, respiratory troubles, disorders of the mucus membranes, lymphatic complaints, indigestion, intestinal disorders and flatulence, soreness of the vagina, troubles associated with fat metabolism, skin disorders, tooth decay, brittle & crumbly nails, lack of energy due to weak suprarenal glands, thyroid deficiency, conjunctivitis, cysts, etc.

22.) Iridium. (The Metal)

The biochemist uses Iridium mainly for psoriasis and sometimes for anemia when other well-selected remedies fail. It is undoubtedly one of the best remedies for psoriasis.

23.) Kali Arsen. (Potassium Arsenicum.)

Although a poison, Arsenic is a valuable constituent of the blood and a lack of it results in great physical and mental exhaustion. When split up biochemically, it ceases to have any poisonous action, for its minute particles are then in a form that can be utilized by Nature. This is true of many substances which in a crude form are poisonous, but which are, in normal quantities, essential to the correct functional activity of the human organism and which are always found in a healthy body. Arsenic employed biochemically is usually in combination with Potassium.

It is indicated for profound prostration and exhaustion (especially with fair types, and frequently for others), heart disorders and weakness, anemia that does not repond to the Schussler salts and Calc. Iod., septic or non-septic disorganization of the blood, all pains and symptoms that are relieved by heat, brain and nervous disorders, and skin diseases. As a rule, people requiring Kali Arsen. have a clay coloured complexion, anxious features, and dark rings around the eyes.

They are lacking in patience and want to change from one remedy to another. Although more suited to fair people this is by no means a fixed rule, and there are many exceptions.

24.) Kali Brom. (Potassium Bromide)

Kali Brom. is a most valuable element associated with brain and nerve functions.

This remedy has a normalizing effect on the intestines and is useful for most affectations of the bowels associated with pain, contraction, and inflammation.

Kali Brom. is indicated in all disorders of nerve and brain cells when there is degeneration and evidence of mental failure, generative troubles, wasting diseases associated with the brain and nervous system, croup, some skin diseases, cysts, etc. People requiring this remedy are better without common salt with their meals.

25.) Kali Bichromicum. (Biochromate of Potash.)

This remedy has a very wide range of action and is often indicated for asthma, catarrh, and disorders of the mucus membranes. In several respects it is similar to Kali Mur. It is of great value in cases of progressive muscular atrophy, cirrhosis of the liver, anemia, nephritis, polypus, and dilation of the heart and stomach. Whenever a catarrhal condition is present, think of Kali Bich. It helps in all respiratory troubles.

26.) Kali Silicatum. (Silicate of Potash.)

Kali Sil. is used for general debility, lassitude, and lack of muscular tone. Many cases of this nature which have failed to respond to other remedies have made excellent progress after a few doses of Kali Sil. However, the suggested dose is once every other day in the 50th potency for two or three weeks. Results are not to be expected from the lower potencies and so are not advised.

27.) Mercurius. (Quicksilver.)

In orthodox medicine this has proved to be a very damaging remedy as it tends to bring about serious degeneration of the bones, teeth, and gums. In fact, Mercurius in Allopathic doses will eventually cause the very conditions to manifest for which it is administered. On the other hand the same remedy in potency is harmless and has the very opposite effects, being a reliable medicine for many troubles associated with the skeletal system and disorganization of the blood. Mercurius seems to affect every organ and tissue, and is an outstanding example of how a medicinal malignant force can be converted into a life-saving preparation by trituration and potentising. It has been used by the orthodox profession for venereal disease (with disastrous effects in countless cases) and will produce constructive results in such troubles when employed in the 6 × trituration upwards. It is good for ulceration of the mouth and gums, tooth decay, rheumatoid arthritis, trembling, foul excretions, colds with ulcerated nostrils, pains in the bones, enlargement of the liver, and skin disorders associated with itching. Mercurius may be tried when the more usual remedies fail to act. An irritated state of the veins may call for this remedy.

28.) Neodynum Oxide. (Oxide of Neodymium.)

This is one of the new remedies. The biochemist employs Neodynum in this form for paralysis agitans, for which disorder it has produced the most desirable results. Not enough is known concerning this preparation for further comment.

29.) Platina. (The Metal.)

This remedy seems to be indicated more frequently for females than for males, and it is to be thought of in all cases of hysteria, especially when of sexual origin. It is a useful remedy for highly emotional states, weariness of life, vaginismus, nymphomania, and ovaritis. For emotional states give the 30th potency once daily for a while. Give the 6 × potency for physical conditions. Platina has been found to be most helpful when the sufferer is very anxious about members of the family and friends, also for inhibited people, and those who find great difficulty in relaxing in mind and body. Another peculiar mental symptom calling for Platina is anxiety over the digestive organs (e.g., fear of malignant conditions being present). A feeling of sexual inferiority may also call for this remedy in both men and women.

30.) Palladium. (The Metal.)

An outstanding remedy for prolapse of the uterus, retroversion and misplacements in general. Also has a favorable action on the ovaries, particularly on the right. States of fatigue related to generative troubles will receive benefit from Palladium. Another use for this metal is for blood disorders associated with staphylococcus; hence it has its uses in obstinate skin disorders, boils, disorganization of the blood, and septic conditions.

31.) Plumbum. (Lead.)

This salt is found in the brain, nerves, and mucous membranes.

A remedy for sclerotic conditions, progressive muscular atrophy, spinal degeneration, mental depression, neuralgia, constipation, amenorrhea, menorrhagia, menopause, chlorosis, and intestinal troubles. Use the 6x potency or higher.

32.) Radium. (Radium Bromide.)

On no account should this form of Radium be employed medicinally below the 16× potency. The 30th is recommended. In all potencies from 16× upwards it is a harmless and potent remedy. It is of undoubted value in cancer and relief of pain in all parts of the body which are made worse by moving about. It has been used with success in the treatment of ulcers and acne rosasea. In diarrhea and dysentery Radium Bromide is a most useful remedy, removing some of the toxic causes and relieving the pain. According to Dr. Guyon Richards it kills a virus found in such conditions. The dose should be once daily in the 16× or 30th potency. Other remedies should be taken separately.

33.) Selenium (The Element.)

Selenium is found in the bones and teeth. It is useful in laryngitis and general debility, senile decay, and impotency. Itching of the skin, acne and alopecia may also call for this element. Perhaps its outstanding action is on the sexual organs and in sexual neurasthenia.

34.) Samarium. (The Element.)

Another of the new remedies whose main action is on the sexual organs of both sexes, and we employ it exclusively for this purpose. For low tone of the testes it is one of the best remedies and is somewhat similar to Selenium. Low tone of the ovaries, with local pain of these glands, may respond to this mineral. When other remedies fail it may be tried in cases of sexual neurasthenia.

35.) Strontia. (Carbonate of Strontia.)

A remedy of profound importance in high blood pressure, arteriosclerosis, arterial troubles, and after effects of surgical operations (shock). Headaches due to congestion and blood pressure may call for this remedy, also the nausea so often associated with these conditions. It restores tone to brittle arteries and also to the heart muscle, and should be considered in cases of auto-toxemia and a morbid state of the intestines. For nervous dyspepsia with great flatulence and excess of acid try Strontia Bromide. This form of Strontia is also good for the vomiting of pregnancy. As a rule the indication for Strontia is high blood pressure with congestion, when it is a very potent remedy. It is unlikely to help in any condition when the blood pressure is low.

36.) Stannum. (Tin.)

Stannum is found mainly in the superficial tissues of the body.

It can be used for respiratory, skin and nervous diseases, violent cough which is excited by talking or laughing, expectoration of yellowish green mucous, sick headache (megrim), defects of the nails, cysts, and pains which come and go gradually. People requiring Stannum are usually sad and anxious; they dread company and meeting others.

37.) Titanium. (The Metal.)

While found mainly in the bones and muscles, we use it for shingles and irritating conditions of the skin and nerve endings. It Has been employed with some success in Lupus. In all these conditions, there is likely to be a call for additional remedies.

38.) Tellurium. (The Metal.)

For eczema (especially behind the ears), catarrh of the middle ear, and mastoiditis. It is the latter condition that usually calls for this remedy. Some cases of sciatica yield to Tellurium when other remedies fail.

39.) Thorium. (The Element.)

To date this new remedy has been employed for chronic disorders of the mucous membranes only. It may be tried with hopes of succes in chronic catarrh when the condition does not respond to the better known remedies.

40.) Thallium Oxide. (The Oxide of Thallium.)

Seems to exert a powerful influence on the endocrine glands and nervous system. It is indicated for muscular atrophy, paralysis (especially of the lower limbs), locomotor ataxia, numbness of the extremities, and alopecia. Cerebral irritation will sometimes respond to the remedy, probably because of its action on the thyroid and other endocrines. Sharp, neuralgic pain may respond to Thallium.

41.) Tantalum. (The Element.)

A new remedy in biochemistry, it has so far been employed as a medicine for the menopause and is of much value for flushes. Until more is known about Tantalum it should be used for menopause symptoms only.

42.) Zincum. (Zinc.)

Found in the blood, nerves and brain, Zincum appears to have an affinity for the nerve endings.

It is excellent in brain fag and works well with Kali Phos. and Mag. Phos., or it may be employed when those remedies do not produce results. Intense fidgetiness may be regarded as a sure indication for Zincum. Neuralgia, pruritus, formication of skin, headache over eyes, burning eyes, neurasthenia, delirium, emaciation, phlebitis, etc. are all indications that Zincum is needed.

43.) Chromium

1× or 3× See Chromium page 58.

44.) Manganese

1× or 3× See Manganese page 65.

45.) Sulfur

1× or 3× See Sulfur page 81.

CHAPTER 10

GLANDULAR THERAPY

In glandular therapy, the philosophy is: "Like cell helps like cells". When a glandular substance is taken in by the body, it immediately goes to the gland in the body that is similar to it. For example, if a Pituitary gland tablet (usually of Bovine nature) is ingested it will immediately enter the blood stream and be used as nourishment for the Pituitary gland.

In 1958 and also in 1972 in a German medical publication, Dr. A. Kemet documented through radioactive isotope tracing, that factors from glandular tissues were taken up by the bloodstream and absorbed by corresponding glands in the recipient. Glandulars are not hormones, but activate the glands to produce hormones. The entire point in glandular therapy is to normalize the affected gland or tissue. Other names used for raw glandular substances are concentrates, extracts, protomorphagens, nucleoproteins, and cytottophins.

Until now it was quite complicated to pin-point the dormant or non-functioning gland, but with the M.R.T. system it is quite simple and accurate. Let me show you how!

The M.R.T. acupuncture point for the Pineal gland is found on the top of the head. (The Hindu "Crown Chakra".)

(See Figure 59)

The Pineal gland is located:

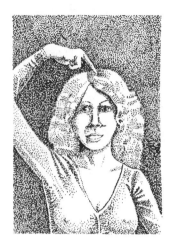

Figure 59

If upon touching this point the extended other arm goes down when pressed, this is showing that the Pineal gland is weak. By placing one (or as many as needed to strengthen the extended arm) Pineal trophic pill in the hand, the arm should become rigid. If too many pills are added and you overdose, the arm will again become weak. The amount that finally shows strong is the amount that is presently needed by that person.

The Pineal gland, spiritually, is the entrance point to the body for divine revelation (Crown Chakra). On a physical level it controls skin pigmentation, mental sanity, and it helps the Pituitary gland to hold the Potassium and Sodium levels in the body.

Other corrective nutrients for the Pineal gland are:

Glandular Concentrate: Pineal Trophic
Herbs: Wood Betony and Gotu Kola
Vitamins: Vitamin E and Vitamin B-6
Minerals: Manganese, Potassium, and Sodium
Amino Acids: Taurine, Ornithine, and Tryptophan

PITUITARY GLAND

The M.R.T. acupuncture point for the Pituitary gland is found on the forehead directly above the nose, one-eighth of an inch below the hair line (approximately one-and-a-half inches above the R.N.A. point).

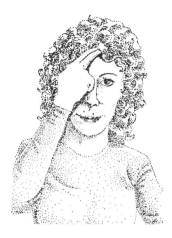

Figure 60

Place one finger on the Pituitary point and extend the opposite arm. Press down on extended arm. If arm goes down or shows weak, this is a sign that the Pituitary gland is malfunctioning.

Place the corrective nutrient in the hand and touch this point with the fingers of the same hand. The extended arm should then be strong when it is "pumped".

The Pituitary is the "Master Gland" because it commands all other glands to function, making it the most important gland in the endocrine system. The Pituitary gland produces at least six hormones that govern a wide range of body processes.

Produced in the anterior Pituitary lobe are: TSH (Thyrotropin), a hormone that stimulates Thyroid functions; ACTH (Adrenocorticotropic hormone) which stimulates activity of the Adrenal cortex; FSH (Follicle stimulating hormone) which regulates the production of sperm or eggs; LH (Leutinizing Hormone) which triggers the manufacture of testosterone in the testes in the male and the Corpus Luteum (ovaries) in females; Prolactin, which stimulates the secretion of milk as well as parental behavior; and GH (growth hormone) which governs cellular metabolism.

Two parts of the brain known as the Hypothalamus and Hippocampus, control the hormone output to the Pituitary gland. Receptor proteins located in the hypothalamus respond to hormone levels secreted by the glands of the body. If proteins are not working properly, the hypothalamus cells will not put out enough of the substance that is normally sent to the pituitary gland to signal it to stimulate the body gland needing stimulation.

Tyrosine Hydroxylase is an enzyme located in the hypothalamus that diminishes with oncoming age. Tyrosine hydroxylase has a very important role to play with nervous system functions and Hormone level regulation. Diminished production of this enzyme causes diminished production of two other substances in the hypothalamus which signals the pituitary to send ACTH (Adrenocorticotropic hormone) to the adrenal gland to put out more Cortisol. These two substances are norepinephrine and dopamine.

With aging and decreased production of Tyrosine Hydroxylase, Dopamine, Norepinephrine, and other substances, there is a loss of control of all glands and the production of hormones because the Pituitary does not get the proper signals. The importance of receiving the proper nutrition to nourish the cells in the proper proportions they require can never be stressed sufficiently.

The Pituitary gland is a cornerstone in the endocrine system as it operates in a feedback system with other glands.

Corrective nutrients used for the Pituitary gland:

Glandular Concentrate: Pituitary substance
Herbs: Gotu Kola, Ginseng
Vitamins: Vitamin B-6, Vitamin E, Vitamin B-Complex
Minerals: Manganese, Selenium, Trace Minerals
Amino Acids: Ornithine, Tryptophan, Taurine

If and when there is a nasal drip or continuous mucous discharge from the nose, it is usually caused by a "leaky" Pituitary gland. This continuous nasal drip can also drip down the throat into the chest while sleeping, causing an excessive accumulation of phlegm in the chest.

The way to check to see if this is the cause is to place a finger over each center of the eyebrows and extend opposite arm. If extended arm goes down when "pumped", this is an indication that the Pituitary gland is discharging into the sinus glands above the eyebrows causing them to drain into the nasal passages.

See Figure 61.

Some of the things that are useful in correcting this situation are Alfalfa and GH Release (Growth Hormone Release; a combination of Vitamin B-6, Pituitary glandular, and amino acids Ornithine and Tryptophan).

NOTE: My own research indicates many illnesses are due to a lack of Potassium and Sodium which I believe are affected by the Pituitary and Pineal glands. When either of these glands are

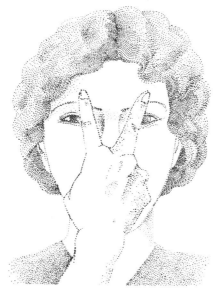

Figure 61

weak there is usually the inability to sustain the Potassium and Sodium levels. Both Potassium and Sodium are passed out of the body through the excretion of urine.

THYROID GLAND

The M.R.T. acupuncture point for the Thyroid gland is located in the hollow of the neck by the joint of the clavicles, about 2 inches below the Adam's apple on the neck. (The same point as the Iodine point.)

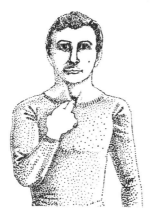

Figure 62

To test this point, have one or two fingers touching it while extending the other arm to be "pumped". If the extended arm goes down when pressed, place a Thyroid glandular capsule or Kelp or Dulse pill in the palm and again touch it to the Thyroid point while pumping the extended arm. Add or subtract the amount of pills in the palm until the extended arm becomes rigid, this will show the proper amount needed to correct the situation.

The Thyroid gland is located in the front part of the neck and consists of two lobes joined by a narrow band of tissue. The Thyroid is the largest of all the endocrine glands, weighing about two-thirds of an ounce.

The Thyroid gland secretes a hormone called Thyroxin which regulates the rate of metabolism of human cells. The mineral Iodine, and the amino acid Tyrosine, are the most important components of Thyroxin. If the Thyroid gland does not absorb enough Iodine from the bloodstream, it will become enlarged in its effort to entrap more, thus becoming a condition called "Goiter".

A properly functioning Thyroid produces just the right amount of Thyroxin necessary to maintain a normal rate of metabolism for the rest of the body. This metabolic rate may be measured by the amount of heat generated within the body. This is called the Basal Metabolic Rate (B.M.R.).

Hyperthyroidism is a condition in which there is an excess of Thyroid hormone. This condition tends to create a feeling of heat and the body will tend to lose weight due to the fact that more fuel is being burned even though there may be a tremendous appetite. Bulging eyes, nervousness, and mental aberrations are also common in this condition.

Hypothyroidism is a condition in which there is insufficient Thyroid hormone (a weak Thyroid or a lack of Iodine or Tyrosine in the system). In this condition, the body tends to feel cold and the individual becomes puffy faced, obese, sluggish, dull-witted, and in extreme cases, a semi-vegetable.

Other hormones produced by the Thyroid are Triiodothyronine, which influences physical and mental growth; and Calcitonin, which prevents a build up of calcium in the blood by balancing the hormone from the Parathyroid, which maintains blood levels of Calcium by drawing Calcium from the bones and teeth.

Through our research we believe that many "weak" Thyroids are actually strong, but their "controller", the Pituitary, is malfunctioning causing the Thyroid to malfunction also. So, in determining the cause of the Thyroid problem, also be sure to check the Pituitary gland. Corrective nutrients used for the Thyroid gland:

Glandular Substance: Thyroid glandular concentrate
Herbs: Kelp, Dulse
Vitamins: Vitamin B-6, Vitamin B-Complex
Minerals: Iodine, Potassium, and Sodium
Amino Acids: Tyrosine

THYMUS GLAND

The M.R.T. acupuncture point for the Thymus gland is located in the center of the upper part of the chest about 2½ inches below the Thyroid point.

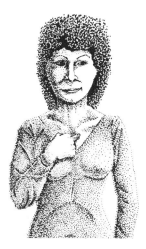

Figure 63

To check the Thymus gland, place one or two fingers on the Thymus point and extend the opposite arm to be pumped. If the extended arm cannot stay rigid, then this is an indication that the Thymus gland is weak.

If the Thymus gland shows weak, place a Thymus glandular pill (or as many that are needed to make the arm strong) and test the arm again. The correct amount has been found when the extended arm stays rigid and does not go down when pressed. Another substance that can be used to stimulate and normalize the Thymus gland is a product called Bee Propolis.

The Thymus gland controls the immunological defense system of the body. It stimulates the production of white blood cells, an important defense against disease and infection. Lymphocytes created in the Thymus migrate into the blood stream and colonize lymph nodes throughout the body. These lymphocytes later begin to manufacture the still more powerful antibodies vital for immunity.

In our research, we have found that the Thymus gland, the key gland in the body's immune system, is affected by a person's thoughts and attitude. What I mean by this is if a person thinks positive, the Thymus gland will test strong!! If a person is a negative thinker (the "woe is me" type), the Thymus gland will test weak.

This can be substantiated by a simple demonstration! Place your finger on your Thymus gland and extend your opposite arm. Have a friend pump the extended arm while you first think a positive thought. The arm should be strong. Now relax, and do the whole thing again, but now think a negative thought. The Thymus gland will test weak this time. This brings about a very important thought. To get well, a patient must think positively!! A person must have a positive attitude in order to get well. If the person doesn't, the practitioner should try to make the client believe the practitioner will help the client get well through the practitioner's direction. This is not giving the person false hopes!! Miracles can and have happened.

God helps people who help themselves. I often teach my clients about faith, hope and charity. Faith in God, Faith in themselves (because God doesn't make junk!), and faith in their friends, among whom their practitioner is.

In regards to hope, a person who is terminally ill should have hope because the situation usually cannot get any worse, but only better! And love (charity) is what life is all about. Love God, love yourself! Loving one's self is very important, for it is impossible to "Love thy neighbor as thyself" if you don't love yourself!!

Many illnesses are caused by a lack of love!! People who feel unloved often "will" themselves to become ill subconsciously, if not consciously, because by being sick they often receive sympathy. They will soon learn, though, that sympathy is no substitute for love. If you want to be loved, start loving! Find goodness in everything—the rain, the sun, the heavens, the convenience of the 20th century! Find goodness in your environment. It is easy to criticize, but hard to do! Do not bring down others to bring yourself up. Rejoice in thy neighbor's wellness, and do not focus on your own illnesses. By doing this you will heal by strengthening your Thymus gland and strengthening your immune system.

If you continually amplify your illness, it will stick with you. By saying "I have this and this, etc.," you will weaken your Thymus gland and your immune system will also become worse. So, Dr. Norman Vincent Peale was and is right on the money when he promoted and still promotes positive thinking!!

Corrective nutrients used for the Thymus gland:

Glandular Substance: Thymus substance
Herbs: Bee Propolis
Vitamins: Niacin, Vitamin B-complex
Minerals: Potassium and Sodium
Amino Acids: L-Phenylalanine and Tyrosine

ADRENAL GLAND

The M.R.T. acupuncture point for the Adrenal gland is found in the center of the body, approximately 2 to 3 inches above the navel (according to the length of the torso). The point is located one-third the distance up the center seam line from the navel to the sternum (breast bone).

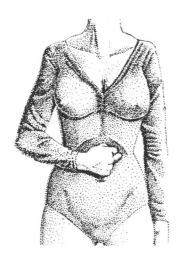

Figure 64

Even though there are two Adrenal glands sitting on top of the kidneys, the point is in the solar plexus area. The Adrenal glands are very small, weighing about ⅛ of an ounce each, and have two main functioning parts: the medulla and the cortex.

The medulla manufactures Epinephrine (Adrenaline) and Norepinephrine (Noradrenalin). The outer portion, which is the adrenal cortex, produces glucocorticoids (steroids) which, among other things, are involved in blood sugar regulation and inflammatory responses. Mineral corticoids, also produced by the cortex, regulate minerals in the body by retention and excretion, especially Sodium and Potassium.

Raw Adrenal substance was the first widely used glandular, and is presently the most popular. For years, it has been specified for carbohydrate dysfunctions (hypoglycemia and diabetes), fatigue, and improving resistance to infection and allergies. In stressful situations, the Adrenal glands must send various hormones to organs that counteract stress. This accelerated pace, caused by stress, cannot be maintained for a long period of time without exhausting the supply of nutrients that feed the Adrenal glands.

In our research we have found that when Adrenal glands become exhausted, the person immediately becomes allergic to citrus fruits (lemons, limes, oranges, grapefruits, tomatoes, pineapple, cantaloupe, and all bioflavonoids). The nutrient that corrects this condition is Vitamin B-5 (Pantothenic Acid), at least 2000 mgs. In my practice I use a product called "Royal Jelly", which is a natural source of Pantothenic acid and Niacin (Vitamin B-3). One 1000 mg. capsule of Royal Jelly has the potency of a 500 mg. Pantothenic acid pill, and a 500 mg. Niacin pill (without the "flush" of Niacin).

Another problem that may occur when the Adrenals are exhausted, is a sinus condition. To check this out, place a finger on each side of the nose about ¾ inches away from the nose with one hand while extending the other arm to be "pumped". If the extended arm goes down when pressed, this is an indication that the sinuses are inflamed. Inflamed sinuses in this case are caused by the citrus allergy because of stress and exhaustion of the adrenal glands. See Fig. 65, next page.

To dry up the sinuses, the things to use are Pantothenic acid (Royal Jelly) and Vitamin C (which cannot have a citrus flavoring or contain bioflavonoids).

To test the sinuses, place a finger on each side of the nose while extending opposite arm to be "pumped"!

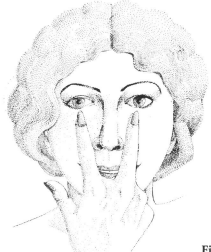

Figure 65

The Adrenals are vital to many life processes, such as regulating the immune response system that allows for quick healing with less pain. The steroid hormones reduce inflammation and help govern the immune response. The adrenals help in the distribution of muscle tissue and coping with day to day stress. Aging has been also linked to stress, causing a gradual deterioration of the glands.

Addison's disease is a result of poor adrenal function. Some symptoms of this disease are weight loss, nausea, low blood pressure, and brownish pigmentation of the skin and mucous membranes. Corrective nutrients used for the Adrenal glands:

Glandular Substance: Adrenal Concentrate
Vitamins: Pantothenic Acid (Vitamin B-5), Vitamin A, Vitamin C
Minerals: Potassium, Sodium, Magnesium, Calcium

PANCREAS

The M.R.T. acupuncture point for the Pancreas is found 2 to 3 inches to the left of the Adrenal point. (According to the size of the person's torso.)

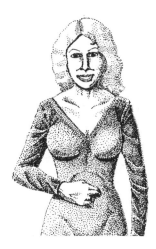

Figure 66

To test the Pancreas, place your fingers over the Pancreas while extending opposite arm to be pumped. If extended arm goes down when pressed, this is showing that the Pancreas may be weak and perhaps malfunctioning.

The Pancreas governs Glucose metabolism by secreting insulin for the metabolism of sugars, and enzyme precursors for the digestion of food components. The Pancreas produces the hormone Insulin, which is necessary for the conversion of Glucose (blood sugar) to Glycogen (stored sugar). The Pancreas also produces another hormone, Glucagon; which converts Glycogen back to blood sugar (Glucose) as needed.

Diabetes results when the Pancreas is unable to produce enough insulin. Diabetes is a carbohydrate dysfunction that is usually treated by oral or intravenous injections of insulin obtained from the pancreatic glands of animals.

Corrective nutrients used for the Pancreas:

Glandular substance: Pancreas concentrate
Vitamins: B-Complex
Minerals: Chromium, Selenium, Manganese, and Sodium
Amino Acids: Isoleucine, Leucine, and Valine (Kreb cycle nutrients)
Herbs: Juniper Berries, Uva Ursi, Saw Palmetto, Golden Seal

REPRODUCTIVE ORGANS

The M.R.T. acupuncture point for the prostate gland is located on the male pubic bone to either side of the penis.

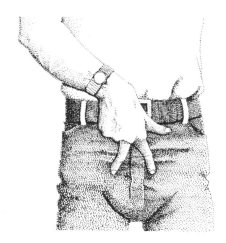

Figure 67

To test the prostate gland, hold two fingers of one hand to this point while extending opposite arm to be pumped. If extended arm goes down when pumped, this is showing that the prostate is weak. The corrective substance for the prostate would be prostate glandular substance or Zinc.

To test the amount needed, place the prostate substance or Zinc tablets in hand while holding to M.R.T. prostate point. Add or subtract amount of tablets until extended arm becomes rigid. This will show you the amount needed at this time.

Many prostate conditions are caused by an absence of Zinc. When the gland is "hungry" for Zinc, it will often swell in size causing a choking effect on the urinary passage way. Sometimes the prostate, like other glands, will become "petrified". This is caused by a lack of Magnesium. Both conditions can be reversed!! This can be done over a period of time nutritionally, and with gentle finger tip massage therapy through the anus.

A prostate problem usually develops because of a Zinc deficiency.

Zinc, along with Selenium, and the amino acid Arginine, are the elements of sperm and semen which are lost through ejaculation.

Many men are misdiagnosed as having a prostate problem if they have nocturnal urinations (over 4 per night); but in reality this could be a lack of GABA (Gamma Amino Butyric Acid), or a lack of Sodium. This could also be caused by drinking liquids before bedtime, especially if the person is allergic to whatever it is they are drinking. For instance, if the person usually drinks milk before retiring, and is allergic to milk, it will cause a nocturnal urination problem because the body is trying to pass the allergic substance out of the body.

Corrective nutrients for the prostate:

Glandular substance: Prostate substance
Vitamins: Vitamin E
Minerals: Zinc and Selenium
Amino Acids: Ornithine and Arginine
Herbs: Damiana, Ginseng

TESTES

The M.R.T. point for the testes is the scrotum. To test this, have the person place one palm on the scrotum while extending opposite arm. This can be done while the person's pants are still on by having him place his hand and arm through his belt into his pants. This will save a lot of embarrassment, especially if the practitioner is a female. I often omit this point if there is no specific reason to test it.

The testes produce the hormone Testosterone and other androgens. These hormones all govern the development of the male characteristics, such as the growth of a beard and body hair, deepening voice, and sex drive, and inhibit follicular stimulating hormone (FSH) from the pituitary in a feedback system.

Corrective nutrients used for the testes:

Glandular substance: Teste substance or Orchic substance
Vitamins: Vitamin B-6
Minerals: Zinc and Selenium
Amino Acids: Arginine
Herbs: Damiana, Sarsaparilla, Ginseng
NOTE: The herb "Yohimba" is known to be a sexual stimulant to men, and so is useful if a male has trouble with an erection.

"Yohimba" is available from many homeopathic pill manufacturers much cheaper than what it is sold for at other sources.

OVARIES

The M.R.T. acupuncture point for the ovaries is located approximately 3½ inches below the navel and about 2½ inches from the middle body seam on both the right and left side of the body.

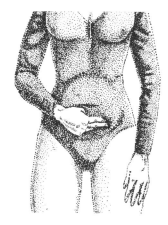

Figure 68

To test the ovaries place two fingers on the ovary point while extending opposite arm to be pumped. If extended arm goes down or shows weak, this is an indication that the ovary is mal-functioning. The corrective substance for the ovaries would be ovarian substance.

To test the amount needed, place the ovarian tablets in the palm while again touching the ovary point and extending opposite arm to be pumped. Add or subtract amount of pills in hand until extended arm is rigid when pressed. This will show the correct amount needed at this time.

Each ovary is composed of two distinct areas: the follicles and the corpus luteum, which have somewhat distinctive functions as well. The follicle produces Estradiol and other estrogens. Estrogen is the female hormone responsible for development of primary and secondary sexual characteristics of the female. This includes development of the breasts, widening of the hips, distribution of body fat, and the onset of menstruation.

GLAND CHART

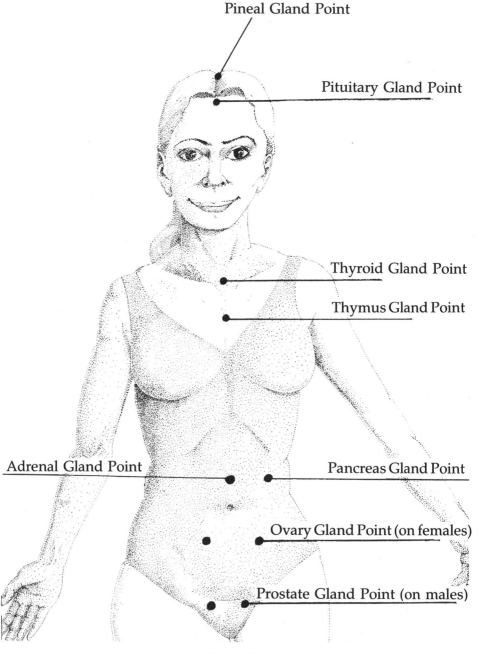

Pineal Gland Point

Pituitary Gland Point

Thyroid Gland Point

Thymus Gland Point

Adrenal Gland Point

Pancreas Gland Point

Ovary Gland Point (on females)

Prostate Gland Point (on males)

Figure 69

The corpus luteum manufactures Progesterone. This hormone stimulates secretions of the oviduct, uterus growth in pregnancy, and also inhibits Leutinizing Hormone (LH) secretion from the pituitary. Both Estrogen and Progesterone interact in the regulation of the menstrual-ovulatory cycle and pregnancy.

The endocrine function of the ovaries is the development and expulsion of the egg or ovum. This is the female counterpart of the male sperm.

Corrective nutrients used for the ovaries:

Glandular substance: Ovarian substance and Uterus extract
Vitamins: Vitamin E
Minerals: Calcium, Magnesium, and Zinc
Herbs: Dong Quai, Sarsaparilla

ORGANS
THE HEART

The first organ we will discuss is the heart. The primary heart M.R.T. acupuncture point is found one inch above the bottom of the sternum (breast bone). The secondary heart point is approximately 2 to 2½ inches below the arm pits on the rib cage of the left side (1.2 inch above the Serta-Magnus muscle).

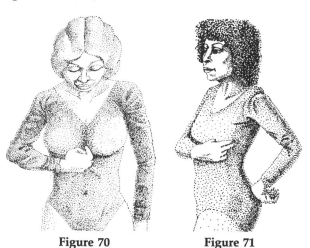

Figure 70   Figure 71

The heart is the circulatory pump of the body. In taking blood pressure, the high number, or systolic pressure, shows the pressure when the heart is contracted, while the diastolic pressure (low number) shows the pressure when the heart is relaxed. We have found that if there is an absence of Sodium, the systolic pressure will be too high, and with an absence of Potassium, the diastolic will also be too high.

We have found that a blood pressure reading can actually be changed by the ingestion of the proper electrolytes (Sodium and Potassium). Nutrients for the heart include:

Alfalfa (rich in Potassium and Sodium)
Bee Pollen (rich in Potassium)
Hawthorne Berries
Heart Glandular substance
Lecithin
Calcium
Magnesium
Selenium
Carnitine
Taurine

If when testing a person the heart shows weak, place the amount of Potassium in the client's hand while touching it to the heart point with opposite arm extended. Press down on extended arm to test strength. The arm should now be rigid while holding the correct amount of Potassium to the heart point.

Never concern a client needlessly by indicating there is something wrong with the heart. The correct thing to tell the client is that there is nothing wrong with the heart except that it is lacking the fuel (electrolytes) that permits it to run!

I often tell my clients that without fuel, the vehicle can't run. For instance, if you were driving a brand new Cadillac down Main Street and it ran out of gas, it would die! That doesn't mean there's something wrong with the engine, it's just out of gas!! The same thing happens with the heart.

Many heart conditions are due to a lack of electrolytes and existing allergies that could inflame the heart.

KIDNEYS

The kidneys can be tested by placing the right hand flat on the side of the waist while extending the opposite arm to be pumped. Use the same hand for both right and left kidney because sometimes the right and left arm differ in strength.

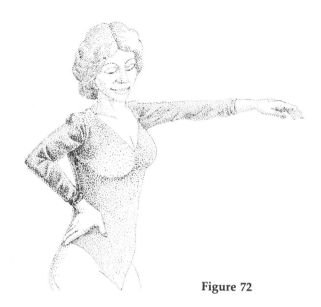

Figure 72

If the arm should go down when testing the kidneys, have the client go to the rest room and empty their bladder then re-test the kidneys. If the kidney is now okay, then test the bladder by placing the open palm over the lower abdomen while extending the opposite arm. If the extended arm goes down when testing the bladder, this means that debris has passed from the kidney into the bladder and will probably be passed out of the body the next time the bladder is relieved. If the kidney still tests weak when they return from the bathroom, this could mean that there is some calcification or a stone forming. This can be corrected by administering Magnesium & cranberry juice over a period of time. To find the amount of Magnesium needed, place the Magnesium in the hand while holding to solar plexus (see Magnesium Page 65.) If the kidneys still show weak after the bladder is relieved, then the kidneys should be checked again while holding the predetermined amount of Magnesium in the hand.
Corrective nutrients for the kidneys:

Magnesium, Golden Seal Herb, Juniper Berries, Uva Ursi, Parsley, Ginger, Marshmallow, Vitamin A, Vitamin B-6, Vitamin C, Vitamin E, and Lecithin.

It should be noted that the adrenal glands sit on the ends of the kidneys, and when there is a pain in the back area of the kidney this could very well mean that the adrenal glands are under stress and causing the pain. In this case, Pantothenic Acid (Vitamin B-5 contained in Royal Jelly) should be administered. Please refer to chapter   on Adrenal glands.

If a stone does exist in the kidney and is being reduced in size by the use of Magnesium and cranberry juice, it could pass into the ureter which carries the urine from the kidneys to the bladder. If this happens, please do not stop administering the Magnesium and cranberry juice until the stone passes into the bladder. Stopping them too soon could cause the stone to lodge and possibly block the passage to the bladder.

BLADDER

The bladder can be tested by placing the "pinkie" side of the hand on the lower abdomen, about 1 inch above the pubic bone, while extending the other arm to be "pumped".

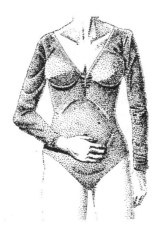

Figure 73

If the extended arm goes down when pumped, it may mean that the bladder contains debris or calcification. To find out if this is the problem, place the predetermined amount of Magnesium in the hand while holding over bladder. If the arm now shows strong, this may mean that the bladder contains a Calcium deposit, stone, or debris. Before

Please see chapter 4 on Magnesium.

alarming the person of this possible condition, ask them to use the rest room to empty their bladder.

After they have emptied the bladder, retest the bladder without the Magnesium. If the bladder now shows strong, this indicates that the debris has passed out of the body and that a condition does not exist and that the debris was probably only in the transitional stage.

If when re-testing the bladder, the extended arm goes down, place the predetermined amount of Magnesium in the hand, hold over bladder, and re-test. If the bladder now tests strong with the Magnesium, this is showing that there is some calcification or stones in the bladder.

To clear the bladder, administer the needed Magnesium along with lots of cranberry juice. Also, withhold any Calcium supplements until the problem has cleared up. Females have less trouble passing stones than males, but males will also eventually pass debris and gravel out in the urine, so do not stop using the needed Magnesium until the gravel and sand have appeared in the urine.

LUNGS

To test the lungs, place the fingertips of the test hand under the last (lower) rib (either side—depending on which lung you are testing). Push the fingertips inward about 2 inches while turning them upward as if to slip the fingertips under the rib cage. To make it easier and painless you can have the person bend forward while doing this, as it will loosen the muscles in the abdomen area.

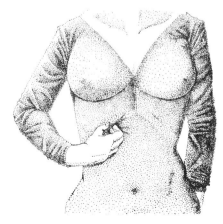

Figure 74

When testing each lung, have the person extend the opposite arm to be pumped. If extended arm goes down when pumped, place a pre-determined amount of Vitamin B-15 in the test hand and insert the finger tips again under the rib cage. The extended arm should now show strong.

GALLBLADDER

The M.R.T. acupuncture point for the Gallbladder is similar to the lung test on the right side, but you would not go under the rib cage and turn the fingers up.

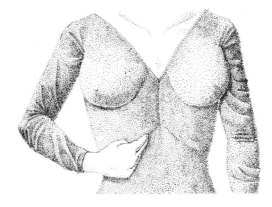

Figure 75

If the extended opposite arm goes down when testing the gallbladder, this may be showing that gallstones are present.

To melt the stones and permit them to fall into the stomach to pass through the intestines, we would use Lecithin, Vitamin C, and Bran. I have also successfully used Magnesium, Methionine, Cysteine, and Taurine to help alleviate gallbladder conditions. I have also found that a gallbladder disorder is usually caused by a "fat allergy". If upon testing, the person does have an allergy to fats, then the gallbladder will probably be cleared up by correcting the fat allergy.

LIVER

The M.R.T. acupuncture point for the liver is

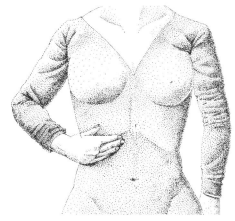

Figure 76

Many nutritionists advocate the use of a cleansing diet for the liver which usually consists of citrus fruits or juices such as lemons. I do not recommend these. The liver is the filter of the blood and if an allergic substance is ingested, it would contaminate the blood and cause it to become acidic instead of alkaline. Therefore, the blood would cause the liver to inflame.

The contaminated blood would also overload the liver and cause toxemia. So the proper way to cleanse and correct the liver would be through *blood* purification, for the blood would then nourish the liver.

Incidentally, one of the dangers of "liver cleaning fasts and diets" involving lemons or citrus, is that a person could be allergic to citrus if the Pantothenic acid level is insufficient, which will do much more harm than good!

ORGAN CHART

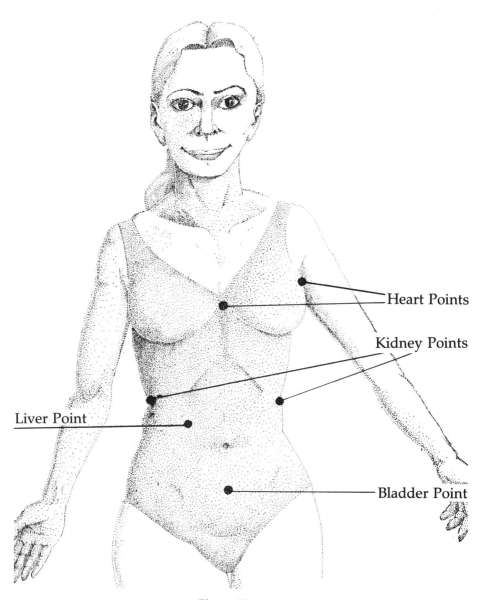

Heart Points

Kidney Points

Liver Point

Bladder Point

Figure 77

CHAPTER 11

DIS-EASE

ACNE

Acne is a condition of the skin where lesions appear on its surface. Usually under the lesion is pus, which is actually dead blood cells. What acne actually is, is a visual detoxification of the body. The body detoxifies in four ways:

1.) Through urination
2.) Through bowel movements
3.) Through breath
4.) Through the pores, by sweating

When there is a toxic substance trying to come through the pores, the condition is called Acne. There are many causations of this condition, but one of the most prevalent is allergies. The acne condition, while it can be arrested by the utilization of topical acne creams, should be approached by the following:

A.) Finding out the person's allergies and food sensitivities.
B.) Taking nutrients which are the antidotes to the allergies which will stop the acne condition.

There are some pharmaceutical products on the market, such as Caladril, which will dry up acne, but unless the condition is changed by correcting the allergies, it will continue in another area. The first thing to do is to check for the allergies to find out what may be causing the condition. To heal the skin lesions and to straighten out the pot holes that were left on the skin from the acne, we suggest Vitamin F and

Vitamin E.* Vitamin F is available to us in the form of oil. Safflower oil and Olive oil contain both Vitamin E and Vitamin F, but people with acne are usually advised to stay away from oils, believing that this is what causes the condition. But what actually causes the condition is a fat allergy. If a fat allergy exists, then there is usually a Sulfur deficiency. The thing to do is to find the antidote to the allergy (refer to chapter on allergies), correct the allergy, and the condition will clear up.

Acne is a tell-tale sign of toxic blood. Purification of the blood by correcting the allergies in it, will correct the acne condition.

Another cause of acne is constipation. Constipation will cause toxins to pass through the colon wall and into the blood stream, which will try to escape the body through the skin! Did you ever stick your hand in a bucket of water for over an hour and notice how your skin has absorbed the moisture?

The pores of the skin are a two way vehicle. They eliminate Uric Acid, Ammonia, Potassium, and Sodium in the form of sweat.

As mentioned before, the body detoxifies in four ways: Through bowel movements, urination, sweating, and breath. With breathing, oxygen comes into the lungs and unites with the Carbon there which the body has created by its intake of sugar and carbohydrates. This expels the toxic Carbons by creating Carbon Dioxide, which the body expels by exhaling.

Remember, acne appears on the skin which we can see, but how about the organs of the body which we can not see? These organs are sometimes inflamed and ulcerated by the blood toxemia which constipation can cause. So in curing acne, it is always important to have good bowel movements.

Urine should never be retained if the person finds it necessary to release it (urinate). Not only because of the physical discomfort urine retention can cause, but because of the toxemia to the blood that it can cause. To help clear up and eliminate this toxemia, a person should drink plenty of fresh, clean water!

A.I.D.S. (ACQUIRED IMMUNE DEFICIENCY SYNDROME).

The problem of A.I.D.S. in the 80s has been found to be caused by a

---

*Vitamin E and Vitamin F in oil form should not be administered until the fat allergy is corrected.

collapse in the immune system. Before 1976 all medical books stated that the "Thymus gland atrophies at puberty", implying that it no longer was needed! However, in the 80s we now realize that the Thymus gland is the "boss" of the immune system!!

Through our research, we have found that the Thymus gland can be strengthened with Potassium and Sodium (which can be found in Alfalfa, Spirulina, and Kelp), Bee Propolis, and Thymus glandular extract. However, the most important ingredient which is necessary for strengthening the Thymus gland is positive thinking!! The most destructive element to the Thymus gland is negative thinking.

Let me show you how this may be demonstrated. Have the person being tested place the right index finger on the Thymus gland point while the client extends the opposite arm to the side to be "pumped" by you. Before pumping the arm, ask the client to think of the most beautiful thought (have client nod head to let you know thought has occurred), and pump the extended arm. The arm should be strong and rigid with a good thought. You should now perform the same test, but have the person think of the worst calamity that could possibly happen while you pump the extended arm. The extended arm should now test weak, demonstrating that negative thoughts have the effect of weakening one's Thymus gland.

So, to strengthen the Thymus gland and rebuild the immune system, people must learn to think positive thoughts only, for negative thoughts are destructive! Supplements of herbs, vitamins and other nutrients can also be used, but they will only be burned up by the negative thinking, so a status quo will occur, but not a regeneration.

In order to place a person in a positive frame of mind, it is necessary that the client realize that worry is a destructive aggressor. Instead of worrying, the client should be encouraged to *pray* and place self in the hands of God!! Prayer is a positive act!! The prayers should be so designed to thank God for forgiveness. This removes all guilt a person may have from "wrongs" of past life styles (Thanksgiving contrition). The prayer should ask for a physical healing (petition), and should express the person's love of God as a parent, for we are all His children (adoration).

Remember, "There are no atheists in a foxhole", and a person with A.I.D.S. is practically in a "foxhole". This mental approach is very important. The person with A.I.D.S. should be put on a total reconstructive nutritional program, checking for allergies and needed nutrients. The A.I.D.S patient should also drink at least 2 quarts of organic vegetable juice four times a day, consisting of one quart of carrot juice mixed with one quart of celery juice (16 ounces, 4 times a day). It is also good for the A.I.D.S. patient to soak in a bath rich in minerals for at least 45 minutes every day before retiring (for more information, please see the chapter on Bath Therapy).

The A.I.D.S. patient would also benefit from the use of biomagnetic therapy and should wear a magnet (north side toward the skin) over the Thymus gland while sleeping to help strengthen the Thymus gland. As mentioned earlier, the use of Bee Propolis and Thymus glandular substance are also very important, and the need for these substances should not be underestimated.

The A.I.D.S. victim on a nutritional program should be re-tested every 5 days to re-shuffle the nutritional program and maintain the correct balance of needed nutrients. If the person is using biomagnetic therapy, do not test the client until you have removed the magnet and waited at least half an hour.

Wearing a gold chain (14k to 18k) around one's neck will also help, more so if a precious stone or metal (gold) were to be used on the chain touching the Thymus area. (Also see chapter on Metal & Gem Stone Therapy for more information.)

We have found that most of the researched A.I.D.S. victims are allergic to everything because of low levels of Sodium in their bodies. With a lack of Sodium, everything they eat is rejected and therefore not absorbed, consequently causing a starvation (Anorexic) situation.

If through testing you find that a person needs a great deal of Sodium, you should begin to use celery juice, alfalfa capsules and Spirulina to bring up the Sodium level. Baths in Kosher or Epsom Salts with Powdered Potassium can also be helpful as the minerals are absorbed through the skin. Spirulina powder can be used orally or added to bath water as a good source of Sodium and other minerals.

A.I.D.S. can be beat, but it must be done on a mental, spiritual and physical level. The A.I.D.S. victim should avoid coffee, black tea (not herbal), sugars (this means ice cream too), and any actual or suspected allergic foods. It is also important for the A.I.D.S. victim to breathe in clean fresh air (mountain or sea areas) to obtain a sufficient amount of oxygen to help in detoxifying the system. Therefore, the A.I.D.S. victim should avoid smoking and people who are smokers. A sufficient amount of sleep is also important and the A.I.D.S. victim should sleep at least 8 to 12 hours per night with the head pointing towards the north to insure maximum charging of the electromagnetic field. For this reason, it is better to sleep in a wood framed or brick building, rather than one which may be grounded in metal and concrete so that the magnetic pole energy is not dissipated prior to affecting the victim's body.

I have also found electro-acupuncture as an adjunct, to be an energizing system to regenerate the immune system, and the A.I.D.S. victim can thus be "charged up" with the use of electro-acupuncture or low voltage electro-therapy.

I believe the A.I.D.S. virus (HTLV-III) feeds on dying cells, so hence we can destroy this virus by starving it and regenerating the dying cells to once again become living, thriving cells. This will cause the HTLV-III virus to become ineffective and burn itself out. Yes, there is hope!!

ANEMIA

Anemia is a condition in which the Iron level of a person is so low that not enough red blood cells are produced, making the person feel constantly tired. One of the secrets I have found in correcting anemia, is to first check the Zinc level instead of the Iron level. When the Zinc level is low, the body rejects Iron, so both the Iron and Zinc levels must be balanced. By bringing the Zinc level up, the Iron will then be absorbed because it will have to keep up with the Zinc level. What will happen then is that the red blood cells will be manufactured and the anemia will eventually be healed.

There are two types of Iron: organic Iron, which is from vegetables, and inorganic Iron, which is from the mines. Most pharmaceutical products are inorganic. We have found the herb Yellowdock to be a very good source of Iron, and also liver and blackstrap molasses to be good sources of organic Iron. By taking these organic Iron substances and raising the Zinc level, you will have an effective remedy to get rid of the anemic condition.

ARTHRITIS

There are two types of Arthritis, Osteo and Rheumatoid. Osteo Arthritis is caused by a deficiency in Calcium and Phosphorus. This is usually caused by the body's inability to absorb Calcium carriers such as milk and cheese.

The body's inability to absorb Calcium is thought to be caused by a malfunctioning Parathyroid gland. However, we do not accept this theory which is held by many medical authorities. We believe that the reason the Parathyroid gland may be considered malfunctioning is because the body is lacking in Potassium which is needed to absorb the milk properly. We have found that a lack of Potassium can cause an allergy to milk (milk products) and cheese which can hinder the absorption of Calcium from foods such as these. This we believe may be one of the reasons a Calcium deficiency occurs in the body. We have found that it is not what the people are eating that's causing the deficiency, but what they are not absorbing.

Many people who cannot tolerate milk are allergic to it because they are lacking in Potassium. But if the Potassium level is brought up, this allergy can be corrected making the milk seem more tasty and more absorbable.

A lack of Calcium can also cause the bones to shrink. They do not shrink in diameter, but in length. That is why with age people will tend to get shorter, because they are unable to absorb Calcium from the foods they are eating. This is one of the reasons we have an aging process. Therefore, the aging process can be corrected by better absorption and youth can be sustained.

Getting back to Arthritis. Osteo Arthritis is usually a degeneration of the bones which can be corrected by the administration of a non-allergic source of Calcium such as Bone Meal. We have also found Oyster Calcium to be satisfactory. Many nutritionists use Calcium Lactate, which is from a milk source, and not absorbable. Bone Meal has a natural balance of Phosphorus and Calcium. When there is a degeneration of Phosphorus in the body and a tremendous abundance of Calcium, you are going to have Calcium oozing through the joints, which can cause Rheumatoid Arthritis. When the bones start to knit together you will get a stiffness in the joints. This is caused by many things, but one of the things it is caused by is lack of Phosphorus.

Why is there a lack of Phosphorus when it is so abundant in eggs? In recent years there has been a scare about egg consumption causing high cholesterol and therefore, contributing to heart disease. This is not true. In each egg there is fourteen percent more Lecithin which neutralizes the existence of Cholesterol making this whole theory false. Eggs have Phosphorus and are good for you!

One of the reasons for the depletion of Phosphorus, is the use of refined sugar in our foods. When the refined sugar is ingested it enters the bloodstream through the saliva glands not the stomach. So if you eat a little candy it does not attack the teeth externally as we are led to believe by the dentist. Instead, it enters the bloodstream directly through the saliva glands and burns up the Phosphorus there. This is why many diabetics with high blood sugar levels will end up with arthritic pains and brittle teeth. The reason for this is that they are burning up the Phosphorus which is the enamel of the teeth. If there is not enough of the nutrient Phosphorus in the body, it is not able to rebuild the enamel on the teeth. So a reduction of sugar in the body will help the Phosphorus level to accumulate to a better density, therefore helping the bones and tooth enamel to become stronger. Phosphorus is the outer bone, Calcium is the inner bone. A lack of Phosphorus will cause softer bones.

There are two other things needed which we will discuss: FLUORIDES and MAGNESIUM. Fluorides help to make the bones stronger so there is also a need for Silica. Silica is a sand that is found in vegetables that helps to regenerate the bones. One of the best sources of Silica is found in the herb Horsetail. Another valuable herb, and a good source of Calcium, is found in the herb Comfrey.

We have found out much about Rheumatoid Arthritis which is found in the muscles and ligaments of the body. We believe that it can be cured instantaneously within days because it is not really a condition, but an allergy. It is usually caused by a lack of Sodium and/or Potassium. Pains on the left side of the body are caused by a lack of Sodium, while pains on the right side would indicate a lack of Potassium. One of the best sources of Sodium is Spirulina. Other sources of Sodium are celery, watercress, Irish Moss, and Dulse.

The best sources of Potassium are: Bee Pollen, the herb Burdock, and Alfalfa.

We have found that Alfalfa contains two parts Potassium and one part Sodium. Therefore, it can be utilized as a tremendous aid in the reduction of Rheumatoid Arthritis, which is not really Arthritis, but a Sodium/Potassium deficiency. By administering these electrolytes to the body, the Arthritis will disappear. One causation of Rheumatoid Arthritis is sometimes heavy metals or impurities in the muscle tissues caused by Toxemia. The way to excrete these would be through anti-oxygen agents such as S.O.D. (Superoxide Dismutase), the herb devil's claw, and amino acid L-methionine. One of the best pain killers would be an herb called White Willow or the amino acid DL-phenylalanine. You might find this very informative and useful.

One of the misconceptions about people who have arthritic pain and stiffness in the joints, is that it is believed to be Arthritis. This is not true. It is called Arthritis, but it actually is a Manganese deficiency which is usually related to a rice allergy. Manganese is a mineral and a nutrient that is food for the connective tissue.

The amino acid L-proline (which is found in beets), along with Vitamin C also helps with the development of collagen (connective tissue). This is why we administer Beet Powder in these kinds of conditions. When people start to get arthritic hands, it usually is not the bones, but the connective tissue. The connective tissue starts to get rigid and stiff because of a lack of L-Proline, Manganese, and Vitamin C. By administering these, the hands will start to loosen. If after a period of time they are still stiff, it may mean that they also need Magnesium which melts the bone spurs that may be connecting the joints.

The herbs rich in Magnesium are Black Walnut and Kelp.

Magnesium's job in the body is to more or less control the growth of Calcium. A Magnesium deficiency can cause the bones to try and knit because of the over-growth of Calcium. The over-growth of Calcium connecting the fingers and joints will make them stiff, but in order for this to change, the Magnesium deficiency must first be corrected.

This condition can be corrected in about three or four weeks by administering the Magnesium to correct the deficiency. So even Arthritis is curable.

ASTHMA

We have found the illness called Asthma to be multi-allergies usually complicated by a trauma or stress situation. As a result of trauma or stress the adrenal glands become depleted of Pantothenic Acid and possibly Potassium and Sodium which are the vitamins and minerals that feed the adrenal glands.

The first thing would be to test for all the allergies to find out what the antagonists are. Then after finding the antagonists, determine what nutrients and supplements are needed to correct the allergies. (The adrenal point of the body can be used for these tests.)

The Adrenal Cortex can be corrected by the administration of Adrenal Glandulars, Pantothenic Acid, the proper balance of Sodium and Potassium, and also with herbs.

A good herb for the adrenals is Licorice Root. However, this should not be given to people with high blood sugar. If the blood sugar is low, it can be given, but if the blood sugar is high it should not be used. Another adrenal gland stimulator would be Wild Yam. This can also raise the blood sugar so should not be used by Diabetics.

The Asthma problem can be caused by allergies, the adrenal glands, and possibly the pituitary gland.

To find out which gland is malfunctioning:

> Place a finger on each side of the nose, on the maxillary sinuses below the eye. (These sinuses are controlled by the adrenals.) If your muscle testing shows weakness it signifies that the adrenal glands are not in good working order.
>
> With the same two fingers, touch above the eyebrows on each side. (These frontal sinuses are controlled by the pituitary gland). Muscle test at this moment and if the arm goes down it means the pituitary gland is malfunctioning.

The pituitary gland can be stimulated by Alfalfa, Pituitary Glandulars, L-Ornithine, and Vitamin B-6. Also beneficial for the pituitary is a product called "GH Release", the herb Gota Kola, and Vitamin E. These products should be used with other nutrients that are needed for the entire system.

The biggest problem with the asthmatic is fear (not believing that he can get well). The body can live forty days and forty nights without food. Jesus showed that when he fasted in the desert. Moses also fasted, but for eighty days instead of forty days. He went back into the mountains after he broke his tablets and fasted an additional forty days. The body can go for six days without liquid and not perish. People survived in the desert in World War II, but after six days it became very difficult.

The body can survive without food and water for this long, but it cannot survive without oxygen for six minutes! The Asthmatic is frightened of dying when unable to breathe. Therefore, when

*SPECIAL NOTE:

Carl J. Reich, M.D. an Orthomolecular Nutritional Physician, from Calgary, Canada, has reported curing 80% of 5,000 asthmatics by giving them large doses (Orthomolecular or optimal) of Vitamins A, and D, and minerals in the form of bone meal. He has published several articles in the *Journal of Orthomolecular Psychiatry*, 1970s.

Elimination of hypoglycemia (low blood sugar) and cerebral (brain) allergies, and neuro-allergies, plus the addition of nutritional supplements of Vitamins A, B, C, D, E, and minerals have been found to eliminate asthma according to research.

Chiropractic adjustments have helped reduce asthma too.

attempting to treat an asthmatic, the tester should not remove the client's medication too quickly (even if it may be negative to the client), as the emotional support that the medicine represents may still be needed.

As the client improves, the biggest problem is to make the client realize that getting well is really occurring! Feelings of the client will fluctuate similarly as the mineral content in the body changes.

It is a very hard road to travel, but it is not an impossible one; we've had many cures of asthma.

HIGH BLOOD PRESSURE

(Hypertension)

High blood pressure is grossly misunderstood. High blood pressure is a tell-tale sign of existing allergies. What happens is that when food that is hostile to the body is ingested, it will enter the blood stream as an antagonist, thereby inflaming the arteries. When the arteries become inflamed, the circumference of the inner bore of the artery tends to inflame, causing a swelling up inwardly, which causes a constriction. Therefore, the pump, which is the heart, must pump harder to send the fluid through a smaller bore. When this antagonist reaches the arteries of the heart, their inflammation and swelling can cause what is termed Angina Pectoris.

We have changed the blood pressure in many ways. One way is to break down the plaque in the arteries which can be done with the use of Lecithin, Phosphatidyl Choline (a super Lecithin), the B-Vitamins, Bee Pollen, and the proper balance of electrolytes. Artery cleaners are Choline and Inositol and anything derived from Lecithin. The plaque in the arteries could also be Calcium deposits which are usually caused by a lack of Magnesium in the diet which controls the body's intake of Calcium.

The first real approach to treating high blood pressure is getting rid of all the allergies. Begin by finding out what the allergies are and then use the antidote to correct them. This is important because if the person is lacking in Potassium, for instance, then there would be an allergy to foods such as milk and soy, and the person would not be able to use Lecithin since it is derived from Soy. Once the Potassium level rises however, and the allergies are gone, the person can begin to use Lecithin safely. I have had clients come to me with a blood pressure reading as high as 185; then after getting rid of their allergies and cleaning up their arteries, have their blood pressure drop down to 140.

To reiterate and to summarize: High blood pressure is usually caused by an allergic reaction within the blood stream causing an inflammation of the arteries which swell up and narrow causing an elevation in blood pressure. High blood pressure is also caused by plaque build-up in the arterial walls.

We have found the plaque build-ups to be Calcium, Cholesterol, and believe it or not, Aluminum sludge. Aluminum poisoning (toxemia) can be caused by the utilization of Aluminum pots and the use of antacids containing Aluminum. Many people take antacids for heart burn or indigestion not realizing that they contain Aluminum. Aluminum is poisonous. The body cannot tolerate Aluminum and it eventually becomes sludged into the liver. If it passes the liver it may also go into the arteries and lay there as a plaque on the arterial wall, being entrapped by Calcium deposits which can accumulate when there is a lack of Magnesium. Deficiencies in Magnesium and other minerals can also be caused by Aluminum Cooking.

Aluminum will divorce certain minerals from food. Some of these minerals are Iron, Zinc, Copper, Manganese, and Magnesium. When food is cooked in Aluminum pots and pans the Aluminum reacts with the food and displaces the metal minerals in the food. The cooked food is then laden with Aluminum, but lacking in all other minerals. Foods heated in Aluminum tinfoil pick up Aluminum. This will cause Aluminum toxemia. This happens because the body is not able to absorb this much Aluminum, so it will lay as sludge in the arterial walls. The way to remove this sludge is with Lecithin, Methionine, Cysteine and Chelation elements. This can take a long time, but it can be cleared up and the Aluminum Toxemia can be removed. Homeopathic doses of Al can chelate out the Aluminum.

As we add Magnesium and break down the hardening of the arteries (Cholesterol and Calcium deposits), there will be a lot of debris floating around in the blood which can eventually cause a headache. The headache is only temporary, and will clear up as long as the program is continued.

High blood pressure can also be helped by the utilization of garlic, which is an antibiotic (natural) and can be used to help normalize blood pressure (Hypertension). Garlic contains two important elements: Sulfur and Selenium. Sulfur is effective in breaking down fats and is also contained in the herbs Sarsaparilla and Dandelion. Sarsaparilla is an important herb which also contains the amino acids Methionine and Cysteine. These amino acids, along with the Sulfur will chelate the heavy metals out of the body and more or less clear up the arteries.

Two other herbs which are effective in the treatment of high blood pressure are Golden Seal and Siberian Ginseng. Golden Seal is an antiseptic which cleans infections and controls secretions. It also burns up triglycerides in the blood and lowers the blood sugar level. This is why I usually advise that it be used at night. When the blood sugar level lowers, this might make a person crave sweets to replace the sugar which was burned up. Thus by using it at night the person will most likely be sleeping and not bother to get out of bed to eat.

Siberian Ginseng is used to help stabilize blood pressure. It works differently, but simultaneously, with the other herbs mentioned to attack the problem and straighten out the situation.

Another advantage of taking Garlic is that it is a good source of Selenium for people who cannot tolerate yeast. The Selenium is contained naturally in the garlic and not mixed with a yeast base as Selenium usually is. Selenium works well with Vitamin E.

Vitamin E is thought by some to cause heart problems. This is not true. Vitamin E comes from different sources. If the Vitamin E is from a wheat based wheat germ oil, which it was originally, then a person with a wheat allergy would have a problem. There have been some studies conducted which have shown that wheat germ E could cause artery problems, but what was not realized was that it was not the wheat germ, but the wheat allergy that was causing the problem. Another source of Vitamin E is soy. Soy is considered non-allergenic by the industry, but we have found that soy can be allergenic if the person is low in Potassium. Potassium neutralizes allergies, so that if the person's Potassium level is high, then a soy Vitamin E may be used safely.

Another factor we have found to help with the arteries is Bioflavonoids. Bioflavonoids are very helpful in strengthening the capillaries to give them more elasticity so the blood pressure can be reduced. However, bioflavonoids can also be antagonistic if there is a Pantothenic acid deficiency, as this would cause an allergy to citrus, which is the source of bioflavonoids.

One thing which should always be considered when checking the blood pressure is the size of the cuff on the blood pressure monitor. This is important because if the person is obese and a regular size cuff is used, the reading will not be accurate.

Many doctors and nurses will check a perfectly healthy obese person and tell them that their pressure is high, not realizing that the cuff they are using is inadequate. The cuff is made in two different sizes; one for normal people and a larger one for heavier people. Many doctors use the smaller cuff. The use of a smaller cuff on a heavy person could show a high blood pressure reading and the patient could panic unnecessarily. This is very important and it should be realized that a person with a fifteen or sixteen inch arm must be checked using the larger cuff so that the reading will be accurate. I have seen healthy heavy people with no problems or pain told they have high blood pressure and put on medication needlessly, only to be injured by it.

Another thing which should be avoided is the use of diuretics. Diuretics should not be used when lowering the blood pressure as they not only excrete water from the system, but also excrete the vitamins and minerals which are the antidotes to the allergies. This causes more allergies and higher blood pressure.

The greatest break-through in normalizing blood pressure to come out of our research, is that if the *systolic is too high, it can mean a lack of Sodium. We have brought down the systolic number twenty points in six minutes by administering five ounces of celery juice (high in Sodium) to a client. After this, we retested him, and the systolic had lowered twenty points, but the **diastolic number remained the same.

We then administered three ounces of carrot juice (high in Potassium) to the client and found that the diastolic number had also lowered ten points. So we deduce that the higher number (systolic) is influenced by the lack of Sodium, and the diastolic is influenced by the lack of Potassium.

BRONCHITIS

Bronchitis is a condition of irritated bronchial tubes. We have found that this irritation can be caused by allergies, and by identifying the allergies and correcting them, the Bronchitis condition will disappear.

Ironically, the same cause can be at the root of many different conditions and so have many different names. Bronchitis is an irritation of the bronchial tubes usually caused by an allergy to something in the environment that is inhaled through the nasal passages. However,

---

*The higher number is the ejection, or pumping phase of the heart.
**The resting phase of the heart beat.

when a person's Potassium level is low, all animal fur and other dander can be allergenic. So when working with bronchitis, it is important to check a person's Sodium and Potassium levels.

We have found that a majority of the time, bronchitis and respiratory problems are caused by a definite Sodium deficiency. However, in today's civilization we are warned against the use of Sodium by the medical profession and are led to believe that it is not good for our health. This is not true. We realize now that it is not the Sodium, but the Chloride that can be detrimental to us. A Sodium deficiency will *cause* respiratory problems. Some organic sources of Sodium are Alfalfa, which also contains twice as much Potassium, Spirulina, and celery juice. We found that drinking more than two glasses of celery juice a day, along with the use of other sources of Sodium such as Spirulina and Alfalfa, will actually help improve a bronchial or respiratory condition if it is caused by a Sodium deficiency.

CANDIDA ALBICANS

Many physicians mis-diagnose an *inflammation* caused by allergies as an *infection* (which it usually is not) and then prescribe antibiotics which in turn will also produce serious side effects in the form of fungal disorders.

The micro organism Candida Albicans is one prevalant example of an infectious overgrowth resulting from the repetitive mis-use of antibiotics. Dr. Orion, M.D., discussed in his book "The Missing Diagnosis" the frequency, scope, and severity of the Candida Albicans infection.

Dr. William G. Crook, M.D., states in his book "The Yeast Connection" that "We all have the Candida Albicans micro-organism in our bodies." In my research, I have found that by elevating the host resistance through a complete nutritional program after determining the person's needs via the Muscle Response Testing technique, that the Candida Albicans condition can be totally controlled and placed in remission. One of the main deficiencies I have found in the metabolism of a person with Candida Albicans is an absence of sufficient Sodium ions, usually accompanied by a parallel Potassium depletion. When the Sodium and Potassium levels are brought up to normal levels, the Candida Albicans fungus condition will usually disappear.

In determining a nutritional program for a person, it is important to first find their allergies through the use of Muscle Response Testing. This is not simple if the person has a Sodium deficiency, because everything will test weak (show allergenic) as long as their Sodium level is very low, and you will not be able to find their true allergies.

To find the true allergies, you must first bring the person's Sodium level up by administering a source of Sodium such as Alfalfa capsules (which also contain Potassium), Spirulina, or celery juice (Sodium) mixed with carrot juice (Potassium). This should be done *after* you have measured their Sodium and Potassium levels and have found out how much Bee Pollen and Royal Jelly they need; because if they were given the Alfalfa or juice first, it would effect the reading of the Sodium, Potassium, and Bee Pollen levels because of the Potassium and Sodium in the Alfalfa and juice.

After you have brought the Sodium level up you can retest the allergenic substances. You will probably notice that after taking the Alfalfa capsules (or juice), the person's extended arm is much stronger when you re-test the allergenic substances. This will at least allow you to do a "semi-true" test. The reason I say "semi-true" is that once the Sodium and Potassium levels are brought up, the grains such as rice, corn, wheat, etc. may not show that they are allergenic, when they really are.

The way to double check this is to wait and see how much of a specific allergy antidote is needed by the person. For example, if wheat checks out O.K. (non-allergenic), but the person needs approximately 800 milligrams of Magnesium, 4×500 milligrams of Histidine, and 4 capsules of Safflower oil (Vitamin F) (all are antidotes to the wheat allergy), then the person is most likely allergic to wheat even though it tested strong (non-allergenic).

Yeast can also react in the same way. For instance, if Yeast seems to check out O.K., but the person needs over 650 milligrams of Zinc and over 2,000 milligrams of L-Lysine (antidotes to the Yeast allergy), then you can almost be certain that the person is allergic to yeast.

Some methods of treatment for Candida Vaginitis include the use of different types of douches. One effective combination is a mixture of 4 aqueous chlorophyll capsules and one tablespoon of vinegar in a pint of water used twice daily. I would also recommend inserting 2 Zyomex wafers (by Standard Process) and 1 Vitamin E suppository (Carlson Labs) into the vagina at bedtime (a pad can be worn to keep them in place).

Zymex wafers are said to contain a strain of yeast known as lactic acid yeast which inhibits Candida. Lactobacillus Acidophilus organisms can also be inserted into the vagina to counter the Candida. A yogurt douche can also be used, but it must contain potent live cultures of Lactobacillus. An herbal douche of Golden Seal, Myrrh, Chaparral, and Comfrey can also be used, but the solution should be checked by using only a small amount to see if the solution is too strong. If the solution is too strong it may burn and irritate the mucous membranes of the vagina so it should be diluted with water.

Researchers at the University of Massachusetts have reported that the internal use of garlic has been successful in killing Candida. Garlic contains Sulfur, a blood cleaner, and Selenium, an anti-oxidant.

Candida can also be suppressed or eradicated by a sugarless diet. Candida Yeast thrives on sugars and a diet high in sugars, honey, etc., only feeds the Candida what it needs to prosper. If Candida is present, there is usually also an allergy to Yeast, so all foods containing yeast should be avoided until the allergy has been abated.

Some effective prescription medications that seem to work well are Nystatin, which comes in a powder, pill, or capsule form; Mycolog Cream, which is used to coat the lesion on the local area; and Flagyl, a relatively new drug that seems quite successful. Before using any drug be sure it is tested to see if it is compatible for the individual who will be using it in order to avoid an allergic reaction. This can be done with the use of Muscle Response Testing as previously described. Remember, everyone is different!!

Another product that is available is the Homeopathic remedy called "Candida Albicans" which comes in a distilled water base in a small bottle with a dropper, available in different potencies from $5 \times$ to $500 \times$. In my research, I have found this to be an unpractical way of treating the condition because if the Candida is already over-abundant, why would you want to contaminate the body with more Candida? It is obvious that the Candida is already running wild! I am aware of the philosophy of Homeopathy, but I hesitate to use it in this case because the immune system is already too weak to respond.

In my research I have also found that birth control pills can have an adverse effect on the Sodium level in the body, thereby permitting the Candida to prosper. Authorities also state that Cortisone and Corticosteroids can also aggravate Candida Albicans.

With the use of optimal nutrition and meticulous hygiene, there is no reason Candida Albicans cannot be suppressed or even eradicated.

CATARACTS

Cataracts can be cured. Some cataracts can be removed with laser surgery and lens implants; however, there is no guarantee that the surgery will be successful. Contrary to medical beliefs, we have found that cataracts can be dissolved. Cataracts are not found on the outer lens, but actually on the second level underneath the outer lens.

Many people believe that cataracts are caused by age, but age is a degeneration caused by a lack of proper nutrition. We have found that Cataracts are caused by a lack of Vitamins B-2, B-6, B-12, and Vitamin D. We have also found that the amino acid L-Glutathione is important, as it regenerates the normal tissue so that the cloudy effect of the Cataracts will disappear.

Research has been done in a hospital in Mexico with a French formula DMSO. DMSO is a federally non-approved drug, but is available in this country as an industrial solvent cleaner. It is also used in this country for arthritis pain. What DMSO does, is take anything from the surface and go right through the tissues of the skin. What they did in Mexico was take the DMSO, put it in distilled water, and dissolve powdered L-Glutathione in it. This is then put in an eye dropper and placed on the lens. The DMSO then carries the L-Glutathione from the lens to the sub-lens where the cataract is formed. By administering this substance over a period of time, the cataracts will disappear.

This substance will probably not be available in this country for about twenty more years from now, but it does help to correct the condition.

Some of the important nutrients used are B-2 and B-6, which are found in Bee Pollen, and B-12 which is abundant in desiccated liver. Two other important vitamins are Vitamin D, which comes from the sun, and Vitamin A.

The fat soluble type of Vitamin A can be found in fish oil. This is the fat soluble type. Another source of Vitamin A is beta carotene, which is found in carrots. I prefer the beta carotene because it is water dispersible, and therefore, non-toxic.

Cataracts can be cured, but it can take up to six months of treatment before the condition is improved, so patience is needed. This approach can also save thousands of dollars in surgery expenses.

I also wish to mention the use of eyeglasses for Cataracts. There is no way a pair of glasses will correct a cataract condition. How can an outer lens amplify the things you are looking at if the inner lens is clouded?

This does not make sense. I do not mean to put the ophthalmologist on the spot, but if the inner lens is cloudy, how could thicker glasses give better sight? Beware of glasses that claim to correct cataracts, for there are none.

It should be remembered that there are three stages to go through before the condition is corrected. The first stage is stopping the degeneration-stopping the growth of the cataracts. The second stage will be a period in which you feel you are not making any progress, but treatment must be continued during this time as the tissue is starting to change. The third stage is a period of regeneration.

It can be as long as two months before the regeneration process begins, as it will take at least two months to stop the degeneration, so have patience.

COMMON COLDS

We believe the cause of the common cold is neither viral nor bacterial. We have found it to be a shortage of one or more of the following: Potassium, Sodium, and Sulfur.

If the colds seem to be causing stuffiness in the right nostril, this would indicate a Potassium deficiency. If the congestion occurs in the left nostril, this would probably mean a Sodium deficiency. To decide which nostril is congested, place one finger on a nostril and blow through the other nostril.

A Sulfur deficiency will manifest itself in the throat area where the Adam's apple is. With a sulfur deficiency, there will usually be a lot of phlegm, especially in the morning. This can be alleviated by eating foods rich in Sulfur such as eggs, onions, garlic, and apricots.

Other sources of Sulfur are the homeopathic Sulfur cell salts (we use the Sulfur 1× tablets), the herbs Dandelion, Sarsaparilla, Fenugreek, and Garlic, and the amino acids Methionine and Cysteine.

Not all sore throats represent a Sulfur deficiency. A sore throat can be brought on by a lack of Sodium which would make everything allergenic. An allergic reaction will make the throat seem sore and look infected, but it is *not infected*, it is *inflamed*!

I believe the tonsils should never be removed, for the tonsils are the Sulfur sack of the body! Sulfur is a blood purifier, and as the blood passes through the tonsils it is purified. So if and when the tonsils become inflamed, what should be administered are sources of sulfur such as: the amino acids Methionine and Cysteine, the herbs Dandelion, Sarsaparilla, and Fenugreek, and the Sulfur IX cell salts. Sulfur cell salts are tablets which are dissolved in the mouth, not in the stomach. Therefore, they penetrate the saliva glands, and go right to the throat, clearing it up in minutes.

Tonsillitis occurs from a lack of Sulfur which can create a fat allergy. It is beyond me how the medical profession used to prescribe ice cream for a person whose tonsils had been removed! Ice cream contains fat, and a person with inflamed tonsils undoubtedly has a fat allergy since there is a sulfur deficiency.

The symptoms a person experiences when there is a "cold" are not actually "cold" symptoms, but allergy symptoms. One of the symptoms a person may experience is a nasal drip, which can drip down the back of the throat and into the chest if the person is lying down. Another symptom is inflamed sinuses.

The nasal drip comes from the sinuses above the eyes which are governed by the Pituitary gland. The nasal drip is actually the Pituitary gland throwing off any mucus which may have formed around it.

Some of the things which can be used to stop the nasal drip are the herbs Gotu Kola and Wood Betony, along with a product called GH release (a combination of Vitamin B-6, Pituitary glandular, and the amino acid Ornithine). By the administeration of the GH Release formula every hour (check for individual need) for about four hours, the nasal drip should stop.

Inflamed sinuses on both sides of the face can be cleared up with the use of a product called Royal Jelly, which is rich in Pantothenic Acid, the vitamin that is needed in this situation.

Another thing that is usually recommended for colds is Vitamin C. Vitamin C works as a catalyst to aid in the absorption of Potassium, Sodium, and other important vitamins and minerals. Vitamin C works well in this way, but we feel that Sodium and Potassium play an important part in this case.

DIABETES

Diabetes is Hyperglycemia, high blood sugar. We have found that diabetes can be cured by getting rid of the allergies that the person has. If sugar is found in the urine or is in high concentrations in the blood, the person is considered diabetic and may be given insulin or hypoglycemic drugs to lower the blood sugar level. High blood sugar is destructive to the eyes, bones, heart, and arteries, so the use of insulin to control sugar is justified. However, taking insulin needlessly can shorten the life span by fifteen years, so it is important to find out the cause of diabetes.

One causation is lack of Chromium, which manufactures insulin in the body. Many health and nutrition-conscious people will advise taking GTF (glucose tolerance factor), which is a combination of Niacin, Chromium, and L-Glutamine in a yeast base. I find this to be dangerous because many diabetics are allergic to yeast. What we use is the amino acid L-Glutamine, Royal Jelly (which contains Niacin), and straight Chromium. These are separate products and not in an allergenic base, so that they are absorbed.

Chromium manufactures insulin in the body, so if this is lacking upon examination of the client, then this is the cause. The first thing is to find the allergies and correct them by using the antidotes. Usually if a person has a wheat, oat, or corn allergy he will be eating these products but not absorbing the nutrients that they contain.

When food is not metabolized properly due to allergies, the blood sugar can rise and simulate diabetes, though diabetes does not really occur. I had a client who came to me who had been on insulin for years believing he was diabetic. What he actually had was Maple Syrup Urine Disease.

Maple Syrup Urine Disease occurs when there is a lack of the amino acids Leucine, Isoleucine, and Valine. If these are not taken in balanced proportions, or one is missing, this disease can occur. Many doctors are not aware of this in adults because it is basically a childhood disease, but it can occur in an adult if these amino acids are lacking, or not balanced. When they are not balanced, sugar will show in the urine and the condition is sometimes mistaken for diabetes. By balancing these amino acids, the urine sugar normalizes, and therefore the presumed diabetes is corrected.

There are many herbs and other substances that can be used to burn up excess sugar in the body. Some of the herbs that can be utilized to burn up sugar are Gentian Root, Raspberry Leaves, Buchu Leaves, Saw Palmetto, Juniper Berries, Huckleberry Leaves, and Uva-Ursi. Two other substances that are helpful in burning up sugar are the enzyme COQ10 (Coenzyme Q-10), and a product called Max Epa, which is a salmon oil that will also burn up Tryglicerides.

I would advise that all of these things be taken at night before retiring because when they start to take effect and burn up the sugar in the body, the person may begin to crave sweets to replace the sugar. So by taking these things before bedtime the person will not likely bother to get out of bed to satisfy this craving for food.

Herbs should not be administered until the medication is gradually withdrawn. The first thing is to treat the whole body and get rid of the allergies, then when the sugar level starts to come down to a normal level, the sugar burning herbs can be substituted.

A good thing to use when working with diabetics are test tapes. These are available in drug stores to show the amount of sugar in the urine. By using these, the person can check the sugar level after using the herbs to see how much the level has changed. If herbs are being used and the person is on Insulin or Diabinese, then these should also be checked to see how much is needed.

To test the medication:

1.) Place substance you wish to test in person's left palm and hold it to the Solar Plexus.
2.) Have person raise the right arm.
3.) When arm is raised, have person resist while you push down on the raised right arm while they are still holding the substance to Solar Plexus.

The results of this test will tell you how much is needed by the body. If the arm goes down or feels weak, it could mean that the substance is too much, or not enough. So if the arm feels weak, add more of the substance you are testing and try again. If the arm feels weaker yet, this means that the substance is too much and should be cut back until the arm shows strong. When the arm feels strong and rigid, this will mean that the person is holding the exact amount required for their body at that time.

It is important that you do not use the sugar-burning herbs while the person is still using Diabinese or Insulin, as this will create too much insulin in the system which might make the person go into insulin shock.

Withdrawing a person from Insulin should be a gradual process, and the insulin amount should be checked regularly. To test the amount of insulin you will use the muscle response testing as mentioned before. Take the type of insulin the person is using and drop around half the amount (if they are taking say 30 ccs of N or P insulin, try 15 ccs) into a cotton ball. Have the person hold this to the solar plexus while you pump the right arm. If the arm still goes down, add more until the arm is strong. When the arm is strong, this means that the amount that is in the hand is what is presently needed by the person.

The next visit (which should be in one week), should be made early in the morning, before the insulin and nutrients have been taken, to get a true count of the insulin. When checking the amount of insulin, put half of what they are presently taking into the hypodermic needle and drop the extract into a cotton ball. By using the same testing procedure as before, you can determine what amount is right for the person at this time. In one week, it is possible to cut the insulin in half, as long as it tests strong.

This should be done over a period of time until the person gets stronger and needs less insulin. It is surprising how the body will start to function normally after the allergies are gone and the Chromium level comes up so that the insulin is no longer needed.

Taking insulin will actually make a person tired. The reason for this is that after the person reaches their normal sugar level, and continues to use the Insulin, their sugar level will then drop lower making the person Hypoglycemic, which is low blood sugar and makes the person feel tired.

It is important to realize that what we are trying to achieve is normalization of the body. Some people are fearful of being without the insulin, as the insulin is a crutch for them. But with the testing method that we explained before, there will be no doubt about how much insulin is needed. As the amount of the insulin needed gets down to two or three drops, you should be able to terminate the insulin and begin to use the herbs such as Golden Seal.

The herbs should not be started all at once, but should be added one at a time so that the sugar level is not dropped too quickly. Another herb which is very effective in helping with diabetes, is Juniper Berries. Juniper berries have also been recommended by Dr. Christopher as an aid to help heal the Diabetic. I have also found that Juniper berries contain a lot of Potassium. This may be one of the reasons that it works so well, as Potassium is the detoxifier of the body.

Diabetes can be healed, but it must be remembered that you can take all the vitamins needed to correct the body's condition, but when working to correct diabetes, the person must also be careful of his diet, being sure not to consume sweets to replace the sugar that is being burned up in his system.

If the person feels a strong craving for sweets during the program, this is a telltale sign that you are giving too many herbs, and possibly over-medicating them to burn up the sugar too quickly. When this happens, reduce the herbs which are burning the sugar and try not to administer them if unnecessary. After the insulin has been withdrawn and the signs of diabetes no longer appear, the herbs should also be withdrawn.

A balanced program would also include minerals such as Chromium which helps to manufacture insulin in the body. Chromium should be administered for a long period of time so that the pancreas can become sufficiently saturated with the mineral in order to start to function by itself.

One thing which should be clarified: although many people feel that diabetes is caused by a weak pancreas, this is not necessarily true. It can be caused basically by a lack of proper diet. We have also found exercise to be very important.

Exercise is one of the best ways of burning up sugar besides Insulin, Diabinese, and herbs. What exercise does is excrete glucose from the muscle tissue so that sugar is burned up. An exercise program can be adapted from any of the existing programs that are offered in the person's area such as Y.M.C.A. aerobic classes, etc. These exercise programs should be investigated and utilized by the diabetic. The only problem with exercise, is that when on Insulin or Diabinese, a person will usually feel tired and not want to exercise. When a person overinsulates there will be a feeling of exhaustion and this is why we do not feel that things such as Insulin and Diabinese are the answers.

We have found stress and trauma to be one of the major causes of Diabetes. Death of a family member, divorce, or other emotionally upsetting problems will set off the Adrenal Cortex which triggers a rise in blood sugar, which in turn triggers the Pancreas to secrete insulin. Even just a visual experience of something upsetting will affect the Adrenals and eventually cause an overproduction of insulin.

If there are not enough of the correct nutrients, the Pancreas as well as the Adrenal Cortex can eventually exhaust the body's supply of substances necessary to create insulin and Corticosteroids. When the Pancreas is strong and there is a stressful situation, the Pancreas will shoot up insulin into the blood causing low blood sugar, Hypoglycemia. Many people who are Hypoglycemic (low blood sugar) can become Hyperglycemic (high blood sugar) because of stressful situations. So at this point I'd like to put in a plug for spiritualism!

Worrying shows a lack of faith. You should have faith in yourself, faith in the Father in Heaven, and faith in your friends. Have hope when things are really bad because they have to get better. As Christ's sermon on the mount said; "Love thy enemy". So when you are in a stressful situation, instead of being angry and uptight, "love thy enemy", and your own illness will dissipate and not generate. So you can avoid getting sick by the proper mental attitude of love, faith, and hope. A lack of faith will give you worry. If you really believe and have faith in the Father in Heaven, you will pray instead of worry. Ask and thou shalt receive! This is no joke! Love and have faith in the power of prayer and you will not suffer as much from these specific diseases.

EPILEPSY

There are many types of Epilepsy, but there are two basic conditions. One is Idiopathic epilepsy, where there is no diagnostic way of knowing what is wrong. The other is known as Symptomatic, which happens when there is a lesion on the brain from an accident or concussion. In the two different types of epilepsy, there are different seizures: Grand mal and Petit mal.

The Petit mal is a seizure in which a person temporarily blacks out. It can happen as quickly as when a person is drinking a glass of water & lifts the glass to their lips, goes into a stare and pours the water on themselves, and then snaps out of it not realizing what happened. Another example is a person ironing clothes who blacks out and burns a hole in the clothing, not knowing how it happened. These are examples of the Petit mal seizure, there are no convulsions and no falling, just a temporary blank out for a second or more. Petit mal seizures usually never last more than a minute.

The Grand mal seizure is when a person falls and goes into a convulsion while all the extremities shake uncontrollably, sometimes there will be a bowel movement or urine will be released. The epileptic often chews, or will bite his tongue, sometimes injuring it enough to cause blood to flow. Sometimes phlegm is emitted from the mouth, giving a foamy appearance. The convulsions can last five minutes and when they subside, the person will either sleep from exhaustion, or awake embarrassed, being aware of what has happened because of the pain from the falling and chewing action.

We have had the fortune of having some of these clients healed. We had an incident in our office where a client we were testing went into a

Grand mal seizure. As this happened, my assistant and I moved the client into a chair and proceeded to use the "surrogate technique" (which is explained later in the book), and located the area in the brain where the electrical storm was originating. In this case, it happened to be in the back hemisphere which is the memory banks which is governed by Choline. By administering Choline, raw brain concentrate tablets, the herbs Gotu Kola and Wood Betony, and a product called "RESPOND" (manufactured by Carlson Labs), we were able to help our client recover enough to withdraw from her medication.

There are many types of medication for epileptics, such as Phenobarbital, which we have found actually slows down the metabolism and creates a slowing down of the energy which builds up and is released through the seizures.

We believe that epilepsy is not a disease, but is actually nature's way of getting rid of the deterioring matter on the brain. The epileptic seizure is like an electrical storm; this is nature's way of giving an electrical charge to correct the malfunctions of the brain which sometimes is scar tissue in the area. So, with these beliefs, we treat epilepy not as a disease, but as a symptom.

The symptom actually indicates that something is not functioning in the brain area. What we have found out is that certain chemicals will affect the brain. We have found that the substances Choline and D.M.A.E. will affect the brain positively so that the brain is fed enough so that the seizures diminish. One of the things which throw out Choline is coffee, so it is important to avoid or cut down on this as much as possible.

Our client was not cured of this disease immediately, but the intensity of the seizures went from Grand mal to Petit mal and also became less frequent, so we believe that there is tremendous hope for recovery.

When working with an epileptic, do not withdraw them from medication that is positive to him. Phenobarbitol, we have found, slows down the energies and, therefore, lessens the electrical storms, but we do not feel that the storm is a threat. The injury from the seizure comes from the fall. By administering the substance Choline, we were able to improve our client's condition enough so that the Grand mal seizures eventually changed to Petit mal, with very few falls. As a matter of fact, our client can now tell when a seizure is coming on so she will be able to safely sit down through the Petit mal seizure.

The other important thing for the healing of our client was Sodium. A lack of Sodium will cause the brain to malfunction. We have found that

Sodium helps the nutrients to absorb, just as Potassium helps the toxins to exit.

One of the important things we have discovered in our research is that when a person has a Sodium deficiency, they will be allergic to almost anything. When Sodium is lacking, almost everything that contains Potassium will be allergenic. This was the case with our client who was tremendously deficient in Sodium. She was allergic to almost everything except foods such as greens, which are rich in Sodium. So what we did was put her on a diet of mostly greens, while correcting the allergies with the proper nutrients which restored the balance to the blood, making the seizures diminish.

Some other products which can be used to awaken the brain are Niacin (Vitamin B-3), the amino acid L-Glutamine, Oil of Choline, and a product called "REMEM", which is an herbal formula made by Nature's Way, to aid the memory.

Epileptics should also drink plenty of fluids, as when there is a Sodium deficiency, water will not be held in the system because of excessive urination, this can cause dehydration.

Another important thing for the epileptic, is bowel movements. The system must be cleared of toxins so that the nutrients are absorbed. The less toxemia in the body, the more nourishment will be absorbed. So when you are trying to neutralize the body it is very important that the person stick to a regular bowel movement schedule.

We feel the causation of Epilepsy is allergies, which do not permit the proper nutrients to be absorbed; so by correcting the allergies, the nutrients will then be absorbed and the condition will improve.

HEART DISEASE

We have found heart disease to be relatively simple to cure. Much of the disease that is diagnosed as heart disease is not really heart disease, but merely allergies in the blood stream which affect the walls of the heart, causing the valves to malfunction. We have healed people with this condition through the use of proper nutrients to correct their allergies to help normalize their valves and gradually correct the condition.

The inner heart can be cleansed in many ways. Some of the important nutrients are Vitamin E and Garlic (which are also good for blood pressure problems) along with other beneficial herbs such as Hawthorne Berries.

Hawthorne Berries is an herb that contains one part Sodium and one part Potassium and works like a roto-rooter in cleaning the heart. Sodium and Potassium are also very important for the heart as the heart runs on Potassium, but is located on the left side of the body, which we have found to be governed by Sodium. In our research, we have discovered that the left side of the body is governed by Sodium and the right side by Potassium. This theory also explains strokes and Bell's Palsy: a stroke on the left side would mean a Sodium deficiency, while a stroke on the right side may indicate a Potassium deficiency.

Although the heart is located on the left or "Sodium side" of the body, it needs and runs on Potassium. The heart is the only organ on the left (Sodium) side of the body that is governed by Potassium. This creates an electro-impulse reaction between the Potassium and Sodium which generates energy to make the heart function. Like a solid wooden ship floating in the sea, your heart is a Potassium vehicle floating in a Sodium base!

Potassium is not readily understood by the medical profession. They often utilize synthetic Potassium (inorganic, pharmaceutically produced Potassium), usually in the form of Potassium Chloride, which can be detrimental to the stomach because of the Chloride. We have found some of the best natural sources of Potassium to be Bee Pollen, the herb Burdock, and Alfalfa, which contains the proper balance of Potassium and Sodium.

Another important mineral for the heart is Magnesium. Many people feel that Calcium is an important mineral for the heart. However, Calcium without the proper balance of Magnesium can cause calcification in different parts of the body including the heart and the valves. Magnesium is useful in cleaning up Calcium deposits in the valves and heart. Some natural sources of Magnesium include the herb Black Walnut and Kelp.

We have also found the amino acids Carnitine and Taurine to be very important in strengthening the heart. Carnitine breaks up fats in the blood which affect the heart. Carnitine, along with the amino acids Methionine and Cysteine are also the antidote to a "fat allergy" which can also cause a heart problem. Carnitine is an important amino acid for the heart as it helps in the metabolism of fats that affect the heart, and thus helps in strengthening the heart.

Heart conditions can come from many different things but the first thing to do is to take away the allergies by administering the proper nutrients. Allergies in the blood will cause inflammation and palpitations. I wish people with heart problems would check this by finding out what they are allergic to by checking the difference in their heart rate pattern after they have ingested the substance to which they are allergic.

I feel that many bypass operations are needless and that probably about ninety percent of heart conditions are mis-diagnosed. The heart can be made healthy again by getting rid of the allergies which aggravate the condition(s), and by administering the proper amounts of Potassium and Sodium along with other nutrients.

I had a person come to me, who after having had a heart attack (seemingly), was brought to a metropolitan hospital where surgeons proceeded to do by-pass surgery on him. Weeks after the surgery he had another attack. They brought him back to the hospital and re-examined him and told him everything was okay. They couldn't understand it. It was then that he came to me and we found out that he was allergic to most of the things he was eating, such as his breakfast of bacon and eggs, bread and butter, orange juice and coffee. So when he consumed his "all American breakfast" he was eating all the things he was allergic to (citrus, fats, dairy, wheat, etc.) and then he suffered from an allergic reaction. When these allergenic foods were eaten, they created a reaction right away, inflaming his arteries and making his heart feel as though it was going to jump out of his chest. This was interpreted as a heart attack, but it really was not. It was actually an allergic reaction.

After we healed this man, he showed me an incision from the operation from the groin up, and with a tear in his eye said, "You mean maybe this was not necessary?" The answer was yes. This man had bypass surgery for a non-existent condition. This man did not have a heart condition, he had an allergic reaction that was interpreted as a heart attack!

Many of the medications that are prescribed for heart conditions have dangerous side effects. Inderal is number one. One of the side effects of Inderal, if not properly administered, is heart failure! Here is a medication used widely by practitioners seemingly without the realization that in the manual printed for it, one of the side effects listed is heart failure. I don't understand this at all! Inderal will slow down the heart, so if it is given to a person who does not actually have a heart condition their heart will become slower and finally stop. Inderal would not be as harmful if given to a person with rapid heart palpitations, but the best thing to do is to take away the person's allergies so he no longer experiences these palpitations and becomes healthy again.

Another popular pill given for heart conditions is Nitroglycerin, which is especially prescribed to improve the supply of blood and oxygen to the heart, and also to relieve pain and prevent heart attacks. This is printed in the manual, but possible side effects are: headaches, dizziness, weakness, nausea, vomiting, skin rash, and flushing. Another drug used is Procainamide which is prescribed to restore irregular heartbeats to a normal rhythm and to slow a rapid heart. Common side effects are diarrhea, loss of appetite, nausea and vomiting. Less common side effects are fever, itching, joint pains, and skin rash.

You see, with all medications there are side effects. So the most sensible approach is to get rid of all the allergies a person may have so that a natural balance is restored to the body with the body healing itself naturally. If a person must take medication, at least test it using the Muscle Response Testing Method so that the person does not take more than the body can handle.

This can be done by having the person place the substance in the right hand (or left) while holding it to the solar plexus. Now have the client extend the opposite arm to be "pumped". Press down on the extended arm while the person resists. If the arm goes down, it may mean that it is too much. Try it with less until you reach an amount where the arm stays rigid. If the arm goes down all of the time, it could mean that the substance is negative to the client. If you do find an amount which seems acceptable to the body, check to see if it will affect the client in other ways, such as depleting the body of certain nutrients or affecting the client in physical ways. For more on this please see chapter

HERPES

Fever blisters, canker sores, and cold sores above the waist are usually considered Herpes Simplex Virus #1, while genital infections are considered Herpes Simplex Virus #2.

It is estimated that 85% of people have had Herpes Simplex Virus #1 usually in the form of canker sores and cold sores. It is believed that 5 million people in the U.S.A. have genital Herpes (#2), and over 500,000 new cases are reported each year. In order to stop the growing incidence of the Herpes disease, active infections must be reversed and then permanently suppressed, since the transmission of the virus takes place when blisters or sores are evident.

R.W. Tankersley discovered that the amino acid L-Arginine accelerated Herpes virus growth, while the amino acid L-Lysine displayed an inhibitory effect. L-Lysine slowed down the viral growth process. The absence of Arginine likewise inhibited the Herpes virus from growing. In 1974, Christopher Kagan at the U.C.L.A. School of Medicine administered L-Lysine immediately after the first visible signs of the disease became evident. The infections rapidly cleared up.

In my own research, my first approach is to find a person's allergies with the use of Muscle Response Testing, because a canker sore or cold sore could be an allergic reaction which could be misdiagnosed as a Herpes Simplex virus. After finding the person's allergies, I would then administer the antidote nutrients to alleviate the allergic condition. (These are described in my chapter on "Allergies and Antidotes".) If the Herpes does not clear up after the allergies have been abated, I would then ask the person to refrain from eating foods that contain Arginine.

The most popular Arginine-containing foods are peanuts and peanut butter. Most vegetarians get their protein from nuts which are also rich in Arginine. Other foods that should be avoided are Cocoa, chocolate, cashews, pecans, almonds, sesame, and all sweets. One should always avoid bleached flour, breads, and cakes. On the other hand, one should be sure to include in the diet foods that are rich in Lysine such as all cheeses, yogurt, milk, fish, chicken, turkey, eggs, organ meats, potatoes, & brewer's yeast (provided they are not allergic to any of these foods).

When the Herpes eruptions disappear, *do not* stop the Lysine foods or Lysine supplements, but continue the anti-herpes diet for at least 3 months so that the herpes will stay in remission. A dosage of at least 1,000 mg. (1 gram) of Lysine should be consumed daily as a maintenance control dose. A preferred amount would be 1400 mg. for a 150 pound adult according to the National Academy of Science's R.D.A. (1974).

Some of the herbs that could be used (internally) in the treatment of Herpes are Comfrey, which is very rich in Lysine and Allantoin (a skin healer), Echinacea, for its blood cleansing properties, and Golden Seal, for its cleansing properties. Vitamins that are especially needed are Vitamin E and Vitamin F (safflower oil) both internally and externally as a skin regenerator.

If a Herpes condition erupts after a stressful experience, it may indicate a need for Pantothenic Acid (Vitamin B-5) and Potassium and Sodium which nourish the Adrenal glands. During this time one should

Comparative potentials of common foods for triggering herpes in the average person.

GROUP 1	GROUP 2	GROUP 3
Foods to emphasize. Especially during active cases of Herpes.	Foods to eat with discretion, these foods must be balanced with L-Lysine & foods in Group 1, during active cases of Herpes.	Foods to avoid
All Cheeses*	Breakfast Cereals (wholes)	Chocolate Peanuts & Peanut
Yogurt*	Whole Grain Flour & Bread	Butter
Kifer*	Whole Grain Pasta Foods	Sugar (increases requirement
Cottage Cheese*	Pancakes (whole grain)	for B complex vitamins)
Sour Cream*	Lentils, Barley, & Other Grains	Cakes & Sweets
Milk*	Soybean Foods	Alcohol (excesses of it deplete
All fish & seafood	Oats	Vitamin & mineral reserves of
Chicken	Corn	some vitamins)
Turkey	Rice	Coffee & Tea (caffeine depletes
Eggs	Peas & Beans	reserve of some vitamins)
Organ Meats	Sprouts	Nuts (Cashews, Pecans,
Potatoes	Foods Containing Seeds (eggplant,	Almonds)
Brewer's Yeast	Tomato, squash)	Seed Meal (Sesame)
	Citrus Friuts (may irritate active canker	Bleached White Flour Foods
	sores, otherwise very good foods)	
	Fruits & Berries (containing seeds	
	which are eaten)	

Other foods containing little or no protein, such as carrots, salad, & butter, display virtually no protential for triggering herpes.

avoid citrus foods such as tomatoes, oranges, lemons, grapefruits, cantaloupes, and pineapples for a short period of time after such an ordeal, and consume Royal Jelly capsules and Alfalfa to replace these nutrients which are burned up by stress. A Herpes breakout in this case is not a true Herpes eruption, but an allergic reaction!!

Another product which is used to treat Herpes and is sold in Health Food Stores is BHT, which is basically a food preservative which inhibits the growth of organisms. BHT should only be taken at bedtime because it can make you very drowsy. To determine the amount or dosage of BHT needed, place the BHT in the palm of the hand and place the same hand to the Solar Plexus while extending the opposite arm to the side to be "pumped" by someone else. Add or subtract the amount of BHT in the hand and re-test until you have found the amount that makes the arm strong and rigid.

If you wish to use biomagnetic therapy to treat the eruption, this could be done by taping a magnet, with the north side towards the skin, on the lesion with a band-aid. This has worked for me in the past, but you should also test both sides of the magnet using the Muscle Response Testing method, as described in the chapter on "Biomagnetic Therapy", to find the correct side for this particular purpose.

It should be noted that to date, nutritional therapy is actually the only known successful remedy for Herpes.

HYPOGLYCEMIA (LOW BLOOD SUGAR)

Hypoglycemia is a condition of low blood sugar causing fatigue, irritability, restlessness, and weakness. In severe cases it causes mental disturbances.

We have found Hypoglycemia easy to treat. We believe it is caused by a weak adrenal cortex which can be activated by the eyes. When an hypoglycemic person sees something that is mentally exciting, the adrenal cortex, causing an increase in blood sugar, stimulates the pancreas to secrete insulin into the bloodstream, tiring or weakening the person by lowering the blood sugar level. Because of this over-sensitivity of the adrenal cortex, the pancreas is constantly activated for insulin needlessly.

Normally, the pancreas is activated to secrete insulin when glucose enters the bloodstream. When the adrenal cortex needlessly causes insulin secretion, the blood sugar drops so abruptly that the person will feel the need to eat something to replace the sugar.

When food is ingested and the blood sugar is normalized, the adrenals will cause another shot of insulin to burn up the newly entered nutrient. Each ingestion of food brings up the sugar level, and at the same time, excites the pancreas to secrete additional insulin.

Part of the solution to the problem first is to find out why the adrenal cortex is malfunctioning. The malfunctioning can occur due to: A.) A lack of Pantothenic Acid in the system causing a citrus allergy; B.) A lack of Potassium causing an allergy to milk, cheese, greens and all Sodium foods. C.) A lack of Sodium which can create allergies to *everything*. With these deficiencies and allergies present, sugars are not absorbed properly by the body.

The adrenal cortex can be normalized by:

A.) Pantothenic Acid (Vitamin B-5), which can be found in abundance in "Royal Jelly".
B.) Potassium, which is found naturally in Alfalfa and Bee Pollen.
C.) Sodium, which is found in Alfalfa and Spirulina.

We have also found the herbs Licorice and Juniper Berries to be useful in this situation. Licorice supplies quick energy to a weak system because it actually raises the blood sugar in the body. Juniper berries are known to have an affect on the pancreas, stabilizing Hypoglycemia and Diabetes. We have also found the adrenal glandular concentrate (manufactured from animal adrenals) to give tremendous strength to the adrenals, but it should be accompanied by Vitamin B-6.

IMPOTENCE

There are two basic types of impotence. One type is psychosomatic, and the other is physical.

Male sexuality is normally on a decline after the age of 21, while female sexuality increases at the age of 30 and peaks at the age of 35. This factor may present another problem of supply upon demand, or sometimes performing under the gun. The fact that we are in a situation of "equal rights" for the female in the 80's is causing a psychological castration of many males in the present social environment. Males who were brought up to believe that they were to be the bread winners and the woman the homemaker, are now being threatened by career women who are presently earning just as much, if not more, than their male companions. This affects the male ego, and will eventually castrate him sexually. This will be the result of his own loss of self love and self role concept.

Male psychological impotence can also be caused by guilty feelings that sex and a desire for sex is sinful, being so taught by many religiously fanatical individuals. Another sexual psychological factor in the causation of impotence, is basically the male's fear of failing!! This would be the ultimate ego devastation, so many males would mentally "abandon ship" by becoming impotent so that penetration would be impossible.

One physical causation of impotence could be "low blood pressure" which is the inability of the heart to pump enough blood into the penis to form an erection. Another physical causation of impotence could be diabetes, whereby sugar crystals block the arteries that feed blood to the penis muscle needed for an erection. Another cause could be a Herpes lesion on the penis gland head making an erection painful so that one is avoided. Over a period of a year or two, the muscles of the penis would lose tone, making an erection almost impossible.

Many approaches are recommended to correct the problem of psychological impotence. Did you ever hear the story of the wife talking to her girlfriend stating "So what if he looks at other women, he can only bark and can't bite!" Little does she realize that she may be the reason that he "only barks and doesn't bite", for another lover, if she's clever, might make him into a "biter". She may be the causation of his failure by her approach, or by her crudeness, lack of tenderness, or basically her attitude. She may subconsciously put a material price on his or her sexuality, thereby turning him off. She may not realize it, but he may be impotent with her because she turns him off. She may be doing it subconsciously because she gets no pleasure from sex because of her own guilt feelings.

The first approach in this case would be a sex counselor who may feel that therapy for both partners or either one might be necessary. You would be surprised how many cases have responded positively. The use of a sex therapist could help stop the male from seeking another marriage-destroying affair.

The physical type of impotence can be helped by the following:

A.) A sugarless diet

B.) Herbs such as Ginseng, Sarsaparilla, Damiana, Yohimba, Saw Palmetto.

C.) Glandular concentrates such as "Testes", "Gonads" (male), and "Prostate".

D.) Vitamins, minerals, and amino aicds. Specifically Zinc, Arginine, and Selenium (these are the chemical components of sperm in seminal fluid).

We have found that the herb Yohimba, which can be found in the form of a homeopathic remedy, is very effective. It enters the bloodstream immediately through the saliva glands and effects the penis within minutes, so it should be administered prior to a sexual encounter to insure success. Find the amount needed by using the Muscle Response Testing Method, but if the amount taken does not seem to take effect, take another dose similar to the one originally ingested or more until the desired results occur.

The herb Sarsaparilla contains Testosterone, the male hormone that effects the gonad area, but it sometimes takes weeks for it to start to take effect.

Last, but not least, I have seen two different devices that can be surgically implanted by a skilled urologist. One device creates a perpetual erection which can be bent into position for usage. Another device is more complex. A pump is placed in the scrotum which inflates the penis until it is no longer needed, then it can be used as a release valve to deflate the penis. Sound wild? This I would consider only as a last resort. I would suggest trying therapy, herbs, glandular substances, supplements, or an exciting partner first!!

One after-thought, another cause of male psychological castration is the fact that after having children, many wives become more of a mother to their children than a wife to the husband. The husband also mistakenly places the wife on a "pedestal" as the mother of the children and forgets that they are husband and wife and starts to view the wife as a mother. It is then difficult to make love to one's psychological mother.

JAUNDICE

Jaundice is a quite visual disease in which the skin and whites of the eyes turn yellow because of an excessive amount of bile pigment in the blood. Jaundice occurs when there is a disorder of the liver.

We have found that Jaundice can develop if a person's Sodium level is very low and allergies are prevailing. When a person's Sodium is low there will be an allergic response to everything (except to most green vegetables which are rich in organic Sodium). The blood will then carry these allergic substances to the liver causing not an infected liver, but rather an INFLAMED liver. This wording is very important because many people believe an inflammation is an infection which is then treated with antibiotics. However, antibiotics will not correct this condition because it is not a problem for antibiotics! As a matter of fact, by correcting allergies the client's blood will then begin to carry healthy blood to the liver to correct the problems there. But, if the blood carries allergenic substances to the liver, which in turn filters the blood, this blood will inflame the liver.

Let me explain this a little further! Did you ever see a strainer for spaghetti? It is usually made out of metal. There are also salad drainers which are similar, but are made out of plastic. One time I had a housekeeper who used a plastic salad drainer to drain hot spaghetti, melting and bending the plastic out of shape. The liver and blood act in the same way! If you put acid blood into the liver, its going to burn and inflame the liver!

The liver purifies the blood, but you must put something in the blood which will be soothing to the liver in order to correct the jaundice condition. So if a person is lacking in Sodium, the thing to do would be to bring the Sodium level up to neutralize the allergies that are inflaming the liver.

In bringing a person's Sodium level up, a good thing to do is have the person stay on a bland diet of greens. A juice fast consisting of perhaps celery juice, carrot juice, cucumbers, lettuce, apple juice, or other greens would also be tremendously helpful at this time. (Also see chapter 16 on juice therapy.) One of the things we have found to contain a good amount of Sodium, along with protein and other vitamins and minerals, is Spirulina. This should also be given to bring up the Sodium level, but always check to see how much is needed by using the M.R.T. method. Spirulina is an algae from the sea and naturally contains organic salt from the sea. However, most literature on Spirulina does not mention its Sodium content because the original research was done on fresh water Spirulina, which is very rare at the present time. Most of the Spirulina that is presently being produced, which is different from the fresh water Spirulina, comes from the seas of Japan and other seas around the world.

Another important mineral we have found to be lacking when there is a Jaundice condition is Sulfur. We have found that one of the most common allergies associated with Jaundice is the "Fat Allergy", which is usually caused by a lack of Sulfur. Sulfur is used to purify the blood and is also the antidote to the fat allergy.

Why is there a lack of Sulfur? Sulfur is destroyed in the body by smoking and exposure to our polluted environment. An over-consumption of fats can also exhaust the Sulfur supply. Our western civilization over-consumes many fatty foods which will deplete sulfur and cause a fat allergy. All fats should be avoided when a Jaundice condition is present. Fats include: Meat fats, pork, mayonnaise, cold cuts, dairy products, ice cream, chocolate, butter, margarine, all oils, vegetable and animal, coconut, and soup fats. Some herbal sources of Sulfur are Sarsaparilla and Fenugreek. The amino acids Methionine and Cysteine are also Sulfur-containing amino acids and should be used to get rid of a fat allergy along with the amino acid Carnitine. So we are talking about two important things: Sodium to remove any allergies caused by a lack of it so that the blood is neutralized and the liver is nourished by it; and Sulfur to purify the blood and correct a fat allergy.

With different people there will be different allergies, and all allergies should be corrected. But when the Sodium level is down a person will be allergic to almost everything. Sometimes if a person is lacking more in Potassium, there will be an allergic response to Sodium foods such as greens. Potassium is also very important and some natural sources of Potassium are the herbs Burdock, which is very rich in Potassium containing approximately 500 mgs. and Alfalfa which contains a good balance of Potassium and Sodium. Many people are low in Potassium and Sodium so care should be taken to bring both levels up, as many different problems are caused by a lack of Sodium and Potassium. Another good herb is Fennel, which is particularly good in this case because it contains Sodium, Potassium, and Sulfur. The herb Dandelion is another herb containing a good amount of Sulfur, plus other vitamins and minerals.

Many books on herbs recommend anti-bilious herbs for liver disorders. However, always be sure to test any herbs you plan to use with the Muscle Response Testing Method. This will show you the exact amount that is needed at the time, or show you if the substance is negative to the person.

To test the herbs you plan to use, place the herb in the right hand (or left) while holding to solar plexus and extending opposite arm to be pumped. Press down on extended arm while person resists. If the arm goes down it could mean that the amount is too much, too little, or not needed by the person. Experiment with different amounts until you find the amount that makes the arm strong and rigid. If the arm does not seem to become rigid at any amount, it could mean that the substance is negative to the person or that the person just does not need it at the time. Always be careful of what you administer when there is a jaundice condition so as to avoid inflaming the liver any more.

Many nutritionists believe that the liver needs to be "flushed" or cleansed, and in so doing, advocate the use of a cleansing diet or fast consisting of citrus fruits and juices such as lemon. We feel that this is not necessary and could be dangerous if an allergy to citrus exist. The liver is not diseased, but becomes inflamed by the acid blood carrying the allergenic substances. This is why we feel that Sodium is very important in healing the liver, as Sodium will alkalize the acid blood and help in healing the inflamed liver.

KIDNEY DISEASE

There are different kinds of kidney disease. One problem is calcification, which can be caused by allergies and a lack of the proper nutrients. Problems such as calcification will not show up on X-Rays as kidney stones do. For example, if you were to paint the inside of a kidney with something like nail polish, it would harden and cover the inside of the kidney. Under X-Rays this would not appear abnormal unlike a kidney stone which shows up as a foreign object in the body.

To test the kidneys, have the person place the right hand (preferably) over the kidney area which is the flat side of the waist (also see chapter 10 on Kidneys) while extending the opposite arm to be "pumped". Have the person use the same hand when testing both kidneys as strength in extended arm will be different in each arm. If extended arm goes down when testing the kidneys, have the person use the rest room to empty the bladder and then re-test the kidneys.

If the kidney now tests okay, then test the bladder by placing the open right palm over the lower abdomen while pumping the extended left arm. If the extended arm now goes down, this is showing that there was debris in the kidney which has now passed into the bladder and will probably pass out of the body the next time the bladder is emptied. If the kidney still tests weak after the bladder has been emptied, this could mean that there is some calcification or that a stone is forming.

Calcification and stones can both be dissolved by the use of Magnesium and cranberry juice over a period of time. To find the amount of Magnesium needed, the examiner should place Magnesium in the hand while holding to the solar plexus and extending opposite arm to be pumped. Add or subtract the amount of Magnesium in the hand until extended arm is rigid. This will show the amount needed at this time. This amount of Magnesium should now be tested while holding to the kidneys and having the extended arm pumped. The kidneys that tested weak before should now show strong while holding the amount of Magnesium needed to correct the problem.

The body was meant to excrete things that are foreign to it, and with the use of the proper nutrients such as Magnesium, the kidney stones and calcification will dissolve over a period of time and pass out of the body. Calcification is caused by a lack of Magnesium in the diet. Potassium is also very important and needed by the kidneys. Potassium breaks down Calcium and makes it more absorbable so that it is used properly, rather than calcifying in different parts of the body such as the kidneys.

A lack of Potassium will also cause an allergy to milk, so if a person who is allergic to milk drinks milk, the Calcium from the milk will not be absorbed properly and may end up in the kidneys, sometimes forming stones or calcification.

A WORD OF CAUTION! Never use the herb Comfrey when a kidney stone is present as Comfrey naturally contains a lot of Calcium. Never use Comfrey with other sources of Calcium such as bone meal or oyster Calcium at the same time. The reason I say this is that within a week, a person will not need as much bone meal as at the beginning of the week, so the extra Calcium will end up in areas such as the bladder, kidneys or bowels. For instance, if Comfrey and other Calcium sources are used at the same time, the extra Calcium may pass into the kidneys waiting to be excreted, and if it remains there overnight it may start to form stones. Comfrey with other Calcium sources has a tendency to make the Calcium knit and clump together. Bone meal with Oyster Calcium are okay together, but NEVER use Comfrey with either one of these at the same time!

We have found that there are many mis-understandings about kidney disease. Sometimes a doctor will find too much Phosphorus circulating in the blood (which is believed to be negative) and will prescribe an Aluminum antacid, such as Digel. Aluminum Antacids (which are harmful anyway because of the Aluminum) are often prescribed to "kidney failure" patients to prevent Phosphorus from being absorbed into the body. What the doctor fails to see is that the only reason the excess Phosphorus is negative is that there is not enough Calcium in the blocJ for the Phosphorus to unite with in order for it to be put to proper use. It is very important for these two minerals to be in constant balance. This ratio is 2 to 1, 2 times as much Calcium as Phosphorus. It is also important for Magnesium to be included in this balance, as without sufficient Magnesium, Calcium is not absorbed properly and can wind up as Calcium deposits in the kidneys (or elsewhere) instead of being useful to the body.

So instead of using antacids to cast out the Phosphorus that is circulating in the blood with no place to go, the best thing to do would be to administer Calcium in the correct proportion with Phosphorus (and Magnesium), and therefore bring the Phosphorus level in the blood down. Phosphorus and Calcium also strengthen the entire skeletal system.

Many doctors believe that a high Calcium intake will cause kidney problems. This in part is true, because if there is not enough Magnesium to work with the Calcium, there will be problems. So, instead of limiting a person's Calcium intake (except in the very beginning of the program), the best thing for you to do is to administer Magnesium, which is the controller of Calcium, in order to dissolve kidney stones and calcification.

Most kidney problems are not infections, but INFLAMMATIONS, unless there has been an accident or blow to the kidneys. Kidney stones and calcification are usually non-functional causes of kidney disease. Pains in the back below the lower ribs are usually a tell-tale sign that calcification or other problems are starting.

Dialysis is an abominable approach to the survival of the kidney patient, for when the blood is passed through the dialysis machine all nutrients and minerals are taken out. Ironically, the function of the blood is to carry the nutrients from the food you eat to different parts of the body. But with dialysis, all the nutrients are removed from the blood so that there is no longer any nourishment contained in the blood and the body will soon die. The harm and the expense are enough to make me question the use of this approach. Many patients go for dialysis three times a week. This can cost anywhere up to $4,000.00 a week, but it is also financially rewarding for the medical practitioners to continue using this approach.

Sometimes a kidney stone will do some damage by scratching internally. This can happen if, for example, a person rolls over during sleep onto the kidney stone causing it to scratch inside the body. This person may then have blood in the urine in the morning.

If a person is experiencing a lot of pain in the beginning, it may mean that the kidney stone has passed into the ureter, which is the tube connecting the kidneys to the bladder. This can be tested by testing the kidney using the M.R.T. method as previously mentioned. If the kidneys now test strong, it could mean that the stone has passed out of the kidney into the ureter.

At this point, it is very important to keep taking the Magnesium, even increase the amount, as what will happen is that the stone or debris will pass from the ureter to the bladder until it is finally excreted by the body. Continue to administer the Magnesium and the bladder will finally emit the debris as a sandlike substance in the urine. This is the dissolved stone or calcification being passed from the body.

One of my clients brought in a few stones she had passed which had a greenish color to them and said, "Doc, these are the stones I gave birth to!", and we both chuckled because we knew that both of her kidneys and bladder were now clear.

I had another case with a woman who had one kidney removed. Her remaining kidney was clogged with stones. It took us approximately six weeks to clear this kidney up. The woman then returned to her doctor for an examination and the doctor was dumbfounded because the kidney was now clear!

We feel that kidney disease is not really a disease, but just an imbalance of different minerals and other nutrients within the body. By administering these nutrients, the biokinesiologist can help the client clear up the condition eventually. So when your kidneys suffer, please listen to what is being said: Magnesium, Potassium, cranberry juice and other nutrients will help. Give your body the things it needs to repair itself.

LUPUS

Lupus is a disease with many clinical manifestations. It is associated with problems of the connective tissue in the vascular system, skin, and the Serous and Synovial membranes.

We have had success treating Lupus by balancing the Potassium and Sodium levels of the body. We had a client who came to us with her Sodium and Potassium completely depleted. By administering Bee Pollen, Alfalfa, Spirulina, and other nutrients rich in these minerals, we were able to help her regain strength.

When the Potassium and Sodium levels drop, allergies arise, and the various symptoms of Lupus will appear. Symptoms such as: joint pains, skin rashes (especially "butterfly" eruptions on the face), inflammations of the heart and lung membranes, neurological problems, gastro-intestinal disorders, and blood abnormalities. I believe all these different symptoms are allergic reactions due to the lack of Potassium and Sodium.

The reason our client had such low Sodium and Potassium levels was that she taught school in a building without air conditioning during the hot months of May and June, which caused excessive perspiration which began to deplete her of these two minerals. Being a music teacher, she was under severe stress in arranging concerts. This stress also contributed to the burning up of the Potassium and Sodium levels of the Adrenal Cortex. She was also found to have a weakness of the Pituitary gland.

We have found that the Pituitary gland controls the fluid of the body. By administering the product G.H. Release (which is the Pituitary glandular, Ornithine, and B-6), we have been able to strengthen the Pituitary gland which then retains the Potassium and Sodium in the blood. By administering herbs rich in Potassium and Sodium, we were able to replace these two minerals in her system, and thus neutralize the Lupus. The other mineral we found our client lacking was Zinc, which created other allergies in her system.

We have found other clients with Lupus to have the same Potassium and Sodium imbalances. Lupus is not as fatal as people believe. By restoring the Potassium and Sodium balances in the body, the solution is quite simple.

The public has not been tuned into the importance of these balances in the body. We hope they soon will be by reading this book.

MIGRAINE HEADACHES

We have found that migraine headaches can be caused by two things: Allergenic foods or Aluminum in the system. When something allergenic is eaten, it will enter the bloodstream and then reach the brain, inflaming it.

We have found that migraine headaches can also be caused by Aluminum cooking.

We once had as a client, a person of the clergy who was scheduled for a C.A.T. Scan. He was found to have dark spots on the brain and was scheduled for brain surgery.

What we did was start chelation right away to remove the Aluminum from his system. It seemed that during the twenty years he spent in the rectory, all the foods were prepared with Aluminum cookware. After years of eating the food, the Aluminum began to accumulate in his system.

After the Aluminum in the system was removed, the dark spots on the brain area disappeared, the pain from the migraine disappeared and the allergies disappeared.

Aluminum cooking displaces important minerals. With these minerals missing, allergies arise and cause problems such as migraine headaches. In this case, the migraine headache was caused by the allergies, but the spots which showed on the brain were Aluminum deposits. These "spots" were cleared out by the utilization of the amino acid L-Cysteine and the herb Sarsaparilla.

When using chelation to rid the body of Aluminum, there may be diarrhea; this is a sign that the Aluminum is being cleared from the arteries and other parts of the body.

Chelation does work, and in this case, the headaches from the Aluminum poisoning disappeared and never returned.

A migraine headache is a definite sign that something is not right in your body. *Where* the pain occurs in the head is also an indication as to what is lacking in the body.

A pain on the left side behind the left eye may indicate a shortage of Zinc.

Pain occurring beside the right eye indicates a shortage of Iron.

Pain in the back of the head may mean a shortage of Choline, which is sometimes depleted by coffee drinking.

Pain behind the right ear could mean a need for Potassium.

Pain behind the left ear could indicate a Sodium deficiency, a need for L-Glutamine which is depleted through alcohol consumption, or a Niacinamide shortage caused by smoking.

Migraine headaches are not a disease, but a symptom that something is wrong with your system. Remember, blood feeds the brain. If anything in the blood is wrong, allergenic, or unbalanced, you are going to get a migraine headache. Taking aspirin only complicates the problem because the temporary relief is going to be compounded by an ulcerated stomach. This is not the solution! What you have to do is take care of the cause of the migraine, which is usually an allergy. Hunt the allergy down, remove it, and the migraine will disappear within minutes! If, for instance you have a rice allergy & get a migraine after eating rice the thing to do to bring relief would be to administer the antidotes to the rice allergy.

The following antidote is the remedy for a rice allergy migraine:

Administer Yucca, Manganese, and L-Arginine instantaneously. You can find out the maximum amount that you can take by utilizing the M.R.T. method. By taking this compound, the migraine will disappear in 15-20 minutes or no longer than 45 minutes, according to how long it takes your stomach to convert the nutrients. The migraine headache will disappear by neutralizing the allergy through the nutrients, because the blood is constantly flowing to the brain, so by putting the antidotes in the blood, they hit the brain and the pain will disappear. This is not a deadening of the nerve centers, this is a correction of the allergies that are causing the migraine.

It's a shame to see people come here who have had a history of constant migraine headaches for thirteen and fourteen years, which we are able to relieve within an hour!

Again, a Sodium deficiency is a primary cause of migraines. We are in the twentieth century where Sodium is considered taboo by doctors who have said for years it is detrimental to the heart. I believe when people read my book recommending so much Sodium, they will think I am really a quack!

However, now researches are discovering it wasn't the Sodium, it was the *Sodium Chloride* that was detrimental. I am not recommending Sodium Chloride. I am selling Sodium, which is found in every green vegetable. I also stress Potassium, which is needed to balance Sodium.

Most of us who refrain from salt need it or we start to sweat heavily. Salt holds water in the body. Potassium relieves water from the body. Do not take water pills (Diuretics), as when body fluids are released many minerals and nutrients are carried off at the same time.

The herb Wood Betony is good to remove a temporary migraine headache on the top of the head. There is a difference between the brain area and the top of the head. The top is not the brain, it is the Pineal gland point. When this hurts, Wood Betony is the nutrient to feed this gland, which is crying out for food. By taking Wood Betony, the headache in this area will disappear.

The food for a headache in the back of the head (where the memory banks are) is Choline. Underneath the front of the head and the top of the hairline lies the pituitary gland, its food is: the herb gota kola, amino acid L-Ornithine, Vitamin E and Vitamin B-6. Alfalfa also nourishes the pituitary because it has the potassium and sodium that will help retain body fluid.

Pain above both eyes indicates sinus trouble governed by the pituitary gland. By administering the above nutrients recommended for the pituitary gland, the pain will disappear.

Another cause of headaches is constipation. Constipation, improper release of waste matter from the body, can cause blood poisoning.

Have you ever washed dishes and soaked your hands in dishwater for a long time? After about half an hour your skin gets a little soft and tender. The pores are a two-way street. You eliminate sweat through them, but you can also absorb through the pores. Your colon works the same way. If you don't eliminate waste out of the rectum, it will start to go through the walls of your colon and poison your blood supply. This creates many conditions, one of which is headaches. We have found the best way to solve this problem is with the herbs Cascara Sagrada and Bayberry, the herbal laxative Swiss Kriss, or even enemas.

Moving the bowels properly is very important in solving blood impurities (possibly caused by allergies) of which migraine headaches are a part.

OBESITY

All experts agree; obesity is caused by over eating, with the rare exception of a thyroid disorder which will affect the rate of metabolism, causing an imbalance. But what causes a person to over-eat? We have found that it is not what they are eating, but what they are not absorbing. Many obese people are highly allergic to the foods they are eating, and, therefore, the body rejects the nutrients in the food they eat, rather than absorb them.

Let me give you an example. A person that is allergic to wheat would not absorb the B-Complex vitamins that it contains, and after eating it, he may still feel hungry because he hasn't gotten any nutrients out of the food he just ate. People needing Potassium or Sodium will also eat a tremendous amount of food in order to get these electrolytes. What I am trying to say is that many people are starving because of mal-absorption.

Many people over-eat because they are searching for the nutrients in the food, and since they are not absorbing all the nutrients in the food they eat, they will feel that they have to have twice as much in order to feel satisfied.

Have you ever seen pictures of children in Biafra with their thin arms and legs and extended bellies? They fill up with fluids because they are starving. Their bodies retain water to protect the tissues from the acid in the blood caused by the allergic food. Many obese people often "Blow up" for the same reason. People with huge appetites are often compulsive eaters because they are searching for the missing nutrients by over-eating.

It is not always a good idea to put someone like this on a fast or starvation diet. They may lose weight, but they may also become ill. The right approach is to correct the allergies and problems of mal-absorption first by finding out what the allergies are using the Muscle Response Testing Technique, and then finding the nutrients needed to correct the allergies.

We have found that many obese people are lacking in Sodium and Potassium. Sodium is usually deficient because they have maintained a low-Sodium diet, believing that the salt will retain water making them bloated. However, what they do not realize is that everything becomes allergenic when there is not enough Sodium in the system. Therefore, everything they eat will bloat them because they are allergic to it.

We have found different herbs that work well as appetite suppressants. One such herb is Fennel, which contains Sodium, Potassium, and Sulfur. The Sulfur in Fennel helps to break down fat, while the Sodium and Potassium provide the nutrients needed by the body to satisfy the appetite. You see, when you give the body what it needs, it will no longer be hungry. The right nutrients and herbs can kill the appetite by *satisfaction*, not suppression.

Another very good herb is Bee Pollen, which is very low in calories compared to the nutrients it contributes to the body. Bee Pollen contains a large amount of Vitamin B-Complex and Potassium. Another very good herb is Alfalfa which is rich in Potassium and Sodium. Alfalfa and Bee Pollen are particularly good for obese people since they are both very rich in Potassium (Alfalfa has twice as much Potassium as Sodium) and obese people tend to be lower in Potassium than Sodium. Many obese people are born with a lack of Potassium which will cause an allergy to milk and cheese. A lack of Potassium will also cause an aversion to greens which contain Sodium and other important minerals.

Presently there are many different approaches for dissolving and burning fat from the body. However, it is very important to correct all allergies before starting any of these programs. The proper approach in helping an obese person lose weight is to put them on a sound program with the right nutrients combined with a controlled low-calorie food intake.

Much research has been done with different amino acids to aid in the burning of fat. One such combination is Arginine and Ornithine which affect the growth hormone levels helping to burn fat more or less while you sleep. However, the amino acid Arginine tends to burn up Lysine so this should always be taken with a balanced amount of Lysine. There are products on the market such as "Trim Tone" and "Triple Toner" which are formulas containing a balanced amount of Arginine, Ornithine, and Lysine. These are usually taken at night to help burn fat while you sleep.

Another very good amino acid which breaks down and burns up fat is Carnitine. Ironically, Carnitine is usually not contained in most of the complete protein pills. The amino acid L-Phenylalanine is also very effective as an appetite suppressant and mood elevator. However, this particular amino acid is not always good for the obese person since many obese people have high blood pressure and besides being an appetite suppressant and mood elevator, L-Phenylalanine also raises the blood pressure somewhat.

There are also other interesting products and herbs that could be used in a weight loss program. Chicory is an herb that helps to dissolve fat in the blood vessels. It also contains Potassium and other nutrients to help eliminate a craving for food. Another product is Metabolase, which involves the use of enzymes in helping to activate the metabolism so that it starts to burn fat.

Many people have an enzyme imbalance, and, therefore, are not digesting their food properly to extract enough nutrients from the foods they are eating. This is why it is very important to correct all allergies, as once the allergies are abated, the stomach will begin to function better. There are many different digestive aids that can be used, depending on the individual's need. Some are papaya, acidophilus, and apple cider vinegar. Many people take apple cider vinegar, believing it to help them digest their food. Apple cider vinegar is great, if you are not allergic to apples! But if you are allergic to apples then the apple cider vinegar is going to be hostile to you!!! Again, this is why it is so important to first correct any allergies that may exist.

Many obese people are lacking in hydrochloric acid so there are products on the market such as KLB-6, which contains Kelp, which has a lot of minerals and Iodine to activate the thyroid, Lecithin, which helps to break down fat, and Vitamin B-6 which feeds the Pituitary gland to also help in losing weight. It is also an enzyme activator and is necessary for the production of Hydrochloric acid, & Hydrochloride, to help break down and extract nutrients from food and supplements. There are also good enzymatic supplements containing Hydrochloride and other enzymes to help break down and extract nutrients. I find these are usually good since the Betaine Hydrochloride is less allergenic than other digestive aids.

Many people believe exercise to be very important when one is trying to lose weight. This is true, but when a person is starving nutritionally, there is usually a lack of electrolytes and nutrients needed as fuel for the heart and muscles, and thus the person will not have the energy to exercise.

The heart can be tested by using the Muscle Response Testing Method. Place 1 or 2 fingers of the right hand on the breast bone in the middle of the chest (Also see "Heart", page 255) while extending the opposite arm to be pumped by another person. If the extended arm goes down when pressed, this is showing that the heart is weak. To correct this, find the amount of Potassium needed by placing an estimated amount of Potassium in the right hand while holding to solar plexus and extending opposite arm to be pumped. If the arm still goes down when pumped, this could mean the person needs more or less. Add or subtract the amount of Potassium in the hand and re-check by pumping the arm until you find the amount that makes the arm strongest. This is showing you the amount that is needed at this time.

Now that you have determined the amount of Potassium needed, place hand holding Potassium back on heart point with the finger touching the middle of breast bone and extend opposite arm to be pumped again. The arm should now be strong and rigid when it is pressed. This is showing that the weakness of the heart is due to a lack of Potassium! People with a lack of Potassium will have a weak heart, and usually don't have the energy to exercise in the first place because they cannot afford to burn up the Potassium they do not have. Potassium is fuel for the heart!

For an obese person, one of the best exercises to start with would be swimming or bicycling. Leg raises and situps are also very good. Sit-ups in the beginning should be done by bringing the arms up over the head while sitting up to touch the toes, adding one sit-up each day to increase the amount to make you stronger. Later on as the stomach muscles become stronger, you can begin to do the sit-ups while folding the arms behind the head to make it a little more difficult.

Ironically, many obese people have trouble getting down on the floor to exercise! In this case it might be easier for them to start doing them in bed. This way they can have their partner or companion hold their feet down while they do their sit-ups. Leg raises are also good for strengthening the stomach muscles. These can be done gradually adding one more each day until you reach thirty a day after thirty days. These, along with the sit-ups done morning and night, will make a difference.

Another advantage of sit-ups and leg raises is that it not only tones your muscles, but it also tones your organs internally by massaging them. This stimulates the digestive system and other organs, kidney, liver, etc., to help rid the body of toxins.

Besides Potassium, many obese people are often deficient in Chromium which plays an important part in the manufacture of Insulin, and when lacking, can cause high blood sugar (Hyperglycemia). High blood sugar will also burn up the "B" vitamins along with Phosphorus making the obese person feel like eating twice as much in order to replace the lost B complex vitamins.

B-vitamins are also necessary for a healthy nervous system. If these are being burned up by an excess amount of sugar in the system, this could cause the obese person to feel edgy and nervous, providing another reason to eat more. If the obese person is deficient in Chromium, *all* sugars should be avoided; this includes honey which also converts to glucose in the system.

Sugar in food also divorces from it any nutrients it may contain. Processed and canned foods should also be avoided as much as possible as processing destroys much of the food's natural vitamins and minerals (Also see Chapter 13 "Man's Ecological Suicide). Canned foods not only lose most of their nutrients through processing, but the can itself is harmful because of the Aluminum, Tin, and Lead solder which can be absorbed by the food making it toxic. Raw vegetables, fruits, and grains are always better for the obese person as they naturally contain the Potassium, Sodium, and other nutrients which are usually lacking in the obese person's diet.

Also, if a person is unaware of having a diabetic condition, this individual will seek out sweets and consume them at a tremendous rate not realizing this is causing a process of self-destruction. One way of checking one's sugar level is with the use of Diastix strips which can be purchased at the drug store. These strips are used to show the amount of sugar contained in the urine and I recommend them for the obese person who believes this problem is present. If the sugar is found to be high, there is probably a good chance you are obese because you are taking in too much sugar.

Many people go on "Grapefruit Diets" believing this will help them burn up fat and lose weight. However, if you are distressed and lacking in Pantothenic acid, you are going to be allergic to all citrus fruits; and diets like the grapefruit diet are going to do more harm than good because the grapefruit is going to be toxic to the person with a citrus allergy, possibly giving a feeling of sickness for days. This is why I say it is so important to get on a nutritionally sound program to correct the allergies. When the allergies have been corrected and the person is nutritionally stable, then a sensible diet to help the person lose weight without any harmful side-effects should be chosen and followed.

People can even be allergic to some of the "diet" foods recommended on the more sensible diets. This is why all foods should be checked for allergies before beginning a program. Sometimes when on a diet, a person may eat something like tuna fish (which is high in protein and also Sodium) and belch and feel sick from this not realizing that because of low Potassium, foods high in Sodium will be difficult to handle. Once, however, the Potassium level has been brought up—in balance with the Sodium, foods like this will not have the same effect. The person will then be able to eat this food without any problem.

The way food is cooked is also important. Avoid all Aluminum pots and pans and eat vegetables and fruits raw as much as possible. Cooking food in a wok is preferred, as it is cooked only briefly and the food retains much of its natural enzymes and nutrients. I once knew some people who had cooked some vegetables in a pressure cooker and became very sick. The reason for this was that it was an Aluminum pressure cooker. The food cooked in it absorbed so much Aluminum that the food was made toxic and the people became sick. So again, always avoid cooking in any kind of Aluminum. (Also see Toxemia, page 319 and Man's Ecological Suicide, page 333.)

Fasting every so often is a good way to help lose weight, but it is better to start fasting after all allergies have been corrected and the person is nutritionally stable. Fasting can be done one day each week, preferably on a day when one does not have to go to work and it is easier to refrain from food. A fast of fresh raw vegetable juices or fruit juices is good as it contains nutrients, but is very low in calories. It is also very important to continue taking supplements while you are fasting to give you the extra nutrients you will need.

PARKINSON'S DISEASE

Parkinson's disease is manifested by uncontrollable shaking and jerking motions. I have had much success in helping people with Parkinson's disease, but feel that the person must have great patience in working to get well. The first step is to take away the causation, which we have found to be basically a deficiency in Calcium and other nutrients; and to try and control the shaking manifestations of the disease.

We have found that Parkinson's disease is the result of a tremendous deficiency in Calcium related to a malfunctioning Parathyroid gland. Many times the person is equally deficient in Potassium which would cause an allergy to milk and cheese products so that the Calcium in these foods is not absorbed properly.

We have seen tremendous improvement after three months on a balanced nutritional program along with the use of non-allergenic sources of Calcium such as Bone Meal and Oyster Calcium. In addition to a complete program of nutrients and supplements to correct other related metabolic imbalances, we have also found the Parathyroid Glandular Substance to be helpful in correcting this condition.

Other deficiencies include a lack of the B-Complex Vitamins which are also needed for a healthy nervous system. Many times a person's allergies will not permit them to absorb the vitamins from the foods they eat so they are deficient in many things. A lot of the manufactured B Vitamins have a rice or yeast base which some people are highly allergic to! This is why I prefer to use a non-allergenic source of the B-Complex Vitamins such as Bee Pollen (also a good source of Potassium) and Royal Jelly which are naturally rich in the B-Vitamins and much more absorbable. Other important herbs are Alfalfa, which is an excellent source of Potassium (and also contains Sodium), and Spirulina as a source of Sodium (also contains vitamins, minerals, and protein).

In working with clients who have Parkinson's Disease, we have found that it is also important to test all medical prescriptions by using the Muscle Response Testing method to find out which ones are negative to the person and which ones are appropriate to help stop the uncontrollable spasms. We also check the amount at each visit because the person's needs can change from week to week.

There are also many different herbs that work well as relaxants to help reduce the spasms. One such herbal combination which we use is the Homeopathic product called Calms Forte. This is a combination of different soothing herbs along with different cell salts to help relieve nervousness and insomnia. Other herbs which act as nerve regenerators and relaxants are Valarian Root, Cat Nip, Passion Flower, Lobelia, and Chamomile. The trick is not to use them all at once! I would spread them out during the day; for instance, taking the Passion Flower in the morning, Lobelia at lunch, Cat Nip at suppertime, Valarian Root at bedtime, etc. This way the person is relaxed throughout the day. Another product we have found to be helpful is Gaba Plus (Gamma Amino Butyric Acid). This helps to stop nocturnal urination so that sleep is undisturbed.

Calcium is also a sedative and relaxant and I would not usually take it during the day. However, a person with Parkinson's Disease is better off taking Calcium through the day with the greater part at night. This way the Calcium works as a tranquilizer during the day to help reduce the shaking, and also helps the person to sleep better at night.

One of the side effects of Parkinson's Disease is skeletal deterioration. I have had a few clients with this problem; one gentlemen had a deteriorating shoulder socket, while another client had a deteriorating hip socket. This problem can also be helped with the use of Calcium.

The sockets can also be most difficult to regenerate if they are inactive, as the Calcium can eventually cause the sockets to fuse, creating a solid piece. For this reason it is also important to institute appropriate physical therapy to create movement in the sockets so the Calcium helps to regenerate the bones, but does not knit them together in the process.

I sometimes use the herb Comfrey as a source of Calcium at the beginning of a program because it helps to bring the person's Calcium level up quickly since it is absorbed easily. However, I hesitate to use Comfrey over a long period of time (especially in this case), as Comfrey contains Allantoin, a cell proliferant agent, and can sometimes cause a clumping or knitting of the bones if it is not used properly. Comfrey should also never be used along with another Calcium supplement such as Bone Meal or Oyster Calcium, as this can also lead to some calcification or knitting of the bones. Bone Meal and Oyster Calcium are non-allergenic sources of Calcium, will help the bones to regenerate, and will not cause the bones to knit; but they should not be used with Comfrey.

Sunshine, because of the Vitamin D it provides, also helps the absorption of Calcium and should be considered as part of a therapeutic approach. It should be noted however, that the sun could also burn up one's supply of Vitamin F, so *after* exposure to the sun the person should coat the skin with an oil such as Safflower Oil, Sunflower Oil, or Olive Oil which are all good sources of Vitamin F to restore the Vitamin F to the body through the skin. This will also regenerate the skin and prevent a wheat allergy.

SCIATICA

Sciatica is the inflammation of the Sciatic nerve with generally severe accompanying pain. The pain will start at the area of the buttock and descend along the back on the outside of the leg. Occasionally there will be pain in the anterior aspect of the thigh, and occasionally, the foot and/or the big toe.

My research has revealed that Sciatica on the left side is governed by Sodium, and the right side by Potassium. When there is pain descending down both legs, this signifies that both the Sodium and Potassium levels are down. Some of the herbs used to elevate the Potassium level are Burdock and Bee Pollen, and some very good souces of Sodium would be found in celery, Spirulina, or common salt.

Most Chiropractors feel that Sciatica is a Chiropratic problem; most medical doctors use pain killers. Both professions are incorrect. The Sciatic nerve will become inflamed due to a lack of the electrolytes Sodium (left side), and Potassium (right side).

Inflammation of the nerve can be accompanied by swelling which would engender bone pressure. This pressure can be relieved by an adjustment by the Chiropractor, but the cause of the pain is in essence, the inflammation and not the bone pressure.

Sciatica is a mystery to most doctors. We have found that it can be improved simply by administering the correct amount of Potassium and/or Sodium over a three to four week period. When the pain is gone, you should continue to administer the treatment for at least three more days, or check daily to see what is needed.

If the weather is hot, Potassium and Sodium can be lost due to perspiration, so the Sciatic nerve can be affected. This is why the levels should be checked daily to see what is needed.

Sciatica is basically a deficiency condition caused by the electrolyte imbalance of Sodium and/or Potassium.

SINUS CONDITIONS

Inflammation of the sinuses is usually caused by an allergic reaction. We have found that the lower sinuses are governed by the Adrenal Cortex and also affected by Potassium and Sodium.

The lower sinuses can be found below the middle of the eyes on the cheek bones:

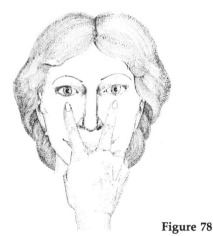

Figure 78

The Adrenal Cortex can be weakened by stress which burns up Pantothenic Acid causing an allergy to the Citrus Group* and affecting the sinuses. If there is a lack of Pantothenic Acid and a citrus allergy is present, the sinuses may become inflamed and discharge mucus through the nostrils.

To test the sinuses, place two fingers of one hand on each sinus point (below middle of the eyes on the cheek bones) and extend the opposite arm to be "pumped" by the other person. If the sinuses are inflamed the extended arm will go down when it is pumped by the other person.

To correct this, place some Pantothenic Acid (or Royal Jelly) in the hand and touch the sinus points again while the other person pulls down (pumps) the extended arm. If there is a sufficient amount of Pantothenic Acid in the hand, the arm will be strong and not go down. If the amount of Pantothenic Acid shows strong, it should now be checked by holding to the Solar Plexus while having the other person pull down on extended arm. If the arm still remains strong it is showing that the amount that is needed for the sinus condition can also be taken by that person at the time. If the arm showed weak when holding to the Solar Plexus, it may mean that the amount may be too much for the person at the time so take one or two out and re-test until you find the amount that makes the arm strong again. This can then be re-tested later on.

I prefer to use Royal Jelly as a source of Pantothenic Acid, as it is naturally rich in Pantothenic Acid and also non-allergenic. Pantothenic Acid will help strengthen the Adrenals and take away a citrus allergy. Other herbs that are good for the adrenals are Licorice Root and Wild Yam.

The *upper* sinus points are governed by the Pituitary gland and can be found directly *above* the middle of the eyebrows:

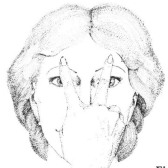

Figure 79

*Citrus Group: Cantaloupe, Lime, Grapefruit, Lemon, Oranges, Tangerine, Tomato, Pineapple.

The Pituitary gland is affected by Potassium and Sodium and if one, the other, or both are lacking, it can create an allergy to different foods causing mucus to form around the Pituitary gland and drain through the nostrils.

For instance, if a person is low in Potassium he may have a reaction to foods that are high in Sodium (Greens). On the other hand, if the person is lacking in Sodium, he could become allergic to foods containing Potassium. A deficiency in both will effect the Pituitary gland causing it to become inflamed because of the need for these nutrients.

We have found Alfalfa to be an excellent natural source of Potassium and Sodium, containing 2 parts Potassium and 1 part Sodium.

Other nutrients for the Pituitary gland are Vitamin B-6, Pituitary Glandular Substance, and the amino acids Ornithine and Tryptophan. A combination of all of these can be found in the product "GH" (Growth Hormone) Release". These nutrients along with the Sodium and Potassium needed for the Pituitary gland, will nourish the Pituitary gland and clear up the inflammation.

The upper sinuses can be checked the same way as the lower. Place the two fingers over each sinus point above the eyebrows as shown in figure 79. Extend opposite arm while another person pulls down (or "Pumps") on the extended arm. If arm goes down it is showing an inflammation. Next, place the antidote for the upper sinuses in the hand and again touch the sinus points above the eyebrows. If the correct amount has been placed in the hand, the extended arm will now be strong when it is pumped. This is showing the amount needed to correct the problem.

A nasal drip or "stuffiness" on one particular side could mean a need for Sodium or Potassium, depending on which side. If the problem is on the right side, this would indicate more of a need for Potassium; while a problem on the left side would mean a need for Sodium. If the nasal drip or inflammation is on both sides, this means that both Potassium and Sodium are needed.

Sinus problems can be corrected by eliminating allergies and administering the proper electrolytes (Potassium and Sodium) and nutrients to nourish the system.

TINNITUS

Tinnitus is a ringing in the ears which can sound like a hissing noise or an avalanche. Through our research, we have found that *what* ear the Tinnitus occurs in is an indication to what is wrong.

We have found that Tinnitus in the *left* ear is usually caused by an allergy to rice and the "rice allergy food group" which consists of cinnamon, blueberries, grapes, rice, strawberry, watermelon, wine, and pumpkin. This allergy can be corrected with the mineral Manganese, Vitamin B-6, and the amino acid Arginine. The herb Yucca is also good for it is an excellent source of Manganese.

A ringing in the right ear is caused by a "wheat allergy" and can be corrected with Vitamin F (which can be found in safflower oil, olive oil, and sunflower oil), the mineral Magnesium, and the amino acid Histidine.

Each ear is affected by a different allergy and we have found that the antidote to each allergy consists of a vitamin, a mineral, and amino acid. By correcting the allergies and replacing these missing nutrients the problem can be corrected. However, if a person has had this problem for a while, I do recommend that they have patience and continue on a complete nutritional program with the proper supplements as a synergistic back-up for the remedies mentioned before. In our experience, we have found that it can take at least one month for every year the person has had the condition before the problem is corrected. So if a person has had this problem for three years, it may take at least three months on this sort of program before they actually begin to notice a difference.

TOXEMIA

Toxemia is actually a poisoning of the body through different substances which make the body toxic. One of the most popular causes of Toxemia is Aluminum poisoning. Aluminum poisoning occurs in many ways. One of the ways it occurs is by cooking with Aluminum utensils. The Aluminum pot will interact with the food being cooked and displace all the important minerals out of the food into the water while the Aluminum is absorbed by the food.

The body can only tolerate so much Aluminum, so what happens is the Aluminum is not absorbed and ends up in the blood stream as a sludge which is then carried into the liver. When the minerals are displaced with the Aluminum, your body will not be getting the minerals it needs to function properly. So when a mineral such as Iron is lost, the result is a diminishing of the red blood cells, and, therefore, Anemia resulting from a lack of Iron. If Zinc is displaced, we have found that problems with the reproductive organs will set in, and possibly problems with the eyes. So by cooking with Aluminum, you are not only displacing all of the important minerals that the body needs, but you will also have food that is laden with Aluminum, and, therefore, toxic to the body.

Aluminum should not be used for cooking at all, this includes Aluminum wrap. If Aluminum wrap is used with any citrus fruit, or tomatoes which have been cut, you will probably notice after a day that the Aluminum is pitted and eaten away. This should give you an example of what is happening!

Beverages, such as the citrus sodas, should never be drunk out of Aluminum cans. Ironically, there is a different taste between the beverages in a glass bottle and an Aluminum can. This is because the Aluminum from the can is now being ingested with the beverage. One of the Cola manufacturers think that the reason the sale of Aluminum cans is ten times more than that of the bottles, is because of the taste, so what they are now doing is pouring liquid Aluminum into the Cola bottles to make it taste the same as the Cola in the can. If this isn't lunacy I don't know what is! Another thing which should be mentioned, is that food should never be stored in Aluminum containers overnight. The toxins from the Aluminum will readily cause a toxic problem in the body.

Toxemia is evident when a person has dark rings showing around the eyes; this shows toxemia of the liver and kidneys. The cooking utensils that are preferred are: stainless steel, Iron, and glass ware such as Pyrex and Corning Ware. These utensils contain Iron and Chrome which are needed by the body.

Teflon products can also be toxic, as it is usually an Aluminum pot that is coated with the Teflon substance which then peels off and mixes with the food causing toxemia. Copper pots and enamel pots should also be avoided. Enamel pots are usually made of Cadmium which is the opposite molecule of the mineral Zinc. Cadmium is also found in cigarette smoke, car fumes, and other urban pollution, and can cause Hypertension if taken into the body. Lead is another toxic substance. Ironically, the government is aware of lead in paint, but not aware of the lead solder that is used in the canned foods that are on the market. Again, if the can contains a citrus food, the acid will dissolve the lead in the can and it will be ingested when the food is eaten.

Frozen foods are treated with a substance called E.D.T.A. which happens to be a chelation factor to make the food look more colorful. What this substance does is hook on to the metal minerals contained in the food and when it unites with water, will wash them out.

Another form of toxemia in the body is Mercury poisoning. Mercury is sometimes found in seafood, but I do not believe that this is the causation of Mercury poisoning in our population. Most of the Mercury poisoning in our population is caused by our dentists. I know I am going to make enemies with some dentists when I say this, but Silver Amalgam, which is used for fillings, is sixty percent Mercury. It is used in fillings because it is less expensive than gold. I have heard of many dentists who have taken the gold fillings out of people's teeth and replaced them with silver fillings. This happens sometimes when Oriental or many Latin people come over to this country and want to be Americanized, so one of the things that they will do is have the gold taken out of their teeth and have it replaced with the silver fillings. This is gross stupidity! Gold is far superior to the Mercury Amalgam.

The Mercury in the Amalgam, if it is too much, will actually go into the gums and then into the blood stream, causing Mercury poisoning. Mercury is highly toxic, and a way you can find out if you have Mercury poisoning is to check for what is called the "Amalgam tatoo" on the gum below the filling. If there is a purple mark on the gum, it is not a Periodontal problem, but actually an Amalgam tatoo.

There are many ways to rid the body of these toxins. One way of chelating the heavy metals out of the body would be with the amino acids L-Methionine and L-Cysteine which are contained in the herbs Dandelion and Sarsaparilla. The heavy metals can also be taken out of the body with Superoxide Dismutase (also called S.O.D.), which will also chelate the metals out of the blood stream and organs.

Aluminum can be very difficult to get out of the system but we have found that Gold Chloride is effective in helping to relieve the Aluminum toxemia. Gold Chloride is a homeopathic formula which is available from any homeopathic wholesale house. Mercury poisoning can be alleviated by Silver Chloride which will neutralize the mercury in the system.

Another form of toxemia in our modern day life is Radiation. Radiation comes to us in many forms. One way is by sitting too close to the television set. I fear that the computer age may be causing more radiation toxemia than in the past. Radiation toxemia can also come from microwave ovens, X-Ray machines, and, believe it or not, by flying above the clouds during the day when there is radiation from the sun. This happens because most planes are Aluminum, so when flying under the sun, you are almost like a potato in an Aluminum casing. We believe that this flight fatigue that is called "jet lag", is not only a time differential problem, but also a solar radiation problem. Therefore, we recommend night flights to day flights if possible.

Unnecessary X-Rays are the major cause of the radiation problem. The medical profession seems to believe in X-Raying everything, even though many times they are not even necessary for the detection of the problem. Many times the X-Rays are not for the purpose of detection or diagnosis, but for the protection of their own practice. It is called practice insurance. It is done so that they will have an X-Ray of the person's condition before it was treated by them to show the condition existed before, in case the person should sue them. It is a defensive practice which is being taught in many medical schools.

Some of the visible physical signs of toxemia are: an acne condition, graying of the skin, darkness around the eyes, and headaches sometimes accompanied by diarrhea, indigestion, or gastritis. Many people who eat food out of Aluminum will have these symptoms, not realizing what it is from.

For more information on Toxemia, please refer to chapter on ACNE.

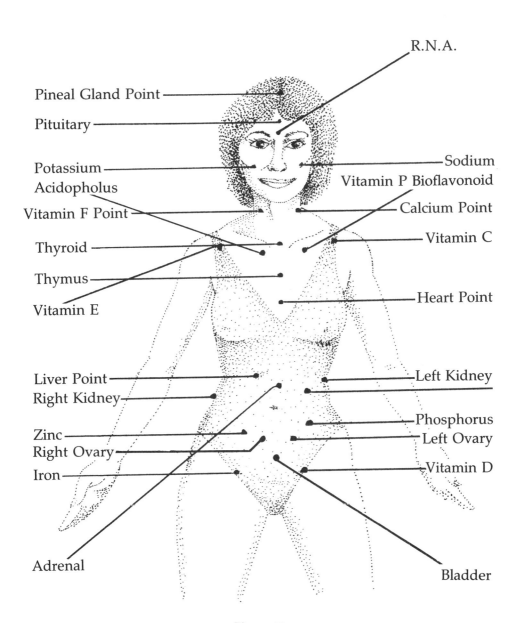

Figure 80

CHAPTER 12

ADDICTIONS

ALCOHOLISM

Alcoholism is a disease. It is usually a physical or physiological disease caused by an allergic reaction to the alcohol substance to which the person tends to be drawn. For instance, a person with an allergy to potato would usually be affected by vodka; rye would probably be the choice of a person with a rye allergy; and people with a corn allergy are usually drawn to most of the colored liquors because of the corn which is usually used as the coloring agent in most of these liquors.

We had an incident where a person was trapped into imbibing two cases of beer each evening. This person could not get to bed unless and until drunk from the beer, and even then, was unable to sleep. It turned out that this man had a Brewer's Yeast allergy and was tremendously deficient in the B-complex vitamins, which he tended to absorb from the beer. We gave him a B-Complex from a rice source, and took away his yeast allergy by giving him Zinc. Within a few weeks, he no longer craved beer and was able to stop his alcoholic need because of the presence of sufficient Zinc to stop the yeast allergy, and enough of the B-Complex Vitamins so that he didn't have to search for them in beer.

We also had a lady who was addicted to gin. We started her on a complete program of nutritional balancing, but we found in her system the need for Juniper Berries. Juniper Berries are used in the manufacture of Gin, but as an herb, they contain Potassium and a natural insulin for the body. What we found basically is that this person needed this insulin, and if she did not get it in the gin, she would feel tired and exhausted. With the gin she was able to get enough insulin to process her sugar properly. Ironically, she started on the program with sixteen Juniper Berries a day, and in a period of three weeks she reduced her intake to two Juniper Berries a day so the gin was not needed by her system. With these results in different situations, we feel that alcoholism is basically a nutritional imbalance by chemicals and allergies.

We did run a clinic to evaluate alcoholics to try and find the missing link and found one of them to be the amino acid Glutamine which feeds the brain and helps make one think clearer and more logically. Alcohol tends to destroy Glutamine in the brain making it very important to replace it. In all cases, the Glutamine was used and was sometimes started out as high as ten 500 milligram capsules. As the dosage dropped down to one 500 milligram capsule, the client's thinking became clearer, the craving for alcohol disappeared, and the person became more or less normal except for one other factor.

In our research we have found that the social climate also has to change. Many alcoholics have spent hours and hours in bars for the greater part of their lives. These types of personalities have to find different places to socialize which can be rather difficult in our present day society. The Alcoholic's Anonymous (A.A.) philosophy is, "once an alcoholic, always an alcoholic". We do not feel that this is always true. We have found that through nutritional programs the biochemical bases of people who are alcoholics can be changed so that they will not become addicted and have to continue drinking after just one drink.

I would like some day for the A.A. group to evaluate the research we have done to see if it is feasible to regenerate the normal chemistry in the body. Therefore the desire for alcohol will no longer be there, so the alcoholic will be free from the constant fear of returning to alcohol.

The Al-anon group, which is a sister group of A.A., is a group which will aid people affected by alcoholics. Alcoholism not only affects the person who is the alcoholic, but those who are family and friends. The Al-Anon group is geared to try to help these people. Their philosophy is "one day at a time", to try to understand the consistency of the alcoholic and the alcoholic's constant denial of being an alcoholic.

It is important that an alcoholic be tested for all of the nutrients, and especially B-Complex (which is used to sooth nerves) and the amino acid proteins to feed body tissues which have become depleted. Zinc, which we have noted earlier, is very important. Many researchers have found that Zinc is depleted by alcohol, but I have found that many times the craving for alcohol is greater if the person is lacking in Zinc. One thing the alcoholic experiences when allergic to what is being drunk, is a hangover or a buzz. One of the important things in treating an alcoholic is after the biochemical balancing has taken place, there is a need for a different social environment. What we found in our experimental group was that some of the people who were cured of alcoholism, could now go into drinking establishments and drink the other patrons (so to speak) under the table without a hangover. Once the allergies are gone, there is no longer a hangover. A hangover is an allergic reaction to the alcohol consumed. We feel that alcoholism can be treated through a proper nutritional environment and a proper social re-adjustment.

Many alcoholics need to face the situation directly, which is very difficult for them to do and, therefore, challenge themselves to succeed. The ratio of success for alcoholics in our experience has been sixty percent. There are people who sometimes want to get well, but still want to drink because of the social implications. This has to be changed along with the nutritional balance.

One of the greatest nutritional deficiencies we have found in the alcoholic population is a Sodium deficiency. Sodium holds water in the cells of the body. Without sufficient Sodium, alcoholics will dehydrate from the loss of water, either through urination or sweating; this is immediately followed by a tremendous thirst for liquids.

Water will usually taste brackish to a person low in Sodium, so water is seldom used as a way to quench the thirst of an alcoholic with low Sodium.

Celery juice would be an excellent beverage to quench the thirst of an alcoholic as it contains a tremendous amount of Sodium, plus much Calcium, which is a sedative and will tend to relax the drinker.

COCAINE

Cocaine is usually administered to the body through a system called "Snorting". Snorting involves the use of a straw through which the cocaine is sniffed into the nostrils. By snorting, the cocaine is pulled through the nostrils directly into the respiratory system.

One of the reactions we have noted with the use of cocaine, is the deterioration of the Pituitary gland, which is the master gland of the body, controlling all other glands. The Pituitary acupuncture point is located at the hair line on top of the skull in the fore front in line with the nose.

We have found that the use of cocaine will also cause the Pituitary gland to "leak". What I mean by this, is that the Pituitary gland will cause a mucus discharge to drain through the nasal passages, causing the classic nasal drip. This nasal drip is actually the Pituitary gland throwing off mucus.

When the Pituitary gland becomes weak, the Sodium and Potassium are not held in the body as they should, but are released through the urine. With the loss of these electrolytes (Sodium and Potassium) the person will feel weak and tired unless he uses more cocaine. This creates a vicious circle.

Some of the corrective nutrients are:

Pituitary glandular substance
Vitamin B-6 and Vitamin E
Amino Acids Ornithine, Tryptophan, and L-Glutamine
The herbs Gotu Kola and Alfalfa

We have found that the herb Gotu Kola is very important for the regeneration of the Pituitary along with the use of Vitamin E. The normal dosage of Vitamin E is about 400 units, but when working with someone with this problem you will sometimes need as much as 1,600 units to start with in order to correct the damage done by the cocaine.

All pharmaceutical drugs, whether they are prescribed or sold over the counter, should be checked for side effects (which can be done by the use of muscle response testing). Many drugs, such as Diuretics, can cause a loss of electrolytes (Potassium, Sodium, and other minerals) which will cause allergies. Any drug that you wish to use should be tested by holding the quantity to the Solar Plexus while having someone pump the extended opposite arm to see if it is acceptable to the body. Even if the substance being tested is acceptable to the body, it does not mean that it does not have side effects.

What I usually do is take the pill the person wishes to use and have them hold it in their hand while extending their opposite arm to be pumped. Have the person place the hand holding the pill first to the top of the skull while pumping their extended opposite arm, then to the sides of the skull while pumping the other arm, then the back of the head while pumping the arm. If the arm goes down when it is pumped this showing you that it could have side effects that would affect the person mentally. The next thing to do is to have them hold the pill to the Sodium point (hollow of check left side) and Potassium point (hollow of cheek right side) while pumping their extended opposite arm. This will tell you if it will affect these levels. Also, it should be noted that a drop in the Sodium or Potassium levels could also cause personality changes. A Sodium loss will cause a depression while a Potassium loss would cause allergies to milk, cheese, and Sodium foods, making the person feel tired and lack energy.

DRUG ABUSE

Two basic drugs being used in this society this century, are Marijuana and Cocaine. In our research we have found Marijuana not be recommended for over-the-counter distribution. Marijuana causes degeneration of the left hemisphere of the brain, which we have found to be the thinking brain. Marijuana tends to throw out the protein and weaken the thinking process of the individual. It is difficult for a person to think clearly if on this drug.

The other thing we have found, is that Marijuana actually destroys the Adrenal Cortex. It depletes the Adrenal Cortex, and the side effect of Marijuana misuse is Hypoglycemia. I do not believe that every hypoglycemic uses drugs, but I am trying to say that a drug user will tend to become hypoglycemic. That is one of the reasons Marijuana users get the "Munchies" and consume a lot of sugar. Perhaps it is hypoglycemia that paves the way for one to become addicted to drugs, but certainly hypoglycemia is an after-effect.

The use of Marijuana can be withdrawn by breaking the addiction with the utilization of the amino acid L-Glutamine and Vitamin B-5, Pantothenic Acid. Pantothenic Acid will feed the Adrenal Cortex and remove the distressful feeling of the dependency for the Marijuana. The amino acid L-Glutamine will start to make the mind think clearly so as to see the real problem.

Marijuana is clearly addictive, contrary to some widely held beliefs; so is cigarette smoking equally addictive. We believe that Marijuana use in this society can be a very dangerous and detrimental instrument.

SMOKING

Smoking is man's abomination to the body, but fifty percent of the population at the present time is still smoking cigarettes! If God wanted you to smoke, He would have built a cigarette on your lip!

Nicotine is the opposite molecule of Niacin. Another name for Niacin is Nicotinic Acid. With Nicotine, the Niacin in the brain is displaced and replaced with the Nicotine, causing an addiction to the cigarettes. When the addicted person is not able to have the Nicotine, irritableness, depression or crabbiness are evident. This individual feels an inability to relax until after procuring "the fix"—a cigarette. The relaxation a person feels after having smoked a cigarette is due to the addiction to the Nicotine which has displaced the Niacin in the body.

If a person wishing to stop smoking does it "cold turkey", usually the body will start to put on weight. The reason for this is that the Niacin now needs to displace the Nicotine which is phasing out. Niacin is one of the "enrichments" in white bread, and this is why many people who stop smoking will start to search out starches which contain Niacin.

By administering Niacin and Niacinamide, the person will not have cravings for starches, so the weight will not be gained if Niacinamide or Niacin is utilized. Another thing smoking does is tar the lungs. It actually tars the holes in the lungs. The best way to demonstrate this would be to visualize a sponge. The function of a sponge is to absorb liquid, but if the sponge is sprayed with something like nail polish, it will harden and solidify and be unable to absorb liquid. By tarring the lungs with cigarette tar, the lungs are not functioning as they should be. Therefore, the blood is not being purified because it is not getting the oxygen that it needs to do so.

Oxygen is very important to the body. The body can go without food for forty days and without water for six or seven days, but the body can not go without oxygen for more than six minutes. This is how precious air is to the body. Oxygen purifies the blood, so when you smoke, you are curtailing your lungs' ability to purify the blood. Therefore, over a long period of time, the blood will become contaminated and start to affect the other parts of the body.

It is said that each cigarette burns up twenty-five milligrams of Vitamin C. The job that Vitamin C does in the body, is basically clean it up, but we have found that it also burns Sulfur. Ironically, the throat coughs which you get are Nicotine demands from the brain, but we have found that smoking also burns up Sulfur in the blood. To replace the Sulfur, we have used the Sulfur-containing amino acids: Methionine and Cysteine and the herbs Sarsaparilla and Fenugreek. When the Sulfur in the system has been burned up, the smoker might experience a sore throat which usually means there is a fat allergy.

The antidote to the fat allergy is Sulfur. When a person with a fat allergy has a piece of bread and butter along with eggs, there will probably be a coughing fit because of the fat (butter), and feel the need to light up another cigarette. By doing this, more Sulfur will be thrown out (remember Sulfur purifies the blood), thus making the situation worse.

Sulfur is the beauty mineral, being used to make beautiful skin, hair and nails. Cigarette smoking throws out Sulfur along with L-Methionine and L-Cysteine, the amino acids which make the cells more flexible. Therefore, cigarette smoking can actually be considered an aging device, causing a person to age faster than normally. One of the first things we recommend to people who enter a Life-Extension Program is to stop smoking.

One of the things which smoking is believed to cause is a Hiatal hernia. We believe this is true because when an allergic substance enters the system, there will be explosions in the stomach affecting the hiatal valve. When the allergic foods are eaten, the acid in the stomach will come up into the hiatal valve of the esophagus and burn it, causing what is known as an Hiatal hernia. One of the most important things to do when this condition occurs, is to stop smoking.

Stopping smoking is much easier said than done, but we believe that if a person's health is restored, that this might make it easier to stop. Some of the things used in our process to cure smokers are:

1.) Niacin, a vaso-dilator, to displace Nicotine in the brain.
2.) Vitamin B-15, to give the body more oxygen so the desire to smoke would be less.
3.) Vitamin E, to utilize oxygen in the body more thoroughly.
4.) The herb Golden Seal, to melt the tar from the lungs.

One thing which should be mentioned about the herb Golden Seal is that it should not be used in the beginning of the program. Since it actually melts tar from the lungs, and acts as an expectorant, it will bring up a lot of green and yellow phlegm from the lungs which might make the person fearful. This herb should be used after the smoking has stopped and the lungs have begun to reconstruct, as if it is done all at once, the person might suffer a traumatic experience and go back to smoking.

Another device that can be used is a special filter that contains a water chamber. What the filter does is lessen the intake of nicotine and tar from the cigarette making it easier for a person to switch to a lower tar and nicotine cigarette, and eventually stop. By using a filter, the person

332 The Ultimate Healing System

will also see the trappings of the tar in the filter which normally enter the lungs. This will hopefully make them think twice about what they are putting into their bodies, and perhaps take an adverse stand against smoking.

A book that we recommend for people who wish to stop smoking is "You Can Stop", by Smoke Enders (co-founder), Jacquelyn Rogers. The book is published by Pocket Books, 1230 Avenue of the Americas, New York, New York, 10020.

CHAPTER 13

MAN'S ECOLOGICAL SUICIDE

ALUMINUM

Aluminum is something that is constantly used in our modern society. Aluminum is used as cookware, as lining in containers, and is also added to things like deodorant and certain antacids. However, Aluminum is a toxic mineral and should never be used as a cooking utensil or ingested in any form.

When food is cooked in an Aluminum pot, a reaction occurs between the pot and the food, causing the Aluminum to displace any of the other metal minerals the food may contain. Minerals such as Iron, Zinc, Manganese, Chrome, Magnesium, and Copper are displaced from the food into the water and replaced with Aluminum. The food may now taste metallic because it is full of Aluminum and poisonous! The body doesn't need Aluminum! Aluminum is harmful to the body! The body needs the other minerals that were displaced by the Aluminum! One of the causes of Alzheimer's disease is too much Aluminum in the blood which lodges in the brain area.

NEVER drink juices or sodas (especially citrus) from Aluminum cans, as the Aluminum in the can will actually be dissolved by the acid of the citrus juices so that the soda or juice will contain traces of Aluminum. Again, this is poisonous! To test this theory, wrap a slice of tomato or citrus fruit in a piece of Aluminum foil. The next day you will see that the Aluminum has become pitted by the acid from the tomato or fruit.

I wonder how much skin cancer is caused by the Aluminum which is used in roll-on deodorants, or how much osteo-arthritis is caused by the taking of antacids containing Aluminum and/or Magnesium Hydroxide which are known to hinder the absorption of Phosphorus which is needed to re-build the outer layer of bone and tooth enamel.

ENAMEL POTS

Enamel pots often contain Cadmium which also is a toxic metal, so enamel pots should also be avoided!

TEFLON COOKWARE

Teflon coated pots could also be dangerous as Teflon itself is a toxic substance, and if it is scraped off it can become mixed in with the food and ingested. Teflon pots are also usually Aluminum pots coated with Teflon.

EARTHEN COOKWARE

One should be careful of using earthen pots because of the possibility of the clay containing toxic substances.

I believe the best cookware to be stainless steel and glass (Pyrex or Corning Ware). Stainless steel is made of Iron and Chrome, both of which the body can absorb; while glassware does not interact with food.

Glass Bottles are also better for storage than plastic bottles. Remember, plastic is not water soluble, but it does react with the food or drink that is stored in it so remember this when you are eating or drinking something that was stored in plastic because you will be getting a little plastic too!

MERCURY POISONING

Many dentists use a Silver Amalgam filling which contains Mercury. Mercury is poisonous!! If you are going to have your teeth filled by the dentist, always request Acrylic or Gold fillings or caps; NEVER Silver Amalgam or Aluminum!! Also be sure that the enamel tooth caps do not contain Cadmium.

Dentists are divided in their awareness of the Mercury poisoning problem. I have actually seen cases of Multiple Sclerosis recover when the Mercury Amalgam fillings were taken out and replaced with Acrylic fillings. The condition can also be helped if a nutritional program is followed and can start to disappear in as little as 3 weeks.

There are different devices that are now available to test for Mercury poisoning, but they can be quite expensive. If you wish to test Mercury Amalgam fillings for possible adverse effects, you can use the M.R.T. method. Have the person that is being tested place the pinky of their right hand in their mouth. Start on either the top or bottom teeth, but however you begin, start on the last molar on either side touching each one individually while pumping the extended opposite arm as each tooth is touched. If extended arm goes down when pumped, it is showing that something is wrong with that particular tooth!

This could indicate a cavity (decay), or it could be toxic from an excess of Mercury. To find out, first use the Homeopathic Substance called "Argent Nit" (Latin for Silver Nitrate) and find out how much is needed by the person using the Muscle Response Testing method. Place some Argent Nit in the hand of the person that is being tested and have them hold the same hand to the Solar Plexus while extending the opposite arm to be pumped. Pull down on their extended arm and add or subtract the amount of Argent Nit until you find the amount that makes the extended arm strongest. This will give you the exact amount needed at the time.

Once you have found the correct amount of Argent Nit, have them again hold it in their hand and extend the pinky of the same hand (as a probe) and put it inside the mouth while touching the pinky to the tooth that showed weak. Re-test the tooth as they hold the hand with the Argent Nit to the tooth and pull down on their extended arm. If the arm now shows strong and rigid while touching this tooth, it is showing that the tooth has a Mercury Amalgam problem.

Another way to visually spot this problem is to look at the gums below the weak tooth. If they have purple blotches (also called Amalgam Tatoos), then there is a possibility that Mercury is seeping out of the filling into the body's blood stream.

PESTICIDES

Man believes that pesticides can protect plant destruction by pests, not realizing that when it rains the pesticides wash off the plant and enter the soil where they are absorbed by the plant and cannot simply wash off since they are now contained within the plant.

This is why (though seemingly more expensive) organically grown foods are preferred. No wonder there is so much illness in the world today. We are eating foods that are saturated with pesticides, and poisoning ourselves needlessly!!

The F.D.A. has now realized the mistake it has made in allowing the use of certain chemicals and is now restricting the use of certain pesticides. But yet, we have sent out our "Peace Corps" to the third world countries to introduce them to the use of chemicals in farming.

We, through our enthusiasm for chemical use in our farming techniques, have screwed up the world and damned the people in it with illness and disease because of this poisoned food.

If you do buy "super market" vegetables and wish to extract any possible pesticides, you can do this by soaking the vegetables in water and clorox. For every quart of water, add ½ a teaspoon and soak the vegetables in this solution for about 20 minutes. After soaking in solution, remove and soak in clear water for about a ½ hour to remove the clorox. This should remove any pesticides that may be in the vegetables.

PROCESSED FOODS

Much of food's nutritional value is destroyed through processing. An example is canned food, which contains only 25% of it's nutritive value compared to fresh food. In vacuum packing, food is usually heated and then sealed so the vacuum will occur when the food cools down. High heat destroys many nutrients and vitamins.

Frozen foods contain only about 50% of their original nutritional value. In order to make the food look more appealing, the substance EDTA is added during processing. This makes the food look great, but when the food is cooked, the EDTA extracts any minerals the food might contain leaving the minerals in the cooking water. So unless the water in which the vegetables are cooked is also consumed, the meal will be lacking in important minerals and nutrients.

Cooking even fresh vegetables can kill the enzymes they contain. Whenever possible, vegetables should be eaten raw, steamed, or cooked lightly in a wok.

COFFEE

We have found that coffee contains properties which destroy Choline in the brain, therefore making one forgetful. The reason many people need a cup of coffee in the morning is that it has the ability to raise the Sodium level in the body, thereby temporarily alleviating all allergies so that the breakfast can be consumed.

TEA

Tea was not meant for human consumption. It contains Tannic acid (Tannic acid is used to remove hair from hides in the leather industry). Because of its toxic effect, it becomes a diuretic for Potassium. Anyone who is low in Potassium should not drink tea, for it could deplete any Potassium one has, thereby causing a heart problem, which is also caused by a lack of Potassium.

MEAT

Many nutritionists believe that red meat is bad for you. I personally am a beefeater. I feel it is probably the best source of Zinc and protein of any food.

What is wrong is the way we permit the livestock breeders (ranchers) and veterinarians to inoculate the herd with hormones (usually female) so that the muscle meat will be soft and tender while the body weight is heavier. Because these hormones are passed on to us, the consumer, we often find ourselves gaining weight.

There was a phenomenon happening in Puerto Rico at one time. Young girls from 3 years of age and up were beginning to develop breasts. This was traced to the consumption of chickens that were raised on feed that was enriched with hormones. When the children stopped eating the hormone fed chickens, the breast growth subsided!!

Again, if you do choose to eat meat, use organic meat from animals that have been raised on organic feed and chickens that have been fed quality feed. Argentinian beef has no hormones added! It is illegal in Argentina to give hormones to livestock!

If a chicken is fed feed that contains pesticides, the eggs from that chicken will also be tainted with pesticides. The egg may also have a Cadmium taste to it. And of course if the egg hatches and grows to be a chicken, that chicken will also be toxic. I guess there is just no end to it!!!

SUGAR

Sugar destroys the B-Complex Vitamins in the body. Sugar also destroys the Phosphorus in the body, causing cavities and osteo-arthritis.

Sugar can also cause deposits in the tear ducts causing Glaucoma. I also believe that too much sugar can cause cancer if a sufficient amount of oxygen is not taken into the body to consume the Carbon caused by the oxidation of the sugar.

CHAPTER 14

DRINKING WATER

DRINKING WATER

What kind or type should you use? There are basically four types of water used for human consumption. One is rain water, which is used in many of the islands such as the Bahamas, Virgin Islands, and Caribbean.

Rain water is very pure, but sometimes is lacking in minerals, and can be contaminated by radiation in the atmosphere. It is not the best source of water to use, but in some cases it is the only available type.

The second type is tap water, which can be pure, but at the same time negative to the human body. Tap water contains purifying chemicals such as Chlorine. From our research, we found that Chlorine is one cause of the heart conditions that exist today. The body needs Hydrochloric acid to help extract nutrients from foods but Chlorine unites with Potassium and Sodium and extracts these electrolytes out of the body.

Before the turn of the century, before the countries in the western world started to chlorinate the water, heart conditions were not so readily prevalent. We feel the chlorination of water causes the electrolytes to be excreted from the body, and this may be the reason for cardiac disease in the twentieth century.

Another problem with chlorinated water is that if a city's water system has old Zinc pipes, Cadmium may have been used to unite the joints of the pipes which could create other toxic minerals in the water.

We usually recommend that our clients drink mineral water. We have found that it can provide certain minerals the body needs to ward off allergies and other conditions. However, if you find yourself choking on mineral water, it is a tell-tale sign that there is something in it that you cannot tolerate.

The mineral content of water tends to vary in different locations. Our home base is on the east coast, in New Jersey, where we tend to need more minerals. When we visited Las Vegas, we had trouble adjusting to the tap water which was highly mineralized because of the limestone in the Colorado Basin. The water we were drinking happened to be from Lake Mead which had run down the Grand Canyon in Colorado picking up so many minerals that it became over-mineralized. This may be the reason why many authorities on the west coast, Utah, and the Colorado area tell their clients to drink distilled water.

Distilled water is considered the purest water, but is also divorced from all nutrients. Since it is so pure, it does not nourish the body, but actually washes it. Distilled water can be used for a period of one to three days to help the body detoxify any excessive minerals. But long term use, without replacing the minerals in the body through food supplements, could cause a tremendous depletion in the mineral resources of the body, which could be detrimental.

It is understandable that many of the authorities recommend distilled water, since most of the herbal authorities are in the western United States, they are aware of the over mineralization of their regular water, so they promote distilled water.

Here on the east coast, our water does not contain as many minerals, so this is why we suggest the use of mineral water. A good compromise would be half a glass of distilled water to half a glass of mineral water.

The conflicts between authorities arise when they evaluate the water from their own prospective areas.

CHAPTER 15

MIRACLE FOODS

BEE POLLEN

Bee Pollen contains an abundance of the B-Vitamins including B-1, B-2, B-3 (Niacinamide), B-5 (Pantothenic Acid), B-6, and B-12. Bee Pollen also contains Vitamin C, Vitamin A, Vitamin E, Folic Acid, and 20% is composed of protein and amino acids.

There are two kinds of pollen, Anemophile Pollens, and Entomophile Pollens. The Anemophiles, from "Anemos" wind, and "Philos" - friend, depend on air for fecundation and are prolific. All conifers (pines, firs, etc.) have Anemophile Pollens. Anemophile Pollens do not contain the necessary desirable nutrients, are not gathered by the bees, and are also allergenic. On the other hand, Entomophile ("friend of the insects") Pollen which is gathered by bees, are of the potent nutritional variety, and are non-allergenic.

Entomophile Pollens, which are collected by the bees, are sticky, some extremely sticky, and cannot be carried by the wind. When the bees form them into pellets, add a little nectar and saliva, this further neutralizes and destroys any allergic principle that may exist. It should be noted that pollen is the male element of the flower. Under a microscope, pollen appears as a fine powder, an infinite amount of grains of very artistic forms and designs representing the specific flower from which it comes. This fine powder, enclosing enormous nutritive and medicinal properties, form the ovules, the starting point of the production of fruits, grains, legumes, and vegetables.

We did use "Riviera" Pollen which is imported from Spain and France because they did not spray insecticides on their flowers as we do in the

United States. But as of April 25, 1986, Chernobyl's Nuclear Power Plant explosion contaminated all of Europe's flowers and herbs with radiation fall-out so as to make us look toward the Southern Hemisphere for pollen.

One thousand milligrams of Bee Pollen (or 2-500 milligram capsules) contain 600 milligrams of natural Potassium!! It also contains the following minerals:

1% - 12%	Magnesium
1% - 15%	Calcium
.05% - .08%	Copper
.01% - .3%	Iron
2% - 10%	Silica
1% - 20%	Phosphorus
1.%	Sulfur
1.%	Chlorine
1.4%	Manganese

The following vitamins are found in 1,000 milligrams (two 500 mg. capsules) of Bee Pollen:

9.2 mg.	Vitamin B-1, Thiamine
18.50 mg.	Vitamin B-2, Riboflavin
5. mg.	Vitamin B-6, Pyridoxine
200 mg.	Niacinamide (B-3)
30 - 50 mg.	Pantothenic Acid (B-5)
3.4 - 6.8 mg.	Folic Acid
7 - 15 mg.	Vitamin C
.5 - .9 mg.	Carotenoids

Also contains traces of Tocopherol Vitamin E

Bee Pollen also contains approximately 17% of Rutin (Vitamin P)

Studies of dry pollen have been done after removing the lipids with Ether, showing 26.88% proteins and 13% amino acids.

The following is the quantitative analysis of these amino acids:

(For 100 parts of dry matter)

Cystine	0.6	Arginine	4.7
Histidine	1.5	Isoleucine	4.7
Tryptophane	1.6	Leucine	5.6
Methionine	1.7	Lysine	5.7
Phenylalanine	3.5	Valine	6.
Threonine	4.6	Glutamic Acid	9.1

It should be noted that bees know and select pollens which are rich in nitrogenous matter (amino acids) and ignore the ones that are poorer in quality. In my research I use Bee Pollen capsules because I have found them to be non-allergenic and also highly absorbable. After three weeks of using Bee Pollen, I have had clients who initially needed as much as 5,000 mg. B-1, 2,500 mg. B-2, 5,000 mg. B-6, etc., drop down to needing as little as 25 mg. B-1, 5 mg. B-2, & 25 mg. B-6! This would have taken months to achieve through the use of a regular B-Complex Vitamin (yeast or rice based).

There is a certain quantity of glucosides in Bee Pollen that acts as a transporter to carry the nutrients into the blood stream and I feel its effectiveness is unsurpassed!! It should also be noted that many olympic athletes use Bee Pollen while in training!

It might also be interesting to note how pollen is collected from the bees. To collect the pollen, the bee keeper uses a pollen trap which consists of a diaphragm, a screen with a mesh barely large enough to permit the bees to return to the hive. Farmers also use a cheese cloth type screen for the same purpose.

As the pollen is collected by the bee, it is stored in little buckets that nature has equipped them with on their hind legs. When the bee returns and tries to enter the hive, their hind legs are caught as they struggle to enter the now screened hive. Through the struggle, the pollen falls from their legs (and sometimes they even lose their hind legs) into another screen through which the bee is not able to pass. The pollen is then passed into a drawer to be retrieved by the bee keeper.

To find out the proper amount of Bee Pollen needed, place the bee pollen in the right hand (anywhere between 3 to 6 or even 10 or more capsules) and hold to solar plexus while extending the opposite arm to be pumped. Have the other person press down on the extended arm to check the arm's strength. If the arm goes down when pressed, it could mean that the amount is too much or too little. Find the correct amount through trial and error, adding or subtracting until you find the amount that makes the arm the strongest. This will show you the proper amount needed at the time.

BEE PROPOLIS

Propolis is used by the bees to "Caulk" up the inside of the hives and to attach the honeycombs to the hives. This propolis is collected from the resinous substance exuded by the buds of trees such as the Horse Chestnut. Propolis is also collected by bees from cracks in the bark of trees such as the Larch, Spruce, and other conifers. Propolis is also collected by the bees from the leaf buds of Poplar trees.

"Propolis" translated from the Greek language means "defences before a town". Propolis is a natural antibiotic. The bees use it not only for construction material in the hive, but also to keep the hive pure and free of pollution from any foreign bodies that may enter it.

Upon entering the hive, the bees must pass through a barrier of propolis which is constructed behind the entrance to the hive as a disinfectant for the incoming bees.

Propolis, the sticky substance which protects the tree's leaf buds to prevent them from drying out, consists of:

> 50 - 55% Resin and Balsam
> 30% Wax
> 8 - 10% Fragrant Essential Oils
> 5% Solid Matter

Propolis is also rich in fats, amino acids, organic matter, composite ethers of univalent alcohols, and trace elements such as Iron, Copper, Manganese, Zinc, and others, Tannic Acid, Phyoncides, and antibiotics. It is also rich in vitamin content, especially those of the "B" group, but also contains Vitamin E, C, H, P, and provitamin A. Other contents include Cinnamic acid; Cinnamyl alcohol; Vanillin; Chrysin; Galangin; Acacetin; Kaempferid; Rhamnocitrin; Pinostrobin; Caffeic acid; Tetochrysin; Isalpinin; Pinocembrin; and Ferulic acid.

The antibiotic properties of propolis are believed to come from the Flavonoids it contains, particularly Galangin. I use Bee Propolis in my practice because it is an immune system regenerator. It has the ability to strengthen the Thymus gland which is the gland that influences the immune system. I also encourage my clients to chew propolis if they have gum, inner mouth, or throat problems as propolis has a soothing effect.

Bee Propolis is also a source of non-allergic bioflavonoids (which is usually from a Citrus source).

For these reasons I have included it in this part of the book.

EGGS

Chicken eggs are very much misunderstood. This misunderstanding may have been caused by the American Heart Association who once proclaimed that eggs were hazardous because of the Cholesterol content. However, in my opinion a diet devoid of eggs is equally hazardous!!

Eggs are a source of complete protein and contain 14% more Lecithin than Cholesterol. The Choline and Lecithin contained in the egg actually cause the H.D.L. (High-Density Lipoproteins) that break up Cholesterol and help clean up the arteries.

Eggs also contain Sulfur, which in my research, has been found to be the antidote to the "Fat Allergy". The Sulfur amino acids in the egg (Cysteine, Cystine, and Methionine) are recognized as being extremely important for cell and tissue regeneration. The egg is the one food that offers hope for proper cell rebuilding and protection against "Cross Linkage" caused by aging. Eggs also contain Vitamin B-1 (Thiamine), B-2 (Riboflavin), B-5, B-6, B-12, Vitamin E, Magnesium, and Selenium. Eggs also contain a healthy amount of Phosphorus (118 mg. per Extra Large egg) which is needed to replenish the enamel of the teeth and outer surface of the bones. The yolk of the egg is also high in Vitamin A.

The eggs one should use are the organic fertilized eggs (usually brown) instead of the kind commonly found in the average store. The reason is not only do fertilized eggs contain more protein, but the chicken that was used to produce the egg was not fed pesticide saturated feed. (Many farms spray their feed to keep it from being eaten by rodents while in storage). This will give the eggs a Cadmium content which can be tasted as one eats the egg.

Eggs should not be boiled in an Aluminum or porcelain pot, as the pot itself can also contaminate the egg. Eggs should not be boiled too long for excess boiling will kill the protein in the egg, leaving a gray, or green ring around the yolk which is the "dead" protein. Such an egg is less nutritious. I prefer a 3 or 4 minute soft boiled egg.

If the egg shell is cracked before cooking, do not eat it, for it might be contaminated. Also, do not wash eggs before storing them. This will wash off Nature's protective coating, making the egg susceptible to contamination.

Eating an egg raw will deplete the body of Biotin. So if you enjoy eating eggs raw, please supplement your diet with extra Biotin.

ROYAL JELLY

I have used Royal Jelly with my clients in place of individual supplements of Pantothenic Acid, Niacin, Biotin, and Folic acid, as we have found Royal Jelly to contain all of these naturally.

Before measuring for the amount of Royal Jelly, I usually measure my client's Bee Pollen first, and then drop an estimated number of Royal Jelly caps into the hand while they are still holding the Bee Pollen. The two contain some of the same nutrients so should be checked together to find out how much can be handled together, so as not to overdose them.

When you have found the correct amount of Bee Pollen needed, add some Royal Jelly capsules while the person is still holding the Bee Pollen. Have them hold this hand to the solar plexus while extending opposite arm to be pumped. Experiment with the amount of Royal Jelly in hand, adding or subtracting from the amount until you have found the amount that makes the extended opposite arm strongest when pumped. This will show you the correct amount of Royal Jelly needed at this time, and that it can be handled with the Bee Pollen.

I have found that by using Royal Jelly, instead of the manufactured individual Pantothenic acid or Niacin pills, that the absorption factor is greatly hastened. I have had clients who at first testing need as much as $9 \times 1,000$ mg. of Pantothenic acid; after 3 weeks on a program including Royal Jelly their need for Pantothenic acid decreased to 25 mg.! This also arrests a citrus allergy, strengthening the adrenal glands, and also causing positive behavior modification (usually noticed by the friends and companions of our clients!). It would have taken months to achieve this level if we had been using individually manufactured Pantothenic acid pills. This also applies to Niacin, which is also contained in Royal Jelly.

The U.S. Department of Agriculture has given the following quantitative analysis on 1 gram of Royal Jelly:

Vitamin B-1(Thiamine), 1.5 to 7.4 micrograms
Vitamin B-2 (Riboflavin), 5.3 to 10.0 micrograms
Vitamin B-6 (Pyridoxine), 2.2 to 10.2 micrograms
Niacin (Nicotinic Acid), 91.0 to 149.0 micrograms

Pantothenic Acid, 65.0 to 200.0 micrograms
Biotin, 0.9 to 3.7 micrograms
Inositol, 78.0 to 150.0 micrograms
Folic Acid, 0.16 to 0.50 micrograms
Vitamin C, A trace
Vitamin E, None

Recently in France, research workers reported having isolated Vitamin E in the jelly. The discrepancy between the French and the American studies seems to show that the quality of Royal Jelly probably varies from hive to hive and from location to location depending on the pollen.

It is interesting to note what Royal Jelly actually is. Royal Jelly is actually Bee's milk which is made by the nurser bees by chewing up bee pollen (without swallowing it) and mixing it with a chemical which they secrete in the glands on the top of their heads. This "milk" or pollen mush is what we call Royal Jelly.

Royal Jelly is fed exclusively to the Queen Bee, which originally was an ordinary female bee, but because of her diet became twice the size of her subjects and grew without pollen baskets, honey stomach, or wax glands. Instead, she grows a larger abdomen which projects far out behind her and acquires a terrific stinger. This Queen Bee lives forty times longer than the ordinary bee and is capable of laying as many as two thousand (2,000) eggs a day weighing two and one-half (2½) times more than she!!

SPIRULINA

Spirulina is a blue-green algae and is truly a miracle food. Sirulina is considered world wide as an immediate food resource. Spirulina has a history of human consumption in Mexico and Africa.

Spirulina can be grown continuously and harvested rather inexpensively on a large scale. Spirulina is more digestable than most algae because it is without cellulose. Spirulina is high in complete protein, Vitamins A, E, F, and B-Complex, along with other vitamins and minerals.

Spirulina contains 65 to 70% of protein and provides all eight essential proteins in the following amounts:

Isoleucine   4.13%

Leucine	5.80%
Lysine	4.00%
Methionine	2.17%
Phenylalanine	3.95%
Threonine	4.17%
Tryptophan	1.13%
Valine	6.00%

In addition, Spirulina supplies 10 of the 12 non-essential amino acids as listed in the following amounts:

Alanine	5.82%
Arginine	5.98%
Aspartic Acid	6.34%
Cystine	0.67%
Glutamic Acid	3.50%
Histidine	1.08%
Proline	2.97%
Serine	4.00%
Tyrosine	4.60%

Spirulina is rich in minerals transformed into a natural organic form by the Spirulina. The minerals in the water become chelated by the amino acids in the Spirulina, and are therefore very easily assimilated by the body.
The following minerals are usually found in Spirulina:

Potassium	15,400 mg/kg
Calcium	1,315 mg/kg
Zinc	39 mg/kg
Magnesium	1,915 mg/kg
Manganese	25 mg/kg
Selenium	Trace
Iron	580 mg/kg
Phosphorus	8,942 mg/kg
Sodium	15,400 mg/kg

Spirulina also contains the following vitamins:

Vitamin B-12 (Cobalamin)   2 mg/kg
(Nature's best source of B-12 from vegetables. Spirulina contains 250% more B-12 than Beef Liver!!)
Vitamin B-3 (Niacin)   118 mg/kg

Vitamin B-5 (Pantothenic Acid)	11 mg/kg
Vitamin B-6 (Pyridoxine)	3 mg/kg
Folic Acid	.5 mg/kg
Inositol	350 mg/kg
Vitamin B-1 (Thiamine)	55 mg/kg
Vitamin B-2 (Riboflavin)	40 mg/kg
Vitamin E (Tocopherol)	190 mg/kg
Beta-Carotene	1,700 mg/kg
(Vitamin A precursor)	

Spirulina also contains Chlorophyll, a green molecule common to plants. Chlorophyll releases ions when struck by the energy of sunlight. These free ions proceed to stimulate the bio-chemical reactions that form proteins, and vitamins.

Chlorophyll increases peristaltic action in the colon, and thus helps to relieve constipation. Chlorophyll regenerates damaged liver cells and increase circulation to all the organs by dilating the blood vessels. Chlorophyll also aids in the transmission of nerve impulses that control contraction. The heart rate is slowed, yet each contraction is increased in power, thus improving the overall efficiency of cardiac work.

Spirulina is only 7% lipid in the form of essential fatty acids that normalize Cholesterol. Essential fatty acids are Vitamin F, Linoleic, Linolenic, and Arachidonic acid. These acids are used in the body to manufacture Prostaglandins, the hormonal regulators of blood pressure and capillary resilience. Essential fatty acids are also oxygen transporters and aid in respiration.

I have also found Spirulina to contain an important amount of *organic* Sodium. For this reason, I have used it in my work!! Most reference materials minimize the Sodium content in Spirulina, but I have found Spirulina to have sufficient amounts of organic Sodium and use it as my Sodium source!!

The correct amount for the individual can be found by using the M.R.T. method. Place the Spirulina in the individual's hand and have them hold it to the solar plexus while extending their opposite arm to be "pumped". If extended arm goes down when it is pumped, this could mean that the amount in their hand is too little or too much. Experiment by adding more or less until you find the right amount that makes the arm rigid and strong when it is pumped. Please read Chapter 4 on Sodium to understand the importance of Spiruline.

CHAPTER 16

JUICE THERAPY

Through my research, I have found juice therapy, in conjunction with a food supplement regimen, to be a most valuable addition. We have found carrot juice, celery juice, and juice from Florence Fennel to be our most important supportive juices. These shall be discussed here. If other juices interest you, please see the attached bibliography and read further into this fascinating world of juices!

We have found carrot juice to be an excellent Potassium booster and celery juice to be an excellent source of organic Sodium. Fennel juice is an excellent source of both Potassium and Sodium and also Sulfur.

When drinking a lot of carrot juice over a period of time, a person may begin to turn an orange color. This orange color is showing that the liver is detoxifying itself through the pores. However, some people do not believe this theory, so I do not argue with them! I just switch them over to Fennel juice which contains Potassium, Sodium, and Sulfur in abundance. If a person needs more Potassium than Sodium, I suggest using a ratio of 2 parts carrot (Potassium) to 1 part celery (Sodium). If a person is equally lacking in Sodium and Potassium, I would use a ratio of 1 part carrot juice to one part celery juice.

I usually ask my clients to drink 4 8-ounce glasses a day in between meals, or before the day's meals. The carrot and celery combination is a great electrolyte builder and should be taken also after exercising, as Potassium and Sodium are both lost through sweating. The heart and muscles also run on Potassium. This is why carrot and celery juice is very important after strenuous exercise or activity, as after drinking it the electrolytes in the juice enter the bloodstream almost immediately, replacing the Potassium and Sodium lost through exercise. Juice should also be "chewed" (sloshed around in the mouth) before swallowing so that one's own enzymes can mix with the juice to aid absorption.

CARROT JUICE:

Carrot juice is rich in pro-vitamin A (Carotene), Vitamins B-1, B-3, B-6, C, D, E, and K. Carrot juice is also very rich in Potassium, Phosphorus, Calcium, Sodium, Magnesium, Iron, Iodine, Chlorine, Sulfur, and Copper. Carrot juice contains 4 times as much Phosphoric acid compared to any other food.

Carrot juice is a valuable aid in the improvement of eyesight, teeth, and bone structures, and it also helps to normalize weight. Raw carrot juice therapy is also an excellent treatment for cancers and ulcers, and also contains an insulin-like compound so is beneficial even to diabetics.

Carrot juice is composed of a combination of nutrients that nourish the entire nervous system. We use carrot juice with infants who have a milk allergy as the abundant Potassium in the carrot juice corrects the allergy to milk.

Because carrot juice also tastes good, it can be used as the basis of many juice combinations. The most popular with us being a combination of celery juice (Sodium) and carrot juice (Potassium). We have found this combination to be very important because of the Sodium and Potassium. To get a therapeutic effect from the juice one should drink one to two quarts of this combination per day!! If a slight discoloration of the skin occurs after drinking carrot juice over a period of time, do not be alarmed, it will disappear!!

Such discoloration should be a welcome sign as it is conclusive evidence that the toxins and impurities which have been clogging up the liver are being dissolved at such a rapid pace that the digestive and urinary systems are unable to cope with the overflow. This is then passed into the lymph glands to be discharged through the pores of the skin causing a temporary skin discoloration. If in effect this disturbs one, please switch over to Fennel juice which is rich in Potassium, Sodium, and Sulfur.

We have found that the organic Potassium in carrot juice can lower the diastolic pressure reading in blood pressure readings. We have experimented by taking a person's blood pressure before and after drinking carrot juice. We have found that the diastolic pressure reading can be lowered as much as 18 points fifteen minutes after a person has finished drinking an 8 ounce glass of carrot juice!! Therefore, the drinking of carrot and celery juice may be a very healthful way of lowering blood pressure.

CELERY JUICE:

Celery juice has the highest amount of organic Sodium. One of the chemical properties of Sodium is to maintain Calcium in solution. Celery juice contains more than four times as much vital organic Sodium as it does Calcium, which it also contains in abundance.

Calcium is one of the most essential elements in our diet, but it should be organic. When food that contains Calcium is cooked or processed, the Calcium is automatically converted into inorganic atoms. They are not soluble in water and they do not furnish the nourishment which the cells in our body require for regeneration.

Sodium plays a very important part in the physiological processes of the body. One of the most important being the maintenance of the fluidity of the blood and lymph fluids in preventing them from becoming too thick. The only Sodium that is of any value in this respect, however, is the vital organic Sodium which is derived from fresh vegetables and some fruits. Celery juice, being rich in Sodium, can also be used to bring down a fever. Celery juice can be used in hot weather as a thirst quencher. This will normalize the body temperature, helping one to feel comfortable while others around him may be sweltering and drenched in perspiration.

Sodium is one of the most important elements in the elimination of Carbon Dioxide from the system. A deficiency of vital organic Sodium results in bronchial and lung troubles, which can be aggravated by the presence of extraneous matter in the lungs such as tobacco smoke.

Celery juice contains Vitamins B, C, E, and also Iodine Potassium and Chlorine in fair amounts, but has Magnesium, Calcium, Iron, and Sodium in abundance. Celery juice is a great help in the treatment of rheumatism, gout, dropsy, and all arthritic disorders as well as dysfunctions of the nervous system.

We have also used celery juice to lower the systolic (high) blood pressure reading. By drinking an 8 ounce glass of celery juice (organic Sodium) we have found that the systolic pressure of a person can drop as much as 30 points in fifteen minutes. We discovered this by taking our client's blood pressure before drinking the juice and then re-tested him fifteen minutes after drinking the juice.

CRANBERRY JUICE

I use cranberry juice with my clients to break down kidney stones and toxic gravel in the urinary tract. Cranberry juice is also a good source of Sulfur. When using cranberry juice it is better not to use the bottled cranberry juice from the store as it usually contains too many sweeteners and corn syrup. It is much better to make your own using fresh cranberries in the juicer. Freshly juiced apples could also be added to the cranberry juice if you like it a little sweeter, although all fruit juices naturally contain their own natural sugar. The juice could also be cut with water. But do not use tap water, use mineral, well, or spring water.

If you do plan to juice your own fruits and vegetables, please use *organically grown* fruits and vegetables!! Most of the fruits and vegetables found in the supermarket usually contain pesticides so it is better to shop for organically grown produce. Some people don't realize that when a farmer sprays his crops with pesticides it just doesn't wash off when it rains, the pesticides then enter the soil to be sucked up by the plant contaminating it. So if you were to juice these products, you will also be getting pesticides in your juice which will probably make you ill!

If you cannot find organically grown fruits and vegetables and cannot grow your own, the next best thing to do is to soak the vegetables (or fruit) you do have in a solution of fresh water using a ½ teaspoon of clorox to every quart of water. Soak the vegetables in this solution for about 20 minutes and then remove them and place them in clear fresh water for about 30 minutes to remove the clorox. This process should remove any pesticides your produce may have. You will also notice that the juice will taste better and sweeter, as pesticide laden juice is bitter!!

FINOCCHIO JUICE (Florence Fennel)

Finocchio juice contains a good amount of Vitamin A, B-Complex, Calcium, Sulfur, Iron, Phosphorus, Potassium, and Sodium. Florence Fennel (Finocchio) makes an excellent juice. The Fennel plant belongs to the celery family, but the juice is much sweeter and aromatic. Some people know it erroneously as "Anise Celery" because it tastes and smells like Anise. Fennel is also used by the Italians to make Anisette liquor.

Fennel alone is good to calm the stomach, and mixed with carrot juice is very good for night blindness or optic weakness. A combination of Fennel, carrot, and beet juice make a good remedy for Anemia, especially the kind resulting from excessive menstruation.

I usually use Fennel juice if the client starts to turn an orange color from drinking a lot of carrot juice. I usually switch them from carrot and celery juice to Fennel and celery juice, this way they are still getting Sodium and Potassium from the Fennel.

BIBLIOGRAPHY

1.) *The Uses of Juices*, by C.E. Clinkard, M.B.E., Benedict Lust Publishing Co., N.Y., N.Y., 1976
2.) *Drink Your Troubles Away*, by John B. Lust, Benedict Lust Publications, N.Y., N.Y., 1981
3.) *Complete Raw Juice Therrapy*, by Susan Charmine, Thorson's Publishers, Inc., N.Y., N.Y., 1977
4.) *What's Missing in Your Body? Raw Vegetable Juices*, by N.W. Walker, Berkley Publishing Group, N.Y., N.Y.

CHAPTER **17**

MISCELLANEOUS THERAPY

COLOR THERAPY

Yes, the color you look at, the color of clothes you wear, the color of the foods you eat, and the color of the rooms where you sleep, eat, study, and relax all effect you physically, mentally, and socially! Color is high frequency energy in motion. Each color has a specific vibration and does effect human cells.

In color therapy the colors that are basically used are the colors of the rainbow which emanate from the "White" sunlight. These colors are: Red, Orange (which is Red and Yellow combined), Yellow, Green (which is Yellow and Blue combined), Blue, Indigo (which is Blue and Violet combined), and Violet. Each colot has a property of its own and can stimulate or depress living cells.

The primary colors are: Red, Yellow, and Blue.
The corresponding life forces which the primary colors represent are:

Red - Physical
Yellow - Mental
Blue - Spiritual

Red:

Red affects the circulation and is therefore believed to enhance physical force, strength, boldness, courage, warfare, sports, power, and sexuality.

The positive aspect of the color Red is that it is stimulating, energizes vitality, healing, and can strengthen will power.

The negative aspect of the color Red is that it can be over-stimulating, primitive, wild, lustful, sexual, and maniacal.

The use of the color Red for healing can stimulate circulation, increase Hemoglobin, raise body temperature, can effect a positive change in the groin area, and is excellent for correcting sexual dysfunctions (the gonads are stimulated by Red).

NOTE: The term "Red Light District" which refers to areas of prostitution is a perfect example!

Orange:

The color orange is created by mixing Red (physical) with Yellow (mental). Orange, therefore, is thought to be the color of wisdom and is so used by certain Yogis and Gurus as the color in their garments.

The positive aspects of the color Orange are that it stimulates energies, relieves depression, is joyful, and brings together physical and mental intunements.

The negative aspect is that it can be over-stimulating and should be used in balance.

The healing aspects of the color Oange effect the lower torso organs of the body, (the Spleen, Pancreas, Stomach, Kidneys), Alleviates gastro-intestinal problems, and helps improve poor assimilation of food. The color Orange also heals gout, rheumatic aches, inflamed joints, Bronchitis, Asthma, and Coughs. Orange can also help to strengthen the mind and alleviate emotional paralysis.

Yellow:

The color Yellow is a primary color and is considered to be the color of wisdom, knowledge, and intelligence.

The positive aspect of the color Yellow is that it enhances inspiration and stimulates a higher mentality by effecting the upper stomach area where the Solar Plexus is.

The negative aspect of the color Yellow is that it can function like a laxative.

The healing aspect of the color yellow helps to stimulate the functions of the stomach, thereby normalizing constipation and diarrhea. The color Yellow will also aid in healing the intestines, liver, and pancreas thereby alleviating Eczema, skin abrasions, and other skin conditions.

The color Yellow, by tuning up the Solar Plexus, stimulates the brain and nerve centers. The Adrenals are also helped by the color Yellow.

Ironically, Orange and Yellow are the colors used in America's most famous and successful fast food restaurants (Yellow effects the stomach, and Orange effects the bowels). Have you also noticed that many classrooms are painted in a light shade of Yellow (stimulating intellect)!

Green:

The color green is created by mixing Yellow (Mental) and Blue (Spiritual). The color Green is considered to be the color of healing, cellular activity, and is sedative and calming. Think of a Meadow where the trees and grass are green, and the feeling that spring gives you when all of Nature comes to life!! This feeling gives you peace, and health.

The positive aspect of the color Green is that it brings balance by calming the sympathetic nervous system.

The negative aspect of the color Green is that it could stimulate malignant growths or tumors.

The healing aspects of the color green can regenerate the sympathetic nervous system, and re-energize the heart, thereby helping to heal cardiac conditions. The color Green can normalize blood pressure, ulcers, neuralgia, influenza, neurosis, exhaustion, fatigue, and can help one to control his temper. The color Green also stimulates the Thymus gland.

One of the reasons we go to the country to become "one with nature" is because of the tonic (healing) effect it has on a person.

I would like to state this: since we spend one third of our lives in the bedroom (8 hours on the average is ⅓ of 24 hours), the color of our bedroom is very important. I personally believe in it and painted my bedroom a light green color and used a Green night light after I was aware that my heart was weak! It is much stronger today than 15 years ago!!

Ironically, surgeons are now wearing Green surgical coats and masks. These were once white. When I am doing a Laying on of Hands healing, I usually wear Green clothes.

Blue:

The color Blue is a primary color and is a spiritually relaxing, cooling color that can induce sleep. This may be why a baby boy's room is usually painted Blue.

The positive apsects of the color Blue are that it is germicidal, antiseptic, astrigent, and can stop bleeding.

The negative aspect of the color Blue is that it is cold.

The healing aspects of the color Blue help reduce fevers and high blood pressure. It can also stop vomiting, headaches, acute rheumatism, hysteria, and insomnia. The color Blue can also correct throat troubles (a very popular mouth wash is blue).

The color Blue affects the throat Chakra. I use Blue clothes most of the time when I teach, lecture, or console people because the throat Chakra being activated by the color Blue gives my vocal directives added power of command, and without raising my voice volume to be dominating, people still listen and obey my suggestion. This I contribute to success which I have achieved in this area. People listen to me!!

One of the reasons people go to the sea shore is that the sea and sky have a cooling effect on the person who views it. It is also relaxing and gives a person a spiritual realization of the grandeur and greatness of God and the Heavens.

Indigo:

The color Indigo is a combination of Blue (spiritual) and Violet (metaphysical). The color Indigo is a purifier, astringent, and is cooling.

The positive aspects of Indigo inspires and helps broaden the mind, and frees it of fears and inhibitions. The Indigo color psychologically clears and cleans the psychic currents of the body. The Indigo color has a powerful effect on serious mental complaints such as obsessions and other forms of psychosis. The Indigo color is a purifier of the blood.

The negative aspects of the Indigo color are that it can be depressing and cold.

The healing aspects of the Indigo color stimulate the Pineal gland which is the king of all glands, it also influences the organs of sight (eyes), and hearing (ears), and smell (nose).

The Indigo color can assist in the recovery from facial paralysis and helps stop bleeding.

Violet:

Violet is a primary color and is said to be the highest vibration of all colors. Violet controls the crown Chakra in the head and is linked with the Pituitary gland which is the center of intuitive and spiritual understanding. The color of Violet enables one to receive divine revelations!

The positive aspect of the color Violet is that it is soothing and tranquilizing.

The negative aspect of Violet is that it is depressing and cold.

The healing aspect of the color Violet has a wonderful neutralizing effect on all forms of neurosis and neurotic manifestations. The color Violet is useful in healing all mental and nervous disorders. Violet is also helpful in concussions, tumors, and serebro-spinal meningitis.

Chromotherapy is a system of using color to heal. Chromotherapy works very slowly, but without any side effects.

The chromotherapist uses three different tools; a light or lights with the 7 different color lenses, foods of the specifically indicated color, and color light "charged" water.

For instance, if the condition indicates a need for the color Red, the chromotherapist will "radiate" the person with a red bulb or light for a period of time. The chromotherapist will also prescribe the consumption of "red foods" such as red tomatoes, berries, cherries, red meat, etc. (Please note: if you do try this system, please make sure that the person is not allergic to any of the foods suggested.)

The chromotherapist will also suggest that the person drink "red charged" water. This is created by placing the water in a red opaque bottle (or a clear bottle with red opaque paper covering it) and letting it stand in the sunlight for 30 to 45 minutes, enough time to permit the sun's rays to pass through the amplified red of the container. Through this process, the water remains clear, but the radiation changes the energy light balance in the water.

This charging technique can be used for all the rainbow colors. If you wish to prove this, place a red lens made from glass or plastic over the groin area of the person to be tested. Now have them extend their left arm and pull down on it or "pump" it. The arm should stay strong because the lens (color) is over the proper area. Now, move the Red lens to the person's neck and test the extended arm again. The arm will now test weak because the proper lens (color) for the neck or throat area is Blue, not Red.

The color of the light would change according to the body area. If a person had a Pituitary problem, a Violet light would be used. If there was a heart problem, a Green light would be used. Different colored clothing would also have the same effect. For instance, if a person has a sore throat a Blue scarf would help, while a Red scarf would only aggravate the condition. Do you see now how the lights could be changed with each different condition in a certain area of the body?! How to select the appropriate color:

The colors enter the body at different points and effect the body in different areas. Here is the way it works:

1.) Red - Groin area
2.) Orange - Lower stomach area
3.) Yellow - Upper stomach area
4.) Green - Chest area
5.) Blue - Neck (throat) area
6.) Indigo - Nose line to top of forehead
7.) Violet - Top of head down to hairline

MUSIC THERAPY

This chapter does not pertain to music therapy as used in hospitals by music therapists in a "sing a long" program, or "music for sociability" as used in a rehabilitation program. What I mean by music therapy is how we as healers can use music as a vehicle of sound wave transmission to affect the physical body positively.

The body as we discussed in the "Color Therapy" chapter has basically 7 color areas:

The lower Chakra center (gonads) is affected by the color Red and is also stimulated by the tonality "C".

The second lower Chakra center which is the lower stomach area (between the navel and the pubic bone) is affected by the color Orange and is also stimulated by the tonality "D".

The third Chakra center which is the Solar Plexus area (between the navel and the thorac arch of the rib cage) is affected by the color Yellow and is stimulated by the tonality "E".

The fourth Chakra center is the heart (chest area) and is affected by the color Green and also stimulated by the tonality "F".

The fifth Chakra center which is the heart (chest area), is affected by the color Blue and is stimulated by the tonality "G".

The sixth Chakra center is the area of the "third eye" and is affected by the color Indigo and the sound vibration for proper stimulation is the tonality of "A".

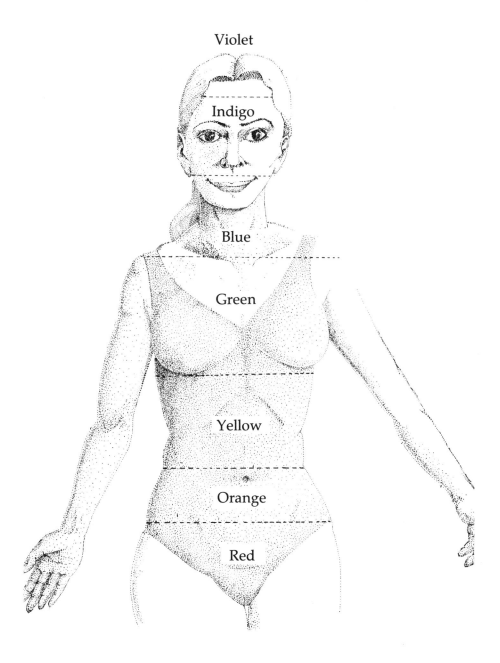

Violet

Indigo

Blue

Green

Yellow

Orange

Red

Figure 81

The seventh Chakra center which is the top of the head (the "crown Chakra") is affected by the color Violet and is stimulated by the tonality "B".

If you have noticed, I have not used the word "tone", but instead the word "tonality" when I described the pitch to be used for each specific Chakra. For it is not only that specific pitch that will affect the body's center, but all the harmonic overtones of that specific pitch (which when reduced would create a scale and harmonic structure with that specific tone as the root).

For example, if I wanted to stimulate the heart area I would use a simple (non-chromatic) folk song in the key of "F". The song should not modulate off the "F" key center. I often suggest to my clients who have heart problems that they listen to "healing tapes" in the key of "F" while driving in their car or working around the house. This actually bombards the heart center with "healing sound vibrations".

A person with a stomach problem would benefit more from listening to music in the key of "E" or "D" as long as it does not modulate into other keys. For an experience, when I taught classes on this subject, I often used a tape with progressing tonalities which would start in the key of "C", then in a few minutes it would change to the key of "D", and then upward to "E", etc. until all tonalities had resonated the body. I synchronized these tapes with my 35 millimeter projector showing the corresponding color for each tonality. For example, as the tape played the key of "C" I would focus the color Red on the front wall of a darkened room so that everyone present could feel the colors and sounds opening and feeding their Chakra centers. This is quite a physical experience. I have used this technique to increase a person's psychic awareness so that they may tune into their own inner health.

A popular song that became a hit was Bobby Darin's "Mack the Knife". Many people were excited by it (not realizing it) because every chorus went up in pitch!! Music can also be checked by the use of Muscle Response Testing to find out if it affects one positively or negatively. This can be done by having the person who wishes to be tested listen to music while they extend their left arm to the side to be "pumped" by another person (other arm should remain at side during testing). The person should now resist as the other person pulls down on their extended arm. You will notice that the extended arm will become weak with something like "Hard Rock" or "Heavy Metal" music, but it will be strong with something like harmonial folk music.

If a person's heart point should test weak you may want to try a

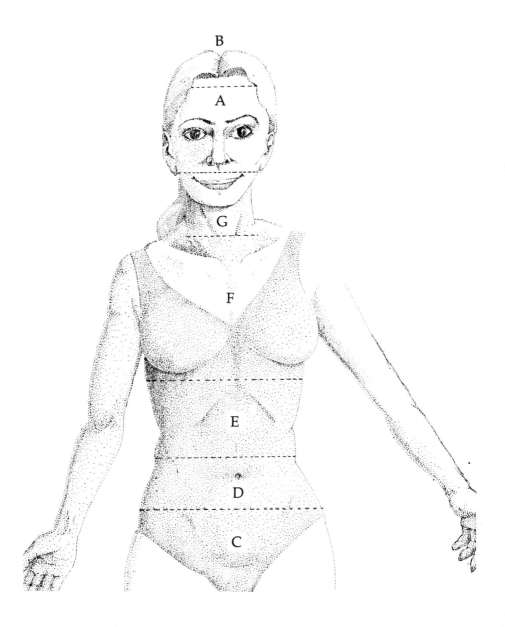

Figure 82

musical experiment to find out what music affects the heart positively. Try playing a tape of something like the "Battle Hymn of Republic" or "Brahms' Lullaby" in the key of "F" and re-test the person's heart point after they have listened to the music for a few minutes at a normal accoustical level. The heart point should now test strong!!

This also applies to every organ and gland in the body when music is played that corresponds to that Chakra area. For instance, the bladder would be affected by the tonality of "C" since the bladder is located in the lower Chakra center, the kidneys would be affected by the tonality of "D" which corresponds to the lower stomach area, the upper stomach would be affected by the tonality of "E", the throat area would be affected by the tonality of "A", the top of the head the tonality of "B", etc.

BIOMAGNETIC THERAPY

In the year of 1976, I had a cardiac arrest and thought my life had come to an end until a friend of mine encouraged me to go to a lecture with him which inspired me enough to bring me back to health, thereby saving my life!!

The lecture was given by Dr. Ralph U. Sierra, Director of the Puerto Rico Scientific Research Laboratory located at 1707 Arkansas Street, San Gerardo, Rio Piedras, Puerto Rico 00926. Dr. Sierra was a research scientist who was working with the healing effects of magnetic fields. After the lecture, I went home and constructed my own magnetic device which consisted of 6 one inch square magnets which I bought for 10¢ each at a local electronic store and some adhesive tape.

I placed the south pole side of the magnets on the glued side of a 3 inch wide (approximately) piece of adhesive tape which I reinforced with three more layers of tape on the opposite side of the tape holding the magnets. I then placed ½ inch pieces of tape (glued side down) on the exposed adhesive areas of the original tape holding the magnets so that all of the sticky adhesive areas were covered but the north side of the magnet remained exposed. This formed a heavy pad into which I added 2 eyelets (one on each side) and attached a ⅛ inch wide length of twill tape to one eyelet, and a ⅛ inch wide piece of flat elastic to the other. Both were long enough for me to place the pad (with north pole side towards the skin) over my heart on the left side with one tape over my right shoulder and the elastic under my armpit where I tied the two together and trimmed the excess so that I was not tickled by the loose ends. This device worked, for my heart started to normalize!!

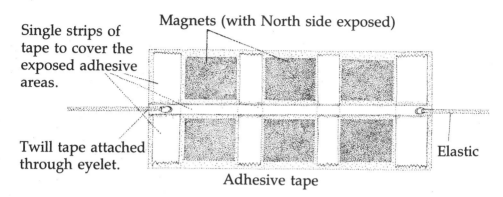

Single strips of tape to cover the exposed adhesive areas.

Magnets (with North side exposed)

Twill tape attached through eyelet.

Elastic

Adhesive tape

Figure 83

A magnet has two sides: A.) North, which is affected by North Pole magnetism. B.) South, which is affected by South Pole magnetism. Both present completely different forms of energy when applied to a biological system. The South Pole emanates positive charged energy, while the North Pole emanates negative charged energy.

We took a sample of blood and separated the fluids (plasma) leaving the red blood cells, and placed it on a slide and inserted it under a microscope. We found that when we put a magnet under the slide that the red blood cells spun around and pointed in one direction. This is called Polarization alignment of the Iron and ions in the red blood cells. As the experiment with the red blood cells showed, when you align any form of energy, you have gathered strength, power, and energy, so that a higher level of energy is created.

Magnetism has been used to arrest certain diseases such as Cancer in laboratory rats and Leukemia in the blood. This was demonstrated to the American Medical Association by Kathy Solis and published in an article in Prevention magazine in February of 1973.

North Pole (negative) energy tends to have a contrasting effect by pulling things together, thereby causing contraction. South Pole energy (positive) tends to cause things to expand, and thereby dissipate energy. During the time when I had heart problems and Angina Pectoris, I wore my magnetic device with the north side of the magnets against my chest to normalize my inflamed heart. If I had something like a blood clot in my leg, I would then use the south side of the magnet to disperse the blood clot.

Many of the books by Dr. Ralph Sierra and Roy Davis tell about the specific application of magnets and which side should be used for specific conditions. For instance, Arthritis can be treated by using North Pole magnetism 20 to 30 minutes per day. The magnet they suggesst is the N-1 model. The N-1 magnet has two flat surfaces, one surface is the north side, and the other side is the south side. The N-1 magnet is 6 inches long, 2 inches wide, and ½ inch thick. This enables the placement only of the north or south side against the flesh, unlike the horseshoe magnet which radiates north pole energy and south pole energy from each tip so that most things are attracted to it.

The N-1 magnet is also usually marked by the distributor so that you can identify the north side from the south side. I used to mark them with "white out".

One way of finding out which side is north is to place a compass on a flat surface and pass one side of the magnet about 1 inch away from the side of the compass. If the arrow *tip* of the compass follows the magnet as you slowly move it past the compass, then the surface of the magnet that is facing the compass is the north side (the tip of the compass arrow is a south pole magnet always trying to face north). If the back (end) part of the compass needle is attracted to the magnet surface, then it is the south side of the magnet because the back of the compass needle is a north pole magnet!

North side of magnet

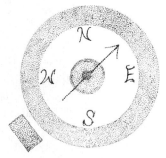

B.) Back end of arrow following magnet shows that side of magnet facing the compass is the *South* side.

Figure 84

South side of magnet

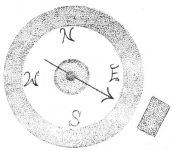

A.) Tip of arrow following magnet shows that side of magnet facing compass is the *North* side of the magnet.

Figure 85

You can also check a magnet's polarity by the use of Muscle Response Testing. Have someone hold an N-1 magnet over their head with one hand while extending their opposite arm to the side to be "pumped". Pull down on their extended arm while they resist. If the arm shows strong, then it is the north side of the magnet that is facing the top of the head. On the other hand, if the arm goes down or gets weak when it is "pumped", then it is the south side of the magnet that is facing the top of the head.

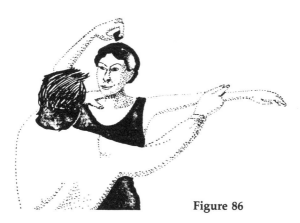

Figure 86

There are many books you can read on the subject of biomagnetics to find out which pole (north or south) energy should be used for specific conditions or specific organs (example: Heart-north pole energy, Lungs-south pole energy), but the best and easiest way is to use the Muscle Response Testing Method, having the person hold the north side of the magnet over the area they wish to energize while extending their opposite arm to be pumped. If their arm goes down when it is pumped by another person, the magnet should then be turned over to see if the opposite side will have a more positive effect. If the arm is now strong when it is "pumped", it means that the side of the magnet that is facing the skin is the correct side of the magnet for that specific condition. Simple, don't you think!!

It should be noted that the Japanese have done extensive research in this direction and that the Japanese Ministry of Health has certified the use of magnetic devices (bracelets & necklaces) as beneficial to the users.

I would also like to mention that I have improved my eyesight with the use of magnetic glasses. This can be done by gluing small magnets which have large north and south surfaces on to a pair of old glasses that you are not using, or even on a pair of cheap sun glasses. The *south side* of the magnet should be glued on to the lens of the glasses so that the north side of the magnet is facing the eyes. Do not try to look through these glasses! They should be worn for 20 to 30 minutes twice a day only when you are relaxing or meditating.

For more information, books on Biomagnetism are available from:

Albert Roy Davis
c/o Roy Davis Research Laboratory
520 Magnolia Avenue
Green Cove Springs, Florida 32043
Phone: (904) 284-5475

METAL AND GEM THERAPY

Metals can affect the body's electromagnetic field either positively or negatively.

Bracelets and necklaces of gold, silver, and copper help to energize the body's electromagnetic field by attracting energy to it. In some instances, jewelry such as this will give the wearer physical strength, energy, and stamina. It can thereby be considered to help a person become healthier.

If one should wear bracelets of gold, silver, or copper, they should be worn on the *left* wrist and not on the right, for the electromagnetic flow of energy flows *in* the left palm and *out* the right palm. This flow of energy also works the same way for the feet, entering the left, and leaving the right. As this flow of energy enters the left palm, it goes up the arm into the left side of the torso, circles in the Solar Plexus, and exits out of the right lower torso down the right leg, and out of the right foot. This energy can also enter through the left foot, flow through the left leg into the lower left torso, circling in the Solar plexus, entering the upper right torso, and then pass through the right arm and out the right palm and fingertips. (See figure 87.)

Metals such as gold, silver, and copper help attract energy because of their purity and electron structure. Metals such as Lead, Iron, Pewter, and Tin tend to short out the electromagnetic field when worn on the body, and should never be worn as "jewelry", because it can make the wearer weak, tired, and eventually ill. The person who says "I just can't wear cheap jewelry", is not just stating an ego position, but a subconscious energy awareness of feeling good when they wear real jewelry, and weak when they wear "Costume" jewelry.

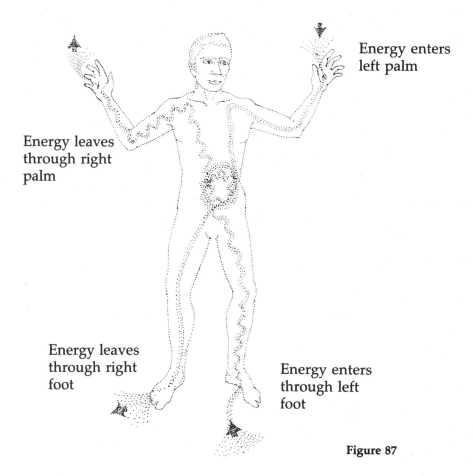

Energy enters left palm

Energy leaves through right palm

Energy leaves through right foot

Energy enters through left foot

Figure 87

To test precious metals and gems, place the metal or gem in the hand and hold it with the fingertips (so that the gem or metal is exposed) on the Thymus gland point while extending the opposite arm to the side to be "pumped" by another person. If the extended arm stays strong and rigid when it is pumped, it is showing that the gem or metal is of true quality.

If an item is made of Iron or Pewter but looks gold (because of a gold plating), it will test weak (the extended arm will become weak when "pumped"). This also goes for testing gems. I have yet to find a diamond that tests weak. They truly are a "woman's best friend"! A diamond worn on the left hand, wrist, or as a brooch over the Thymus gland area, will give the wearer strength and health. However, to be really effective, the metal mounting of such a gem should be such that the gem is able to touch the body. For example, if a brooch is worn over the Thymus area, the diamond or gem should be mounted in gold or silver (or whichever one tests stronger to the wearer) in such a manner as not to cover the stone so that the stone is still touching the body.

This can be achieved by having the surface beneath the gem mounting open so the gem can touch the skin.

All gemstones do not affect everyone in the same way, this is why the stone should be tested to see if it suits the individual. This can be done with the use of Muscle Response Testing as mentioned before. If a gem should test weak when it is held against the Thymus point, then it is showing that the gem is possibly detrimental to that particular person at this period in their life so they should not wear it at this time, because it may have a negative effect on them. The gem can be re-tested in about 6 months as the person's intunement vibration may have changed and the gem may have a different effect on them.

Many people believe that their "Birth Stone" gem, or the gem that corresponds with their astrological sign is good for them. I have found that this is not always true. The best way is to test different stones to find out which stone's vibrations are complementary to that particular person.

The Birth Stones by month:

January	Garnet
February	Amythest
March	Aquamarine, Bloodstone
April	Diamond
May	Emerald
June	Pearl, Moonstone
July	Ruby
August	Peridot
September	Sapphire
October	Opal, Tourmaline
November	Topaz
December	Turquoise, Lapis Lazuli

The following is a list of descriptive attributes & properties of the precious metals and gem stones:

Metal	Traditional Attributes and Curative Properties	Modern Attributes
Copper	Promote generosity, remove uneasiness, rheumatism, gout. Prevent contagion, sterility.	Conductor of energy through the body. Useful for energy blocks or distortions. Does not have spiritual qualities.
Gold	Strength, cure, melancholy, heart disease, asthma, sexual dysfunction, cleanse blood. Symbol of the sun.	Positive energy structure of highest vibration. Attracts physical and spiritual energy.
Platinum		Metal of highest vibration. Energy conductor. Raise vibration from physical to spiritual. Beneficial to most people.
Silver	Metal of the moon, head, brain, epilepsy, rheumatism.	This physical energy conductor benefits many but not all. Does not have the high vibration of gold.
Stone		
Alexandrite		(Chrysoberyl) Attracts & focuses energy. Greatly increases body's energy field. User should be in good mental and physical health.

Metal	Traditional Attributes and Curative Properties	Modern Attributes
Amber	Infection, protect from sorcery, rheumatism, deafness, jaundice, headache, goiter, bleeding, teeth, digestive problems.	Low intensity energy stone (substance) heals affairs of the heart, despair, sorrow, desolation, and broken love.
Amethyst	Preserve sobriety, calmness in danger, infection nervousness, charm against witchcraft.	High vibration energy stone, spiritual high minded. Healing for some. Counters negativity. Helps one look forward to a brighter day. Beneficial to many.
Aquamarine	Stone of purity, preserve married love, sharpen intellect, stone of seers, mystics, clairvoyants, charm for sailors & adventurers.	Energy stone, high vibration. Stone of spiritual seekers. Can raise energy from material to spiritual level. Affects 5th chakra. Best color is clear blue.
Bloodstone	Endurance, courage, constancy, wealth, success, gall stones, digestion, hemorrhage, insect bites, longevity.	Earth stone, grounding, Keep one's feet on the ground. Can help those tending toward schizophrenia.
Carnelian	Soothing, cool blood, stomach problems, inflammatory diseases, hemorrhages, anger, discord.	Earth stone, grounding, can help one with trouble thinking things through. Can help cases of sexual dysfunction.
Citrine	Cheerfulness	Energy stone, can lift personality

Name		
	from depression to joy. Counters negativity. Not to be used by those with severe heart conditions, liver problems, or toxemia.	
Cat Eye-Chrysoberyl	Energy stone. Heightens psychic awareness. Aids in controlling others. Good if used properly. DANGER if used to gratify one's ego.	Bringer of wealth, prevent loss of wealth, talisman for gamblers, asthma, mental balance, foresight.
Chrysoprase	Earth stone with refined vibration. Balancing. Can put some acutely in touch with nature. Healing, soothing.	
Coral	A material from nature with pure vibration. White coral lifts vibration, clears negativity & anger coming from outside oneself. Red dispels anger and negativity.	Charm against sterility, witchcraft, intestinal disease, spleen disorders.
Diamond	Energy stone. Possessive vibration. Can help prostate problems & degenerative diseases of old age.	Courage, daring, fortitude, mental health, constancy in love, strengthen friendship.
Emerald	Energy stone. High vibration. Can heal and cleanse aura. Can be great aid to healers. Balancing for chakras. Stone of the heart chakra.	Faith, memory, foresight, courage, eyesight, childbirth. Talisman for sailors & against contagious disease. Represents immortality.

Metal	Traditional Attributes and Curative Properties	Modern Attributes
Garnet	Health, cheerfulness, remove discord & anger, hemorrhages, inflammatory diseases	Energy stone. Used to accumulate power & possessions. Green Garnets more like Tourmaline.
Heliodor		Energy stone. High vibration. Can greatly aid spiritual growth once body is cleansed of toxins. In tune with vibration of the pituitary gland.
Iolite		High vibration energy stone. Useful to spiritual seekers. Especially useful to one feeling trapped, searching for answers. Raises vibration.
Ivory	Symbol of purity	Calming, lifting, purifying. Energy buffer. Can help despondant persons & those feeling unworthy.
Jade (Jadite)	Brings wisdom, protects against accidents, kidney & stomach problems.	High vibration earth stone. "The wisdom stone". Stone of sages & seers. Calming, soothing. Can clarify mental processes.
Jade (Nephrite)	Brings wisdom, protects agbainst accidents, kidney & stomach problems.	Pure vibration earth stone. Calming, soothing, mentally clarifying. Heals certain internal toxic conditions. Gives feeling of rootedness & solid relationship to the world.

Lapis Lazuli	Succes in love, cure melancholy, timidity, stone of Virgin Mary, apoplexy, epilepsy, skin diseases, spleen.	High vibration earth stone. Emanates powerful spiritual vibration while grounding.
Malachite	Talisman for children and the young, preserve health, sound sleep, depression, protection from lightning, cholera, colic, rheumatism, witchcraft.	Healing earth stone, grounding, balancing, favorable for those with schizophrenic tendencies. Strengthens blood.
Morganite		(Beryl) Energy stone. Radiates love and compassion. Can aid those attracted to one who does not reciprocate. Love is gentle & kind to he who respects it; fire & danger to one who flaunts it.
Moss Agate	Strength, Vigor, Success, eloquence, friendship, good temper, sharper sight and mind.	Earth stone, cooling. Brings down fever, can ease one's temper, grounding. Brings energy and clarity of mind.
Osbidian		Earth stone. Attracts energy. Can draw negativity out of a person & eliminate it. Draws aura close to body. Helpful if one is scattered, overextended, or needs protection.
Opal	Strengthen eyesight, memory, clarify mind, good fortune in	High vibration energy stone. Attracts energy like a magnet attracts

Metal	Traditional Attributes and Curative Properties	Modern Attributes
	travel and business, prophecy. Will not bring misfortune to wearers whose birthstone is not opal.	Iron. Promotes energy & leadership. Not for nervous people.
Pearl	Preserve, purify, restore reason, stomach problems.	Living matter. Symbolizes & emanates purity & clarity.
Peridot	Divine inspiration, eloquence, foresight, protect from witchcraft, melancholy.	Energy stone. Medium vibration. When very clear & fine can balance energy centers & radiate harmony.
Quartz Crystal	(Rock Crystal) Used by seers, said to contain hidden secrets of the future, kidney problems.	A pure energy stone. Prism effect cleanses & expands aura. Stimulates all energy center.
Ruby	Confer invulnerability, shield from ill fortune, love, friendship, health, happiness, foretell danger, spleen, liver.	Highly charged energy stone. Develops sense of power and gives possessor the means to it. Benefits those who need power to do their job properly. Rulers.
Sapphire	Bring spiritual insight, peace, happiness, promote spiritual climate, morality, discovers plots, eye problems, contagious disease.	High energy stone. Clear blue variety radiates high spiritual vibration. This pure piercing vibration stimulates highest energy centers (6th chakra). Aids spiritual development.

Stone		
Tiger Eye	Used by seers	An energy stone used by psychics to enhance clairvoyance. More earthy than most gems. If used for general good and not personal ego, is beneficial while grounding.
Topaz	Cheerfulness, foresight, mental clarity, dissolve spells of witchcraft.	High vibration energy stone. Lifting, purifying. Yellow variety will not benefit persons with diseased or toxic conditions. Clear blue topaz stimulates man's highest ideals.
Tourmaline	Inspiration, favors from the great, friendship.	High vibration energy stone. Green and blue varieties similar to Sapphires but gentler. Promotes qualities of optimism, helpfulness, gentleness & perseverance. Reds more like rubies.
Turquoise	Represents true affections, horseman's charm, protection from injury. Relieve tension, antagonism, headaches.	High vibration earth stone. Both grounding and lifting. Benefits those susceptible to negativity as protection. Soothing, healing, would benefit nearly everyone.
Zircon	Success, riches, honor, wisdom, restlessness, contagious disease, jealousy, digestion, weak heart, fever, appetite, witchcraft.	High energy stone. Brings self assurance & confidence. Radiates peacefulness and feeling that one is doing well. Blue & white are especially beneficial.

The Birth Stone by Astrological sign:

Aquarius	Zircon, Garnet
Pisces	Amethyst
Aries	Diamond, Bloodstone
Taurus	Sapphire, Turquoise
Gemini	Chrysoprase, Agate
Cancer	Moonstone, Pearl, Emerald, Rock Crystal
Leo	Topaz, Amber, Onyx
Virgo	Jade, Carnelian
Libra	Peridot, Opal, Coral, Lapis Lazuli
Scorpio	Aquamarine
Sagitarius	Topaz
Capricorn	Ruby, Malachite

It is not necessary to have a stone cut to obtain the necessary vibrations from it. An inexpensive source of stones is the "Lapidary shop" which would have most stones in a "raw" state.

TESTING INFANTS AND INVALIDS BY USING A SURROGATE

To test an infant using M.R.T. you must have a surrogate whose arm you will use instead of the infant's.

The easiest way of testing an infant that is awake is to sit the child on the lap of the surrogate. Place the substance to be tested in the surrogate's hand while they hold it to the child's solar plexus and extend their other arm to be "pumped".

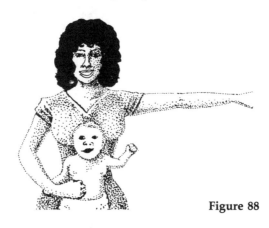

Figure 88

If the arm remains rigid when testing the substance, this shows that it can be tolerated by the child. If the arm goes down when pressed, it shows that the substance is negative or that the child is allergic to it.

Always test for allergies first (food), and then test the nutrients. This way you will know what nutrients to test the child for in order to abate the allergies and regain a sound constitution.

Another way of testing a sleeping child, or a person who may be incapacitated or in a coma is to have the surrogate stand near them while holding the substance to the person's solar plexus and extending their opposite arm to be pumped.

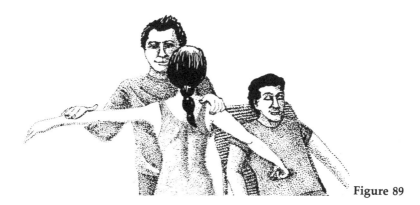

Figure 89

Again, if the arm goes down when pumped, this is showing that the person is allergic to the substance you are testing. If you are testing nutrients, remember that if the arm gets weak and goes down when pressed, it could mean they need either more, or less of the nutrient you are testing.

I once went to a hospital for a client of mine and found that he was in a coma because he had become allergic to the intravenous saline solution he was on. The reason for this was that he needed Potassium, and not Sodium. By changing the solution to Potassium, the client survived!! You see, they don't test for allergies in the usual hospital setting!!

TESTING PETS

There are two ways in which you can test a pet:

1.) To test a domestic pet such as a cat or dog, place the pet in the owner's lap (or assistant surrogate). Have the owner hold the

substance you wish to test to the animal's stomach area while they extend their opposite arm to be "pumped".
See Figure 90.

2.) Another way of testing, if the animal is too large to hold on the lap, is to place him on the floor while having the owner sit next to him to place the substance being tested to the animal's stomach (solar plexus) while extending their opposite arm to be pumped.
See Figure 91, next page.

If the owner's extended arm remains rigid when it is "pumped", this is showing that the substance being tested is okay. If the extended arm goes down when pumped, this is showing that the substance is negative to the animal, or that he is allergic to it.

When testing an animal (as with a person), always test for the allergies first, then for the nutrients needed as the antidote to the allergies. To test for nutrients, have the owner hold the specific nutrient to the animal's solar plexus (stomach) while extending their (not pets!) arm to be pumped. If extended arm is weak when pumped, increase (or subtract) the amount of nutrient in hand until arm is rigid.

Place animal on owner's lap while holding substance to animal's stomach area with opposite arm extended:

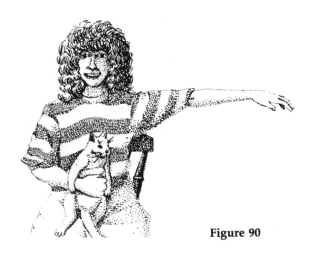

Figure 90

With a large animal, have him sit or lie on the floor with owner sitting near to hold substance to animals stomach with opposite arm extended:

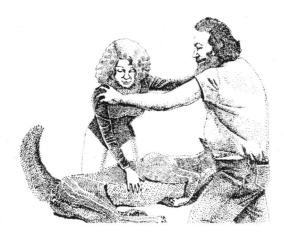

Figure 91

If arm does not become rigid with nutrient, this may be showing that the initial amount of the nutrient was too much and that you should re-test with less. An overdose of anything will also make the arm weak!!

Remember, animals are people too!! They can have allergies just like people and could also be allergic to their food, especially if they are fed the same brand of food over an extended period of time.

Please refer to chapter 2 on "Allergies and Antidotes".

THERAPEUTIC MINERAL BATHS

In my research I have found that nutrients can also be absorbed through the pores of the skin. You see, the pores are a two way street. The pores release sweat containing Sodium, Potassium, Ammonia, and Urea, but they can also absorb minerals and nutrients to nourish the body. One way of doing this is through the use of mineral baths.

If I find that a person is lacking in Potassium, Sodium, Sulfur, or Magnesium I usually recommend (in addition to a nutritional program) that they soak in baths of lukewarm water containing one or more of the following (2 cups is sufficient): Epsom Salts (Magnesium Sulfate), Kosher Salt, or Potassium Phosphate or Gluconate Powder (liquid can also be used). The reason I usually recommend Kosher Salt is that it is the most water soluble because it is basically ground up rock salt and is the best source of Sodium Chloride. Spirulina can also be used in the bath as it is rich in minerals and protein and most beneficial. There are also some commercial products on the market that are very good!

Do not use hot water with these baths as the person will sweat and lose more Sodium and Potassium. We want to raise the level of electrolytes, not lower them by sweating! However, if the purpose of the bath is to detoxify the body, then a hot bath which would induce perspiration would be appropriate. I have found that mineral baths are a very good way to nourish the body through the pores and are also very useful in correcting allergies, fevers, and headaches that are allergenic in origin.

The best time to take such a bath is prior to bedtime because it will also relax the muscles, and is therefore conducive to sleep.

I once had a case with a child who was running a constant fever. The child was extremely low in Sodium, so I instructed her mother to give her Celery and Carrot juice to bring up her level of electrolytes, and to bathe her in a luke warm bath containing Kosher Salt. After 15 minutes of bathing, the child's temperature had dropped back to normal!

If ever a Vitamin A overdose occurs, put 2 oz. of Vitamin C crystals (powder) in the bath, it will help neutralize the overdose.

LIFE EXTENSION TECHNIQUES

"Age is not chronological, but it is the condition of the entity". It is a known fact that many people who are low in years can be aged way beyond their years. Is it true that youth is wasted on the young?

A good approach to anti-aging and life extension is the preventative approach which is multi-faceted. The first thing to do would be to avoid smoking or inhaling smoke. We have found that smoking not only robs the body of Vitamin C, but also of Sulfur. Cysteine, a Sulfur based amino acid helps maintain the elasticity of the cells. When Cysteine is destroyed by smoking the cells become less flexible and more rigid causing the texture of the skin to "age". So if you want to stay young, do not smoke!!

One should also avoid an over consumption of alcohol as alcohol will throw out certain minerals such as Zinc which is very important for maintaining the cell's youth. Sugar should also be avoided as it destroys the B-Complex Vitamins in the body which can cause a loss of hair color and also effect the nervous system. Sugar also burns up Phosphorus which is important for the preservation of tooth enamel and the outer coating of the bones.

White flour and overly refined foods should also be avoided as they only leave you starving for nutrients, which will not only ultimately end with premature aging, but eventually with an early death.

Diet is a very important part of the anti-aging program and it should consist of nutritional natural foods only. Vegetables should be eaten raw and uncooked whenever possible. Steaming is also okay if you prefer. Avoid fruits and vegetables that may have been grown with pesticides as the pesticides wash off the plant with rainfall, enter the soil, and are absorbd by the plant. Avoid eating meats that may have been injected with hormones or raised under improper conditions. Eat organically raised vegetables, fruits, eggs, and meats only, to avoid poisoning your system!

An anti-aging program should also include a customized nutritional supplement program which can be simple with the use of the Muscle Response Testing technique shown in this book. The nutritional program should be used to first curtail and arrest all allergies that may be present, stop the degeneration process, normalize weight, and then geared towards life extension and anti-aging with the utilization of specific nutrients.

I have found one of the most important nutrients to be Bee Pollen. Bee Pollen contains a tremendous amount of highly absorbable B-Complex Vitamins (50 mg. per 500 mg. capsule) and it also contains a phenomenal amount of Potassium. I have also found Royal Jelly (another product of the bee) to be very valuable as it is a tremendous source of Pantothenic Acid and Niacinamide. Pantothenic acid affects the adrenal glands, thereby activating the glands output of hormones that are necessary to keep the body young. We also recommend Bee Propolis which helps to activate the Thymus gland which in turn will up-grade the body's immune system.

Bee Pollen, Royal Jelly, and Bee Propolis can be found in a product called *"Natural Energy" which combines all three products of the Bee in one capsule.

I have found that when I use "Natural Energy" with a person who needs as much as 12,000 mg. of Vitamin B-1 and equally high levels of the other B Vitamins on their first visit, that their need for the B Complex Vitamins will reduce to approximately 25 mg. B-1, 5 mg. B-2, 25 mg. B-6, etc. after two weeks on the Natural Energy. When this level is maintained with the use of a non-allergenic multi-vitamin and mineral

*"Natural Energy" is manufactured by MIRACLE FOOD PRODUCTS, 172 Manhattan Avenue, Jersey, City, N.J. 07307.

capsule along with a Natural Energy capsule, the body seems to stop aging. My own hair which was "salt and pepper" turned back to its natural dark brown color!

I have also found that the endocrine system must be fed the proper amounts of Potassium and Sodium in order to produce needed hormones; and when the body begins to regenerate, a greater need for Sodium arises. Sodium acts as a nutrient transporter helping other nutrients enter the blood stream through the walls of the stomach.

Celery juice contains a tremendous amount of organic Sodium and when mixed with carrot juice, which is very rich in vitamins, minerals, and beta-carotene (an important anti-oxidant), the absorption level of nutrients is remarkable. For this reason a knowledge and use of juice therapy is very important for the person interested in a life extension program.

A trip to the seashore where salt water bathing is available is also beneficial as the Sodium and minerals contained in the sea water can be absorbed by the bather through the pores of the skin. Sun bathing, if done in moderation with the proper sunscreen, is also very important. A PABA type sunscreen lotion should be applied before being exposed to the sun while safflower or olive oil should be applied *after* exposure to the sun. Safflower and olive oil both contain Vitamin F which is used for skin regeneration, and when applied to the skin after exposure to the sun helps regenerate the skin and keep it soft.

Many authorities advise you to avoid the sun which I believe is bad advice. Sunshine is a source of Vitamin D which is needed to help the absorption of Calcium and to hold Sodium ions in the body. The skin cancer which we are warned is caused by the sun, only happens because the victim's diet does not include a proper amount of fatty acids.

Vitamin F which is necessary for skin regeneration exists in fats (oils), but people are instead told to avoid fats and to stay out of the sun. This is bad advice! What they should be told is to use a sunscreen and sunbathe gradually.

Sunbathing should start out gradually at 10 to 15 minutes a day, adding on 5 minutes a day until the skin is tanned. After exposure to the sun, a coat of safflower, olive, peanut, or almond oil (any one will work) should be applied to the skin. All sun-screens and lotions should be first checked with Muscle Response Testing to make sure that the person is not allergic to it. To test the lotion place the bottle in hand while holding it to the solar plexus and extend the opposite arm to be "pumped".

Lotions should be checked daily as the body's sensitivity can also change. What checked out O.K. one day may not be right the next. Also, when using oils on the skin one should check their need for the amino acids Carnitine, Methionine, and Cysteine to avoid an allergy to fats.

Sufficient exercise is also important on a life extension program. One of the best exercises is walking which uses all the muscles of the body. If you should choose walking as your means of exercise be sure you are equipped with the proper shoes. Proper fitting sneakers are good as they have enough padding to avoid discomfort and injuries.

Another very good exercise is swimming. However, chlorinated pools should be avoided as the Chlorine in the water can be absorbed through the pores of the skin and deplete the body of Sodium and Potassium. The best swimming areas are oceans, streams, ponds and lakes. The reason I feel that swimming is so good is because there is no gravitational pull on the spine and the body floats in a horizontal position. This has a positive effect on the body.

Another exercise I encourage is bicycling. Bicycling gets the legs moving and the blood pumping through out the body while also bringing oxygen into the body. I prefer bicycling to running or jogging because there is no skeletal damage caused by the pounding of the feet on the ground. I have seen too many damaged hips, knees, and ankles on joggers who run until it hurts. With any exercise always be sure to replace the Sodium and Potassium that is lost by drinking a sufficient amount of carrot (Potassium) and celery (Sodium) juice, or have someone test you for Alfalfa capsules (which contain 2 parts Potassium and 1 part Sodium) after you have exercised.

A very famous jogger who wrote a book on jogging recently died of a heart attack. Why? Because he did not realize that the muscles run on Potassium and the heart is a muscle! When you sweat you loose *Potassium*, *Sodium*, Uric acid, and Ammonia.

If you had a brand new car and drove it down Main Street and it ran out of gas, it would die! There is nothing wrong with the car, it's just out of gas! Our bodies are the same way!! If we exercise we need to make sure we have enough fuel (Potassium & Sodium). If not, our hearts will also die!!

Other forms of exercise such as aerobics, calisthenics, and weight lifting are all worth investigating for the person interested in body building. Dancing, believe it or not, is an excellent exercise. If you doubt me try doing 3 polkas in a row!! My favorite exercises are leg raises and sit ups, of which many variations exist. In the beginning these can be done right in bed when you wake up. I often tell my older clients to do no more than 5 of each the first day and add one more every day until you reach 20. These exercises can then be done in the morning, noon, and night.

The reason I favor these 2 exercises is not only because they remove the "spare tire" effect, but they also have a massaging effect on the torso to stimulate the internal organs. The internal massage that the exercise gives the body is priceless and rejuvenating!!

GH3 and KH3 are procaine products believed to have a rejuvenating effect on the body. GH3 originally was manufactured in Romania at Dr. Ana Aslan's rejuvenation clinic. KH3 was originally manufactured in West Germany.

One KH3 capsule is twice as potent as 1 GH3 capsule. KH3 is now legal and manufactured in Nevada and GH3 is now manufactured in the Bahamas and is available in Miami, Florida.

Do these products really work? I have found that people who come to me after being on procain therapy have a tremendous deficiency in Pantothenic acid (Vitamin B-5) which causes a "citrus allergy" and a starved adrenal gland. This can be remedied by balancing the amount of GH3 or KH3 with the proper amount of Pantothenic acid.

To balance the KH3/GH3 with Pantothenic acid you must first find out how much of the KH3 or GH3 the person can tolerate. This can be done with Muscle Response Testing. Place the GH3 or KH3 in the person's palm while they hold it to their solar plexus and extend their opposite arm to be "pumped". You should now pull down on their extended arm to test the strength. If the arm shows weak, it could mean that the person is holding too many or too few pills in their hand so you should add more or subtract some until you find the proper amount.

When you have found the proper amount of KH3/GH3 add a capsule of Royal Jelly (50 mg. or 100 mg.) to the KH3/GH3 they are holding and re-test the arm. Add more until the arm becomes strong. The Royal Jelly contains the Pantothenic Acid that will be needed to feed the adrenal glands once the procain activates them. Pantothenic acid will burn up Sulfur so when you are taking KH3 or GH3 along with Pantothenic acid (Royal Jelly) you must also take the proper amount of Sulfur. Sulfur can be found in the herb Sarsaparilla which contains the Sulfur bearing amino acids Methionine and Cysteine. If Pantothenic acid is taken without a sufficient amount of Sulfur, a "fat allergy" will occur.

To find the proper amount of Sulfur, place the Sarsaparilla (capsules or pills) in the hand with the pre-tested KH3 or GH3, and Royal Jelly and re-test until you have found the proper balance.

When checking one of my clients who had recently come back from Ana Aslan's Romanian clinic, I discovered (through the use of *M.R.T.) that their adrenal glands were exhausted due to the procaine therapy. My client, upon returning to the Romanian clinic presented my findings, research and solutions. They are now also aware of the side effects of procain therapy and have presently altered their therapy to utilize the information which we developed and offered them.

In our practice we have found a product called "Placentaglan" to be very effective in anti-aging therapy with no side effects.

A drug called "Hydergine" manufactured by Sandoz Pharmaceuticals is said to prevent or reverse aging in the brain. Hydergine increases protein synthesis in the brain (required for memory), stabilizes electrical activity, increases the brain's Oxygen supply, prevents the formulation of degenerative pigment in the brain, and stimulates the growth of neurites (nerve cell connections). Required for learning and memory, Hydergine is also highly effective as a treatment for hearing loss caused by disease or injury. Hydergine can improve memory, concentration, and intelligence in young adults.

Another anti-aging drug is Vasopressin, which is actually a hormone produced by the Pituitary gland that helps you to incorporate new information into your memory. Every time you see, hear, or touch something that is meaningful to you, Vasopressin is released by your pituitary gland. Vasopressin is marketed as a nasal spray manufactured by Sandoz.

Vasopressin enables you to learn more effectively. It plays a critical role in the "imprinting" of new information within the memory centers of your brain. Vasopressin also plays an important role in the retrieval of information from your memory into your conscious mind. Vasopressin can improve learning dramatically when inhaled into the nasal passages while studying for a test. Vasopressin can also improve test scores significantly when taken just prior to a test. Vasopressin can significantly reverse memory loss in normally aging subjects. Vasopressin is manufactured by Sandoz Pharmaceuticals under the trade name Diapid.

Centrophenoxine is another popular rejuvenation drug. Its primary clinical use is for the treatment of mental deterioration in the elderly.

*M.R.T. - Muscle Response Testing

390 The Ultimate Healing System

Clinical studies have shown that the drug is highly effective in reversing mental disorders such as confusion, psychosomatic asthenia, and memory and intellectual disturbances. The drug consists of two compounds: P-Chlorophenoxyacetic Acid (a type of plant hormone) and DMAE (Diemethylaminoethonol), a precursor to acetylcholine the brain chemical that regulates memory and intelligence. Both of these compounds work together to produce profound rejuvenation effects in patients.

Centrophenoxine improves mental functions by rejuvenating the synaptic structures of brain cells. The synapse is the region of communication between brain cells where nerve impulses pass from one cell to another. Treatment with Centrophenoxine has led to a significant reduction of lipofuscin (brown age spots) in the skin of geriatric patients.

L-Dopa (Levodopa) is one of the most potent life extension therapies. L-Dopa (an amino acid), is the direct nutrient precursor to the brain chemical Dopamine, which plays a major role in muscular coordination and sexual function. Scientists have found that L-Dopa can boost sex drive dramatically (particularly in aging men), and stimulate the growth release hormone to help in weight loss and muscular development. L-Dopa can greatly improve physical endurance and athletic performance. L-Dopa is used by many medical practitioners in the treatment of Parkinson's Disease. Dr. George Cotzins of Brookhaven National Laboratory found that L-Dopa therapy extended the lifespan of mice by up to 50%. L-Dopa is marketed by Merck Pharmaceuticals as Sinemet.

SUNLIGHT THERAPY

Psychologists, medical researchers, lighting engineers, and numerous others are coming to understand that sunlight has a profound impact upon our well-being. Studies have confirmed that sunlight is a major factor in Calcium absorption, the maintenance of biological rhythms, the secretion of hormones, and even emotional stability.

How does sunlight banish the BLUES?

Most experts believe the PINEAL GLAND is involved. The Pineal Gland is an obscure gland deep in the brain which secretes the hormone MELATONIN.

MELATONIN times the onset of Puberty, acts as an internal time keeper, induces sleep, and influences moods.

Melatonin secretion follows a regular daily rhythm.

The Pineal secretes high levels of Melatonin at night and low levels of Melatonin during the day.

In 1980, Alfred Lewy discovered that bright lights put the brakes on Pineal function while darkness accelerates it. So Melatonin's cyclic nature was explained. The light of the day suppresses the secretion of Melatonin, while the darkness of night increases its production. This is how man's hormonal nature is controlled by environmental light. Sunlight can improve our moods and even affect our emotional health.

There are many other physiological reactions that result from light impulses traveling into the brain via the eyes. When the retina is stimulated by visible light, some of the nerve impulses produced travel along the optic nerve to the visual area of the brain which interprets what we see. Other impulses, however, detour from the optic nerve and travel to the Hypothalamus deep in the Forebrain. The Hypothalamus, the major controller of the body's internal environment, responds by regulating the "master" Pituitary Gland, and therefore, the entire endocrine system. In this way, the cycles of light and dark emanating from the Sun influence nervous, metabolic and hormonal pathways.

A blind individual often suffers from a host of metabolic disorders and hormonal imbalances. Since a non-functioning eye is unable to direct light impulses into the brain, biological rhythms run amuck.

Also the body manufactures Vitamin D3 when sunlight strikes the skin. Vitamin D is needed to absorb Calcium and other minerals from the diet. A deficiency leads to Rickets and Osteomalacia, both characterized by weak, porous and malformed bones.

Now there are those who are fearful of exposure to sunlight, as they have been misinformed that it is the cause of skin cancer. It is not!! What is the cause of skin cancer is the absence of a source of Vitamin F, which usually is taken into the body in the form of fats and oils, and the absence of enough P.A.B.A (Para-Amino-Benzoic Acid) internally.

To avoid any skin condition, before exposing one's skin to the sun put on a sunscreen lotion that contains sufficient P.A.B.A. After exposing one's skin to the sun, rub on a vegetable oil such as sunflower, peanut, safflower, or castor bean oil. These are rich in Vitamin F whose job in the body is to regenerate the skin. Many people who suffer from skin cancer have omitted fats such as butter, cream, or salad oils from their diet to keep their cholesterol down so the skin is being STARVED of the Vitamin F it needs for regeneration.

Aloe Vera gels and juice are also good for skin regeneration because they contain ALLANTOIN, a cell proliferator, and a chemical debrider of necrotic (dead) tissue. ALLANTOIN also serves to clean up the area of skin to which it is applied.

Another reason Vitamin F may be missing is that the person having the skin problem may be allergic to fats and oil thereby rejecting the Vitamin F which is usually carried by the fats. This condition can be cured by taking Sulfur (Methionine, Cysteine and Taurine), Carnitine, Threonine and Sarsaparilla. The Sun also corrects a Fat Allergy, so that it can start to be absorbed and thereby start to regenerate the skin from within.

A Vitamin D overdose can cause diarrhea and the desire to sleep. This can be counteracted by the administration of Vitamin E.

Correspondence Course Information

Our correspondence course is designed to coordinate the information that is in this book with more incredible information contained in another text, with a series of exams on both. Upon which successful completion, one will be eligible for a practitioner's certificate of accreditation as a biokinesiologic nutritionist.

The course will include a video tape of Hands On Technique and audio tapes of specific information.

Students will be eligible to purchase a test kit of nutrients and allergy antigens. Also students will be eligible to purchase "Miracle Food Products" at 50% discount.

Outstanding students will be eligible to do an internship at the Life Extension Research Center in Jersey City, N.J., U.S.A. or Rodney Bay, St. Lucia W.I.

For further information on fees and requirements write:

Dr. Don Lepore N.D.
Life Extension Research Center
359 New York Ave.
Jersey City, New Jersey 07307

INDEX